The SAGES / ERAS® Society Manual of Enhanced Recovery Programs for Gastrointestinal Surgery

The SAGES / ERAS® Society Manual of Enhanced Recovery Programs for Gastrointestinal Surgery

Liane S. Feldman, MD, FACS, FRCSC
Professor of Surgery, Director, Division of General Surgery,
Steinberg-Bernstein Chair in Minimally Invasive Surgery and Innovation,
McGill University, Health Centre, Montreal, QC, Canada

Conor P. Delaney, MD, MCh, PhD
Chief, Division of Colorectal Surgery, Vice Chairman, Department of Surgery,
University Hospitals Case Medical Center, Cleveland, OH, USA

Olle Ljungqvist, MD, PhD
Professor of Surgery, Faculty of Medicine and Health, School of Health
and Medical Sciences, Department of Surgery, Örebro University, Örebro, Sweden

Affiliated Professor of Surgery, Metabolism and Nutrition,
Karolinska Institute, Stockholm, Sweden

Francesco Carli, MD, MPhil
Professor of Anesthesia, Professor in the School of Nutrition, Montreal General
Hospital, Department of Anesthesia, McGill University, Montreal, QC, Canada

Editors

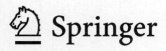 Springer

Editors
Liane S. Feldman, MD, FACS, FRCSC
Professor of Surgery
Director, Division of General Surgery
Steinberg-Bernstein Chair in Minimally
    Invasive Surgery
    and Innovation
McGill University, Health Centre
Montreal, QC, Canada

Olle Ljungqvist, MD, PhD
Professor of Surgery
Faculty of Medicine and Health
School of Health and Medical
    Sciences
Department of Surgery
Örebro University
Örebro, Sweden

Affiliated Professor of Surgery
Metabolism and Nutrition
Karolinska Institute
Stockholm, Sweden

Conor P. Delaney, MD, MCh, PhD
Chief, Division of Colorectal Surgery
Vice Chairman, Department of
    Surgery
University Hospitals Case Medical
    Center
Cleveland, OH, USA

Francesco Carli, MD, MPhil
Professor of Anesthesia
Professor in the School of Nutrition
Montreal General Hospital
Department of Anesthesia
McGill University
Montreal, QC, Canada

ISBN 978-3-319-20363-8   ISBN 978-3-319-20364-5   (eBook)
DOI 10.1007/978-3-319-20364-5

Library of Congress Control Number: 2015945652

Springer Cham Heidelberg New York Dordrecht London

Printed on acid-free paper

Springer International Publishing AG Switzerland is part of Springer Science+Business
Media (www.springer.com)

Foreword

Two major changes have improved outcomes in elective surgery: the introduction of minimally invasive surgery (MIS) revolutionized abdominal surgery, significantly lessening the impact of major surgery, reducing complications, and accelerating recovery. For many surgeons, interest in laparoscopic techniques was fueled by this desire to improve outcomes, especially recovery after surgery. There is a limit, however, to what can be accomplished using surgical techniques alone, and factors that keep people hospitalized and delay their return to normal functioning are multiple and complex. These include the surgical stress response, pain, postoperative nausea and vomiting, limited mobility, fluid overload, fatigue, and deconditioning, even in the absence of surgical complications. Enhanced Recovery After Surgery (ERAS) pathways are coordinated, multidisciplinary care plans incorporating evidence-based interventions along the entire perioperative trajectory and represent the second major step to improved outcomes after surgery. Traditionally, surgeons, anesthesiologists, and nurses have delivered care from individual silos. ERAS pathways represent a paradigm shift from traditional care, instead integrating multiple individual elements of perioperative care from these stakeholders, as well as empowering patients and caregivers to better understand the recovery process. By leveraging the gains achieved by MIS techniques with ERAS pathways, the goal is to further improve recovery, decrease complications, and decrease variability in practice, which in turn will be reflected in shorter hospital stay, lower costs, and improved patient satisfaction improving value for surgical procedures.

The SAGES/ERAS Society Manual of Enhanced Recovery Programs for Gastrointestinal Surgery represents a collaboration between two societies committed to improving surgical outcomes, from two unique but overlapping perspectives. SAGES has promoted the introduction and expansion of minimally invasive surgery, while the ERAS Society was created to promote implementation of evidence-based perioperative care. Both societies aim to improve patient recovery, decrease morbidity, and educate others in proven techniques and interventions.

While information is available in the scientific literature, there is no single source providing information on creating these programs across the wide array of procedures in GI and abdominal surgery. This book is designed to fill this gap and present a comprehensive, up to date and practical approach to creating an ERAS program for GI surgery. The first part, "The Science of Enhanced Recovery: Building Blocks for Your Program," reviews the evidence underlying individual elements of ERAS, including evidence from laparoscopic procedures, when available, or pointing to evidence gaps where more research is required. These are written by experts in the field, including surgeons, anesthesiologists, nurses, and physiotherapists. The format of the chapters is a narrative evidence review, concluding with a table with "take home messages" and 3–5 key references for readers interested in more depth in each topic. Chapters also address management of common complications and patient selection or exceptions, when relevant. The second part, "Creation and Implementation of an Enhanced Recovery Program," addresses practical concerns, including creation of a pathway team, addressing barriers, project management, and engaging administration. In the final part, experts will contribute real-world examples of their pathways for a variety of procedures, including colorectal surgery, bariatric surgery, upper GI and hepatobiliary surgery, enabling the user to have a starting point for creating their own programs.

The manual grew out of the first Enhanced recovery postgraduate course given by SAGES in April 2014 in Salt Lake City, UT, and involves international experts who draw on experiences from a myriad of practice settings. Many authors are contributors of original research in their fields. We hope the book will be of use to anyone involved in perioperative care, including surgeons or surgical trainees with various subspecialty interests, anesthesiologists and anesthesia technicians, perioperative physicians, nurses involved in all phases of perioperative care, and medical administrators. Whether you are beginning your own program, addressing barriers as you are implementing a program, or are expanding an existing program, we hope this manual will prove a useful and practical reference. Of course this is a constantly evolving field, and the ERAS Society and SAGES SMART Enhanced Recovery websites remain valuable resources, curating new knowledge towards improving the trajectory of recovery for patients.

Montreal, QC, Canada   Gerald M. Fried

Contents

**Part II   Creation and Implementation
of an Enhanced Recovery Program**

x   Contents

Contributors

Rajesh Aggarwal, M.B.B.S., M.A., Ph.D., F.R.C.S.
Associate Professor of Surgery Director, Arnold & Blema Steinberg
Medical Simulation Centre, Faculty of Medicine, McGill University,
Montreal, QC, Canada

Sherif Awad, Ph.D., F.R.C.S.
The East-Midlands Bariatric & Metabolic Institute (EMBMI), Derby
Teaching Hospitals NHS Foundation Trust, Royal Derby Hospital,
Derby, UK

School of Medicine, University of Nottingham,
Nottingham, UK

Gabriele Baldini, M.D., M.Sc.
Department of Anesthesia, McGill University Health Centre, Montreal
General Hospital, Montreal, QC, Canada

David Bergqvist, M.D.
Department of Surgical Sciences, Section of Vascular Surgery, Uppsala
University, Uppsala, Sweden

Karen M. Brady, C.N.P.
Division of Colorectal Surgery, Department of Surgery, University
Hospitals Case Medical Center, Cleveland,
OH, USA

Francesco Carli, M.D., M.Phil.
Department of Anesthesia, McGill University,
Montreal, QC, Canada

Bradley Champagne, M.D.
Division of Colorectal Surgery, Department of Surgery, University
Hospitals Case Medical Center, Cleveland,
OH, USA

Kyle G. Cologne, M.D.
Division of Colorectal Surgery, Department of Surgery, Keck School
of Medicine of the University of Southern California,
Los Angeles, CA, USA

Benjamin P. Crawshaw, M.D.
Division of Colorectal Surgery, Department of Surgery, University
Hospitals Case Medical Center, Cleveland,
OH, USA

Andrew Currie, M.B.Ch.B. (Hons), M.R.C.S.
Department of Surgery, St. Mark's Hospital and Academic Institute,
Harrow, UK

Elizabeth A. Davis, R.N., M.S.N.
Department of Nursing, Royal Victoria Hospital, McGill University
Health Centre, Montreal, QC, Canada

Conor P. Delaney, M.D., M.Ch., Ph.D.
Division of Colorectal Surgery, Department of Surgery,
University Hospitals Case Medical Center, Cleveland, OH, USA

Nicolas Demartines, M.D., F.A.C.S., F.R.C.S.
Department of Visceral Surgery, University Hospital of Lausanne,
Lausanne, Switzerland

Jonathan E. Efron, M.D.
Department of Surgery, Johns Hopkins Medicine, Baltimore,
MD, USA

Kenneth C.H. Fearon, M.B.Ch.B., M.D., F.R.C.S., Ph.D.
University of Edinburgh, Edinburgh, UK

Liane S. Feldman, M.D., F.A.C.S., F.R.C.S.C.
Division of General Surgery, Steinberg-Bernstein
Chair in Minimally Invasive Surgery and Innovation,
McGill University Health Centre, Montreal, QC, Canada

Lorenzo E. Ferri, M.D., Ph.D.
Department of Surgery, Montreal General Hospital, Montreal,
QC, Canada

Julio F. Fiore Jr., P.T., M.Sc., Ph.D.
Department of Surgery, McGill University, Montreal, QC, Canada

Tong Joo Gan, M.D., M.H.S., F.R.C.A.
Department of Anesthesiology, Stony Brook University, Stony Brook, NY, USA

D. Hahnloser, M.D.
Department of Visceral Surgery, University Hospital Lausanne, Lausanne, Switzerland

Martin Hübner, M.D.
Department of Visceral Surgery, University Hospital Lausanne, Lausanne, Switzerland

Robin Kennedy, M.S., F.R.C.S.
Department of Surgery, St. Mark's Hospital and Academic Institute, London, UK

Department of Surgery and Cancer, Imperial College London, London, UK

Lawrence Lee, M.D., M.Sc.
Steinberg-Bernstein Centre for Minimally Invasive Surgery and Innovation, McGill University Health Centre, Montreal, QC, Canada

Chao Li, M.D.
Steinberg-Bernstein Centre for Minimally Invasive Surgery and Innovation, McGill University Health Centre, Montreal, QC, Canada

Olle Ljungqvist, M.D., Ph.D.
Department of Surgery, Örebro University, Örebro, Sweden

Metabolism and Nutrition, Karolinska Institutet, Stockholm, Sweden

Dileep N. Lobo, D.M., F.R.C.S., F.A.C.S.
School of Medicine, University of Nottingham, Nottingham, UK

Gastrointestinal Surgery, National Institute of Health Research, Nottingham Digestive Diseases, Biomedical Research Unit, Nottingham University Hospitals, Queen's Medical Centre, Nottingham, UK

Timothy E. Miller, M.D.
Department of Anesthesiology, Duke University Medical Center, Durham, NC, USA

John R.T. Monson, M.D., F.R.C.S., F.A.C.S.
Division of Colorectal Surgery, Department of Surgery, University of
Rochester Medical Center, Rochester,
NY, USA

Allan Okrainec, M.D., M.H.P.E., F.R.C.S.C.
Division of General Surgery, Department of Surgery, University of
Toronto, Toronto, ON, Canada

Robert Owen
Northeast Ohio Medical University, Rootstown, OH, USA

E*mily Pearsall, M.Sc.*
Department of General Surgery, Mount Sinai Hospital, Toronto, ON,
Canada

Yanjie Qi, M.D.
Department of Surgery, University of Rochester Medical Center,
Rochester, NY, USA

William S. Richardson, M.D.
Department of Surgery, Ochsner Clinic, New Orleans,
LA, USA

Thomas N. Robinson, M.D., M.S.
Department of Surgery, University of Colorado, Aurora,
CO, USA

Timothy Rockall, M.B.B.S., F.R.C.S., M.D.
Department of Surgery, Royal Surrey Country Hospital
NHS Trust, Guildford, Surrey, UK

Director of Minimally Access Therapy Training Unit (mattu),
Guildford, UK

Didier Roulin, M.D.
Department of Visceral Surgery, University Hospital of Lausanne,
Lausanne, Switzerland

Colin F. Royse, M.B.B.S., M.D., F.A.N.Z.C.A.
Department of Surgery, The University of Melbourne, Melbourne,
VIC, Australia

Celena Scheede-Bergdahl, M.Sc., Ph.D.
Department of Kinesiology and Physical Education, McGill Nutrition
and Performance Laboratory, McGill University, Montreal,
QC, Canada

Michael Scott, M.B.B.S., M.R.C.P., F.R.C.A.
Department of Anaesthesia and Perioperative Medicine, Royal Surrey
County Hospital NHS Foundation Trust, Surrey, Guildford, UK
Surrey Periop-erative Anesthesia Critical Care Research Group
(SPACeR), University of Surrey, Guildford, UK

Anthony J. Senagore, M.D., M.B.A., F.A.C.S., F.A.S.C.R.S.
Division of Colorectal Surgery, University Hospitals Parma Medical
Center, Parma, OH, USA

J.C. Slieker, M.D.
Department of Visceral Surgery, University Hospital Lausanne,
Lausanne, Switzerland

Monisha Sudarshan, M.D., M.P.H.
Division of Thoracic Surgery, Department of Surgery, McGill
University Health Center, Montreal, QC, Canada

Deborah J. Watson, R.N., B.Sc.N.
Department of Nursing, McGill University Health Centre, Montreal
General Hospital, Montreal, QC, Canada

Elizabeth C. Wick, M.D.
Division of Colorectal Surgery, Department of Surgery, Johns Hopkins
Medicine, Baltimore, MD, USA

Tonia M. Young-Fadok, M.D., M.S., F.A.C.S., F.A.S.C.R.S.
Division of Colon and Rectal Surgery, Mayo Clinic, Phoenix, AZ, USA

Yuliya Y. Yurko, M.D.
Division of Colon and Rectal Surgery, Mayo Clinic, Phoenix,
AZ, USA

1. Introduction to Enhanced Recovery Programs: A Paradigm Shift in Perioperative Care

Liane S. Feldman

What's the Issue?

Despite improvements in surgical and anesthetic techniques, a significant proportion of patients experience complications after major gastrointestinal surgery [1], there is significant variability in care processes and outcomes between practitioners [2–4], full patient functional recovery requires weeks or months, even after ambulatory surgery [5–7], and costs of care continue to rise without resulting in better population health [8]. Achieving higher value care for patients, defined as health outcomes *that matter to patients* achieved per dollar spent, must become the goal [8].

Recovery after surgery is an outcome that matters to all stakeholders involved in perioperative care [9]. Obstacles delaying recovery include preoperative organ dysfunction, surgical stress and catabolism, pain, postoperative nausea and vomiting, ileus, fluid excess, semistarvation, immobilization, and surgical traditions or culture [10]. For many surgeons training in the last 20 years, minimally invasive surgery was the answer to improving recovery. However, even after low-impact procedures such as laparoscopic cholecystectomy, full recovery of physical activities takes longer than most surgeons think [5]. Outside of the traditional purview of the surgeon, many other interventions have the potential to delay or accelerate recovery through their impact on the surgical stress response. These include afferent neural blockade, pharmacologic interventions, fluid and temperature management, nutrition, and exercise [11] (Fig. 1.1). There is abundant evidence to guide best practices in perioperative care [12–14].

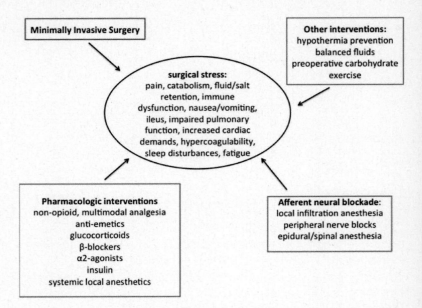

Fig. 1.1. Approaches to reduce surgical stress and improve surgical recovery: There are many developments in perioperative care that are outside the traditional purview of the surgeon that have significant potential to accelerate or delay recovery after surgery (adapted from Kehlet H, Wilmore DW. Evidence-based surgical care and the evolution of fast-track surgery. Ann Surg. 2008;248:189–98, with permission).

The issue is not lack of evidence or even lack of guidelines. The issue rather is how can care be organized to make it easier to get this evidence into practice and improve outcomes for our patients. To make progress, we have to introduce new interventions that are proven beneficial, and, perhaps as importantly, stop doing things that are not beneficial and may even be harmful. But there is an estimated time lag of 17 years between research and the time it takes to benefit society [15].

What Is an Enhanced Recovery Pathway?

An enhanced recovery pathway (ERP) is an evidence-based, multi-modal, integrated consensus on perioperative care that reorganizes care around surgery. The goal is to combine multiple evidence-based interventions, each of which may have modest impact in isolation, into

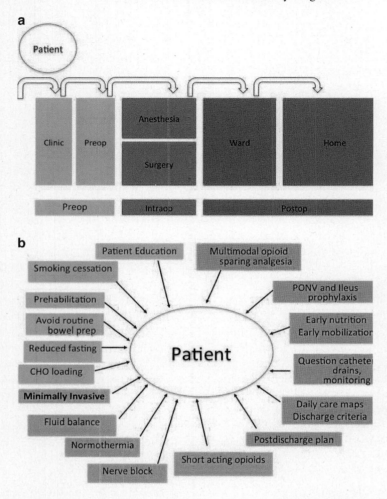

Fig. 1.2. In the conventional approach (**a**), providers work in expertise silos and the patient moves between these silos. ERPs instead look at the entire trajectory of perioperative care to standardize processes and integrate interventions into a cohesive package around the patient (**b**).

a coordinated, standardized package with synergistic beneficial effects on reducing physiologic stress and supporting early return of function. ERPs represent a paradigm shift from a clinician-focused system, where each stakeholder functions in an expertise silo with significant variability between providers, to a patient-centered system integrating each step along the perioperative trajectory into a single pathway (Fig. 1.2). It is not simply a set of standard orders; in addition it should address patient preparation, intraoperative management, and audit. This approach helps introduce evidence into practice and results in less morbidity, less need to remain in hospital, less variability between practitioners, and lower resource use [16–19].

The ERP approach is a philosophical shift from traditional management in several important ways. First, it provides a consistent approach to perioperative care for all patients undergoing a particular procedure, regardless of clinician. This standardizes processes and decreases unwanted variability between practitioners, facilitating decision making for nurses and for trainees. This requires that the team members arrive at a consensus for "how we do it" during creation of the pathway. Routine patients will progress along the predetermined trajectory without the need for the team to write daily diet, pain, catheter, mobilization, fluid, and monitoring orders. Patients who are informed of daily milestones beginning in the preoperative period are more engaged and empowered in their own care. Second, the pathway is geared towards accelerating recovery for patients without complications, which is the majority of patients. Rather than keeping all patients fasting because the minority of patients will not tolerate early oral intake, it allows more patients to benefit from early nutrition. Of course the team must continue to monitor and intervene for patients who develop complications. Although surgeons are very tuned to the "harms" sometimes resulting from surgery, pathways help us better care for the majority of patients without complications, and in many cases decrease the risk developing certain complication in the first place.

It is important for the program to address common contingencies or complications that may occur. For example, absence of voiding after removal of a urinary drain is best investigated and managed using a bladder scan-based protocol, in order to avoid automatic reinsertion of an indwelling catheter [20]. Similarly, intolerance of oral diet is relatively frequent with early feeding after abdominal surgery, and occurs in up to 35 % of patients to some degree [21]. However, NG tube insertion is required in less than 10 % of patients, so a stepwise approach should be outlined.

The ERP approach is applicable across a wide variety of procedures, in both the inpatient and outpatient settings. It should include key interventions in the preoperative, intraoperative, and postoperative phases of care (Table 1.1). Multiple elements of care are addressed in a procedure-specific manner and follow evidence when available. The expression of each element may differ between institutions depending on available resources, experience, and skill, but a standard consensus should be

Table 1.1. Key elements to address and include in development of enhanced recovery pathways. This approach is applicable across a variety of procedures, but the expression of each element may differ between procedures and between institutions.

Preoperative	Preoperative risk assessment and optimization of organ dysfunction
	Patient education
	Exercise/prehabilitation
	Smoking abstinence
	Examine use of routine bowel preparation
	Modern fasting guidelines
	Carbohydrate drinks (when evidence based)
Intraoperative	Avoid fluid excess
	Regional anesthesia (when evidence based)
	Minimally invasive surgery
	Short-acting opioids
	Maintain normothermia
	Glycemic control
	Antiemetic prophylaxis (evidence based)
Postoperative	Multimodal, opioid-sparing analgesia (evidence based and procedure specific)
	Anti-ileus prophylaxis
	Examine use of drains, tubes, catheters, and monitoring (evidence based)
	Early nutrition
	Early ambulation
	Daily care maps, predefined discharge criteria
	Postdischarge rehabilitation plan (evidence based)

From Kehlet H. Fast-track surgery-an update on physiological care principles to enhance recovery. Langenbecks Arch Surg. 2011;396:585–90; with kind permission of Springer Science + Business Media

reached within an institution. For example, there are multiple ways to deliver opioid-sparing multimodal analgesia with one institution relying on thoracic epidural, whereas others will integrate nerve blocks, while still others might use intravenous lidocaine with patient-controlled analgesia. The ERP team can also help change routine procedures for the entire operating room, like introducing modern fasting guidelines, not only for "pathway" patients.

It is not clear which elements of ERPs are most important, and many different approaches, ranging from relatively simple to more complex, can be successful [19]. Development and implementation of an ERP approach is best accomplished by a multidisciplinary team including surgeons, anesthesiologists, nurses involved in all phases of care, nutritionists, physiotherapists, pain service personnel, and administrators. This team should meet routinely and have clear deliverables, following a time line and general principles of project management. Creation and implementation of a new ERP requires review of evidence or guidelines for each step in the perioperative trajectory for a specific procedure; reaching consensus between practitioners on how each care element will be delivered within the local context; creating patient education materials with daily milestones, standard order sets, nursing flow sheets, and discharge criteria linked to milestones with a target discharge date; and training of perioperative personnel. The team should audit selected processes and outcomes and revise the program as needed as well as re-scan the literature for new evidence every 2 years. Although there is nothing particularly complex about elements of ERPs, it is a change in approach and as with other quality improvement initiatives, enthusiastic surgical, anesthesia, and nursing champions, as well as appropriate administrative support, are critical to the success of the initiative.

Several specialty societies have developed an interest in educating their members about enhanced recovery. The ERAS Society has developed an implementation program including an interactive audit that has coached many centers through implementation. The American College of Surgeon's National Surgical Quality Improvement Program (NSQIP) has an ongoing pilot project to help centers adopt an ERP for colon surgery, including the ability to monitor care processes in addition to outcomes. Enhanced recovery courses and workshops are available through SAGES, the ACS, and others. We at McGill have an annual workshop addressing ERPs, bringing together over 100 multidisciplinary professionals annually. Many centres involved in ERPs are happy to mentor colleagues including through e-mail, phone calls, or site visits to facilitate implementation.

Outcomes of the ERP Approach

In 2000, Kehlet published a seminal paper describing a multimodal rehabilitation program for 60 patients (average age 74, 20 patients ASA III–IV) undergoing elective open colon resection. The postoperative care program included thoracic epidural, enforced early nutrition, and mobilization, with a median 2-day hospital stay and 15 % readmissions [22]. This was the beginning of the "fast track" concept, with significant comparative research since then investigating the approach. A systematic review from 2014 identified 38 randomized trials in colorectal (18 studies), genitourinary (5 studies), joint (5 studies), thoracic (3 studies), and upper GI (6 studies) surgery. The review concluded that the use of an ERP was associated with reduced hospital stay (standard mean difference 1.14 days) without an increase in readmissions. ERPs were also associated with a 30 % reduction in complications at 30 days, with no increased risk of major complications or death. The effect was similar across different disciplines and for laparoscopic versus open colorectal surgery [19]. A separate meta-analysis of 13 randomized trials in colorectal surgery also found a shorter hospital stay by about 2 days, without increased readmissions. This is related to better organization of care [23], but also to fewer "general" complications and faster return of bowel function (by about 1 day) [16]. A systematic review of economic evaluations of colorectal ERPs found that eight of ten studies reported lower costs with ERPs [24]. When taking the full care trajectory into consideration, as well as implementation costs for the ERP, overall societal costs were lower when an ERP was used, with patients requiring less time off work and had less care-giver burden [25].

At the McGill University Health Centre, we created a multidisciplinary team to create and implement ERP-prevalent procedures across the department of surgery, building on previous institutional experience with pathways for laparoscopic foregut surgery [26] and laparoscopic colon surgery [27]. Working with clinical experts for each procedure, the team, led by a full-time nurse coordinator, has introduced 11 clinical pathways into practice, ranging from relatively simple ambulatory procedures to very complex in-patient procedures like esophagectomy. In our institution, all patients start the pathway in the preoperative clinic where standard educational information is reviewed by the preoperative nurses. Outcomes have been consistent in terms of reductions in hospital stay for prostatectomy [28], esophagectomy [29], colorectal surgery [25, 30] and lung resection [31], earlier time to achieve recovery milestones [25, 31], reduced infections [31], and lower costs [25, 32].

Take-Home Messages

- ERPs facilitate introduction of evidence-based practice.
- ERPs foster interdisciplinary collaboration and culture.
- ERPs decrease unwanted variability between practitioners.

- ERPs decrease hospital stay by improving care organization, supporting function, and decreasing morbidity.
- ERPs reduce costs and improve the value of surgical care for patients.

References

1. Schilling PL, Dimick JB, Birkmeyer JD. Prioritizing quality improvement in general surgery. J Am Coll Surg. 2008;207:698–704.
2. Lassen K, Hannemann P, Ljungqvist O, Fearon K, Dejong CH, von Meyenfeldt MF, Hausel J, Nygren J, Andersen J, Revhaug A. Enhanced Recovery After Surgery Group Patterns in current perioperative practice: survey of colorectal surgeons in five northern European countries. BMJ. 2005;330(7505):1420–1.
3. Lassen K, Dejong CH, Ljungqvist O, Fearon K, Andersen J, Hannemann P, von Meyenfeldt MF, Hausel J, Nygren J, Revhaug A. Nutritional support and oral intake after gastric resection in five northern European countries. Dig Surg. 2005;22(5): 346–52.
4. Cohen ME, Bilimoria KY, Ko CY, Richards K, Hall BL. Variability in length of stay after colorectal surgery: assessment of 182 hospitals in the National Surgical Quality Improvement Program. Ann Surg. 2009;250(6):901–7.
5. Feldman LS, Kaneva P, Demyttenaere S, Carli F, Fried GM, Mayo NE. Validation of a physical activity questionnaire (CHAMPS) as an indicator of postoperative recovery after laparoscopic cholecystectomy. Surgery. 2009;146(1):31–9.
6. Lawrence VA, Hazuda HP, Cornell JE, et al. Functional independence after major abdominal surgery in the elderly. JACS. 2004;199(5):762–72.
7. Tran TT, Kaneva P, Mayo NE, Fried GM, Feldman LS. Short stay surgery: what really happens after discharge? Surgery. 2014;156(1):20–7.
8. Porter ME. What is value in health care? N Engl J Med. 2010;363(26):2477–81.
9. Feldman LS, Fiore Jr J, Lee L. What outcomes are important in assessment of Enhanced Recovery After Surgery (ERAS) Pathways? Can J Anaesth. 2015; 62(2):120–30.
10. Kehlet H, Wilmore DW. Multimodal strategies to improve surgical outcome. Am J Surg. 2002;183:630–41.
11. Kehlet H, Wilmore DW. Evidence-based surgical care and the evolution of fast-track surgery. Ann Surg. 2008;248:189–98.
12. Gustafsson UO, Scott MJ, Schwenk W, Demartines N, Roulin D, Francis N, McNaught CE, MacFie J, Liberman AS, Soop M, Hill A, Kennedy RH, Lobo DN, Fearon K, Ljungqvist O. Enhanced Recovery After Surgery Society. Guidelines for perioperative care in elective colonic surgery: Enhanced Recovery After Surgery (ERAS®) Society recommendations. Clin Nutr. 2012;31(6):783–800.
13. Nygren J, Thacker J, Carli F, Fearon KC, Norderval S, Lobo DN, Ljungqvist O, Soop M, Ramirez J. Enhanced Recovery After Surgery (ERAS) Society, for Perioperative

Care; European Society for Clinical Nutrition and Metabolism (ESPEN); International Association for Surgical Metabolism and Nutrition (IASMEN) Guidelines for perioperative care in elective rectal/pelvic surgery: Enhanced Recovery After Surgery (ERAS®) Society recommendations. World J Surg. 2013;37(2):285–305.

14. Lassen K, Coolsen MM, Slim K, Carli F, de Aguilar-Nascimento JE, Schäfer M, Parks RW, Fearon KC, Lobo DN, Demartines N, Braga M, Ljungqvist O, Dejong CH. ERAS® Society; European Society for Clinical Nutrition and Metabolism; International Association for Surgical Metabolism and Nutrition Guidelines for perioperative care for pancreaticoduodenectomy: Enhanced Recovery After Surgery (ERAS®) Society recommendations. Clin Nutr. 2012;31(6):817–30.

15. Morris ZS, Wooding S, Grant J. The answer is 17 years, what is the question: understanding time lags in translational research. J R Soc Med. 2011;104(12):510–20.

16. Zhuang CL, Ye XZ, Zhang XD, Chen BC, Yu Z. Enhanced recovery after surgery programs versus traditional care for colorectal surgery: a meta-analysis of randomized controlled trials. Dis Colon Rectum. 2013;56(5):667–78.

17. Coolsen MME, van Dam RM, van der Wilt AA, Slim K, Lassen K, Dejong CHC. Systematic review and meta-analysis of enhanced recovery after pancreatic surgery with particular emphasis on pancreaticoduodenectomies. World J Surg. 2013;37(8):1909–18.

18. Dorcaratto D, Grande L, Pera M. Enhanced recovery in gastrointestinal surgery: upper gastrointestinal surgery. Dig Surg. 2013;30:70–8.

19. Nicholson A, Lowe MC, Parker J, Lewis SR, Alderson P, Sith AF. Systematic review and meta-analysis of enhanced recovery programmes in surgical patients. Br J Surg. 2014;101(3):172–88.

20. Zaouter C, Kaneva P, Carli F. Less urinary tract infection by earlier removal of bladder catheter in surgical patients receiving thoracic epidural analgesia. Reg Anesth Pain Med. 2009;34(6):542–8.

21. Maessen JM, Hoff C, Jottard K, et al. To eat or not to eat: facilitating early oral intake after elective colonic surgery in the Netherlands. Clin Nutr. 2009;28(1):29–3.

22. Basse L, Jakobsen DH, Billesbolle P, Werner M, Kehlet H. A clinical pathway to accelerate recovery after colonic resection. Ann Surg. 2000;232(1):51–7.

23. Maessen J, Dejong CH, Hausel J, Nygren J, Lassen K, Andersen J, Kessels AG, Revhaug A, Kehlet H, Ljungqvist O, Fearon KC, von Meyenfeldt MF. A protocol is not enough to implement an enhanced recovery programme for colorectal resection. Br J Surg. 2007;94(2):224–31.

24. Lee L, Li C, Landry T, Latimer E, Carli F, Fried GM, Feldman LS. A systematic review of economic evaluations of enhanced recovery pathways for colorectal surgery. Ann Surg. 2014;259(4):670–6.

25. Lee L, Mata J, Augustin B, Ghitulescu G, Boutros M, Charlebois P, Stein B, Liberman AS, Fried GM, Morin N, Carli F, Latimer E, Feldman LS. Cost-effectiveness of enhanced recovery versus conventional perioperative management for colorectal surgery. Ann Surg 2014 Nov 3 [Epub ahead of print].

26. Ferri LE, Feldman LS, Stanbridge DD, Fried GM. Patient perception of a clinical pathway for laparoscopic foregut surgery. J Gastrointest Surg. 2006;10:878–82.

27. Carli F, Charlebois P, Baldini G, Cachero O, Stein B. An integrated multidisciplinary approach to implementation of a fast-track program for laparoscopic colorectal surgery. Can J Anesth. 2009;56(11):837–42.
28. Abou-Haidar H, Abourbih S, Barganza D, Al Qaoud T, Lee L, Carli F, Watson D, Aprikian AG, Tanguay S, Feldman LS, Kassouf W. Enhanced recovery pathway for radical prostatectomy—implementation and evaluation. Can Urol Assoc J. 2014;8(11–12):418–23.
29. Li C, Ferri LE, Mulder DS, Ncuti A, Neville A, Lee L, Kaneva PP, Watson D, Vassiliou M, Carli F, Feldman LS. An enhanced recovery pathway decreases duration of stay after esophagectomy. Surgery. 2012;152(4):606–16.
30. Kolozsvari NO, Capretti G, Kaneva P, Neville A, Carli F, Liberman S, Charlebois P, Stein B, Vassiliou MC, Fried GM, Feldman LS. Impact of an enhanced recovery program on short-term outcomes after scheduled laparoscopic colon resection. Surg Endosc. 2013;27(1):133–8.
31. Madani A, Bejjani J, Wang Y, Sivakumaran L, Fiore J Jr, Mata J, Mulder DS, Sirois C, Ferri LE, Feldman LS. An enhanced recovery pathway reduces duration of stay and morbidity after lung resection. Submitted to Surgery, Mar 2015.
32. Lee L, Li C, Ferri LE, Mulder DS, Ncuti A, Carli F, Zowell H, Feldman LS. Economic impact of an enhanced recovery pathway for oesophagectomy. BJS. 2013;100(10): 1326–34.

Part I
The Science of Enhanced Recovery: Building Blocks for Your Program

2. Preoperative Education

Deborah J. Watson and Elizabeth A. Davis

Preoperative patient education is an essential element in an enhanced recovery program. It has been associated with lower levels of anxiety [1], less postoperative pain, improved wound healing, and shorter hospitalization [2]. Preoperative education provides patients with the tools they need to manage the stress of their surgical experience and become partners in their own recovery. Guidelines from the Enhanced Recovery After Surgery (ERAS®) Society consistently recommend "routine, dedicated preoperative counseling" [3, 4].

Since the enhanced recovery approach may be different from what patients expect or have previously experienced, they need information about how to participate. This should be provided using clear written guidelines, including specific goals for each day of the perioperative period, the expected length of hospital stay, criteria for hospital discharge [5], and how to continue their recovery following discharge.

While print materials are frequently used to provide pre- and postoperative instructions, these materials are often written at a reading level beyond the ability of most patients and contribute to confusion and poor health outcomes for patients with low literacy skills [6]. Many people are unable to understand and act upon available health information, due to low health literacy [7].

In this chapter, we explore the concept of health literacy, discuss ways to improve patient understanding, identify strategies to create patient-friendly print materials, and describe the preoperative education model supporting the enhanced recovery program at the McGill University Health Centre (MUHC) in Montreal, Canada.

L.S. Feldman et al. (eds.), *The SAGES / ERAS®*
Society Manual of Enhanced Recovery Programs for
Gastrointestinal Surgery, DOI 10.1007/978-3-319-20364-5_2,
© Springer International Publishing Switzerland 2015

Health Literacy

Health literacy refers to a set of abilities that allow people to read and evaluate information, fill out forms, understand and follow directions, navigate health care facilities, communicate with health professionals, and use information to make decisions about their health. Low health literacy has been linked with poor health outcomes [8]. Ratzan and Parker describe health literacy as "the degree to which individuals have the capacity to obtain, process and understand basic health information and services needed to make appropriate health decisions" [7]. The Canadian Expert Panel on Health Literacy defines it as "the ability to access, understand, evaluate and communicate information as a way to promote, maintain and improve health in a variety of settings across the life-course." The panel recognizes the role of education, culture, language, the communication skills of professionals, the nature of the materials and messages, and the settings in which education is provided as important factors in the uptake of health information [9].

In the USA it has been estimated that nearly 50 % of the adult population, or 90 million people, have trouble reading and understanding health information [10]. Six out of ten Canadians do not have the skills to obtain, understand, and act upon health information and services, or to make appropriate health decisions on their own [11]. Canada's Expert Panel on Health Literacy estimated that more than half of working-age adults in Canada (55 % or 11.7 million) have inadequate health literacy skills and seven out of eight adults over the age of 65 (88 % or 3.1 million) are in the same situation [12]. In 2011, the European Health literacy survey reported that among the eight participating European countries, nearly one of two individuals had inadequate or low health literacy [13]. Those most vulnerable are the elderly, minority groups, immigrants whose first language is not the language of the majority, the less educated, and the poor [7].

Health care professionals tend to underestimate the prevalence of low health literacy because it is not possible to identify this patient population by appearance. Most people with low literacy skills are of average intelligence and able to compensate for their lack of reading ability. People with low functional health literacy may have feelings of shame and inadequacy, so may not admit their lack of understanding or ask for help [14]. While it is not possible to predict low health literacy from a person's behavior, certain clues may point to it. Patients may fill out forms incompletely or inappropriately. They may be unable to name their medications or the indications for taking them. They may bring someone with them to do the reading or they may avoid having to read in front of others by saying, "I forgot my glasses" or "I'll read this later" [10]. Although low levels of literacy predispose people to low health literacy, people who are good readers may also have low health literacy skills. In the context of health care, they may not be able to translate medical jargon and terminology into standard English that makes sense to them [15].

Strategies to Improve Understanding

Communication between health care providers and patients can be improved. Weiss suggests that clinicians slow down, use plain, non-medical language, show or draw pictures, limit the amount of information, use the teach-back or show-me technique, and create a shame-free environment [6]. Other strategies include prioritizing clear communication within one's organization and using a "universal precautions" approach to communication.

Universal Precautions

Health literacy affects every patient interaction in every clinical situation. People of all ages, races, income levels, and educational backgrounds are affected by inadequate health literacy and many are unlikely to admit that they need clarification. If patients do not understand the information provided by health care professionals, they are at risk for poor health outcomes. The Canadian Council on Learning reported that without adequate health literacy skill "ill-informed decisions may be taken, health conditions may go unchecked or worsen, questions may go unasked or remain unanswered, accidents may happen, and people may get lost in the health-care system" [11]. Just as health care providers use universal precautions to protect against the spread of infectious organisms, we should use universal precautions to protect against inadequate communication with patients and families [16]. Most people, regardless of their reading or language skills, prefer medical information that is easy to understand.

Teach-Back Method

One strategy to reinforce learning and optimize understanding is the teach-back method. Having patients restate their understanding of key points in their own words is linked with improved health outcomes [17]. Asking patients *whether* they understand the information will not confirm their understanding. Patients may answer affirmatively, even if they do not understand, because of embarrassment or intimidation. Instead, health care providers should say, "To be sure I have explained clearly, please tell me in your own words what you understand." Giving patients sufficient time to explain their perceptions, and repeating or clarifying information when needed, may optimize learning.

Internet Resources

Many patients are turning to the Internet for health information. Recent statistics indicate that 2/3 of Internet users seek health information online. It is considered the third most common Internet activity [18]. Not all websites are reliable. Some sites may be misleading and confusing for the average health care consumer. There is a plethora of website evaluation tools available and health care providers should become comfortable assessing health information websites in order to recommend reliable ones to their patients. At our institution, patients seeking more information about their surgical procedure, anaesthesia, becoming fit, or smoking cessation are referred to appropriate websites in our printed material.

Patient-Friendly Print Materials

Patient-friendly print materials are essential tools in the preoperative education toolkit. A procedure-specific patient guide increases consistency for the messages received throughout the perioperative period. It reinforces the verbal messages patients receive from members of the health care team. Lists of daily goals create realistic expectations about such things as postoperative nutrition, mobilization, and length of hospital stay. Two elements of information identified by patients as particularly valued are explicit plans for the day and knowing their recovery goals [19]. These messages reduce anxiety and allow patients to play an active role in their own recovery. The use of images helps patients to visualize their progress (Fig. 2.1).

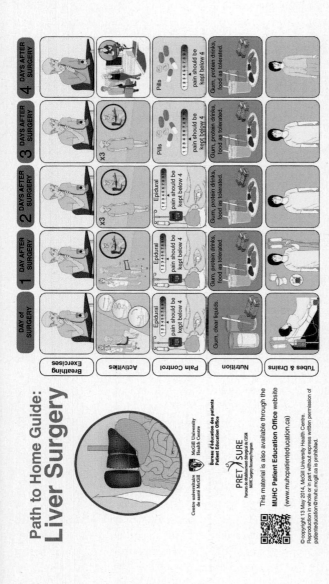

Fig. 2.1. Example of patient-friendly information illustrating daily goals for nutrition, pain management, drains, and exercise after liver surgery. This was created by the McGill Surgical Recovery Group and the McGill University Health Centre (MUHC) Patient Education Office. It is given to patients as part of the information package discussed in the preoperative clinic and is available on the surgical wards as large posters. For each pathway, the same template is used to create patient-friendly materials aligned with procedure-specific daily goals (courtesy of the McGill University Health Centre Patient Education Office).

Plain Language

The use of plain language, instead of technical language or medical jargon, will improve the clarity of communication. Plain language is a way of organizing and presenting information so that it makes sense and is easy for everyone to understand [20]. It uses logical organization, simple words, short sentences, active voice, and friendly tone, to make written material easier to read. An essential feature of writing in plain language is testing the material with the target audience to determine whether the audience understands the intended message.

Plain language is a patient-centered approach to writing. It uses familiar words and a conversational style to convey information clearly so that it can be understood by as many people as possible. For example, instead of saying, "Participants should register prior to the start of the program," it is clearer to say, "Please sign up before the program begins." Writers of plain language materials must make choices about what to include in each document to keep them from being too long. It is best to identify one primary message and support it with a limited number of key points. A strategy for selecting these points is to consider what the reader should know, do, and feel as a result of reading the material [21].

A difference of opinion exists about what grade level should be the target for writing in plain language. Grade level is an estimate of readability as it relates to years of schooling. The higher the grade level, the more difficult it is to understand the text. The Canadian Public Health Association recommends, when writing for the general public, that material should be written between grade levels 6 and 8 so that it has a better chance of being understood by all readers [22]. Researchers have established that the literacy demands of most health materials exceed the reading abilities of the average adult [23]. Regardless of grade level, the main focus should be on whether materials can be understood by the target audience. Evaluation by the target audience is an essential part of development.

Writing in plain language is a skill that requires time and effort to master. It involves a thorough understanding of the readers' needs, and the ability to explain complex medical information in a clear, meaningful way. Many health care professionals have become accustomed to writing for their colleagues using complex vocabulary and a more formal style. This "professional" style of writing is actually a barrier to communication with patients [10].

Critics of plain language suggest that it may offend people who have strong reading skills. However, research shows that people actually prefer materials that are easy to read [6]. Plain language accurately explains concepts and information in a way that eliminates barriers to understanding and demonstrates respect for the audience [10].

Clear Design

Clear design refers to the layout of a document. For educational materials, design features should be chosen to make the information look attractive and easy to read. Design should be simple, well organized, and consistent throughout the document. It should guide readers through the material and help them find and remember information [10]. Elements to be considered are font, type size, line length, white space, bullets, and images.

A font size of at least 12 points is recommended for patient education material [24]. The use of upper and lower case letters improves readability since it is more difficult to read words that are written in all capital letters. Using plenty of white space makes the text more inviting and allows the reader to see how the material is organized. Dense, crowded text can be intimidating to readers [25]. The use of boxes will draw attention to materials that should be emphasized. Vertical lists of words or statements, using bullets, are easier to read and remember than lists written in paragraph form. However, lists should be limited to no more than seven items or the reader will be overwhelmed [24].

Images

Images should facilitate learning [26]. Pictures should illustrate and reinforce the text, be simple and realistic, include captions, and be culturally appropriate. When body parts are pictured, they should be shown in the context of the whole body [10, 21].

Preoperative Education Model

A shift in organizational culture to one that values preoperative education is fundamental. Making patient education an organizational priority and creating a shame-free environment that encourages patients to speak up and ask questions should be the first step when setting up an enhanced recovery program. All health care providers must be sensitized to the concept of health literacy and understand its impact on health outcomes. In many cases, nurses' knowledge of health literacy is limited and organizations do not prioritize it [27].

In our organization, the orientation program for preoperative nurses includes information about health literacy. Nurses who work in the preoperative clinic are selected not only for their critical thinking ability, but also for their educational skills. We use a multidisciplinary approach to developing patient education materials, so that information is less fragmented. A preoperative visit is scheduled at least 2 weeks before the date of surgery, and a nurse, physician, and nutritionist meet each patient individually. For colorectal surgery, the enteral stoma nurse is also part of the team, meeting with future stoma patients preoperatively for their first education session. We prefer a unique preoperative clinic visit separate from when the patient was given initial information about their diagnosis, and recommend the presence of a caregiver during the education session if possible.

All patients receive a procedure-specific booklet to guide them through their perioperative journey. These materials are created alongside the creation of each new pathway in our department. We do not introduce a new pathway into clinical practice without having the patient materials. The preoperative clinic nurse reviews the booklet with the patient and asks them to bring it with them to the hospital when they come for surgery. A poster with the key daily milestones is included and also printed in poster size for the surgical wards. Evaluation of patient booklets is done on an ongoing basis and materials are modified based on patient and staff feedback and new evidence. Patients respond positively to the booklets, using them as a resource before, during, and after their surgery. Enhanced recovery patient materials are also available on the Internet for patients who prefer to access them on a computer, tablet, or phone. The booklets and poster inserts are all available for download in pdf format by the MUHC Patient

Education   Office   (www.muhcpatienteducation.ca/surgery-guides/
surgery-patient-guides.html?sectionID=31).

Patients who are expected to have an ostomy are given the link to an
online learning module to help them prepare for surgery, manage their
stoma, and reinforce the verbal information they receive (information
available   at   http://www.muhcpatienteducation.ca/surgery-guides/
ostomy.html?sectionID=132).

Conclusion

In order for an enhanced recovery program to be successful, it is
necessary to include patients as informed participants in the process.
Preoperative education should be provided by an interprofessional team,
using clear communication and patient-friendly teaching materials. This
has been shown to reduce anxiety and improve surgical outcomes.

Take-Home Messages

- Preoperative education is an essential component of an enhanced
  recovery program.
- Health care providers should understand the prevalence of low
  health literacy and its impact on patient outcomes.
- Printed materials using plain language and clear design may
  improve patient understanding of health information.
- Pictures linked to written or spoken text may increase patient
  attention, understanding, recall, and adherence to instructions.

References

1. Alanazi AA. Reducing anxiety in preoperative patients: a systematic review. Br J
   Nurs. 2014;23(7):387–93.
2. Keicolt-Glaser JK, Page GG, Marucha PT, et al. Psychological influences on surgical
   recovery. Am Psychol. 1998;53:1209–18.
3. Gustafsson UO, Scott MJ, Schwenk W, et al. Guidelines for perioperative care in elective colonic surgery: Enhanced Recovery After Surgery (ERAS®) Society recommendations. World J Surg. 2012;37:259–84. doi:10.1007/s00268-012-1772-0.

4. Nygren J, Thacker J, Carli F, et al. Guidelines for perioperative care in elective rectal/pelvic surgery: Enhanced Recovery After Surgery (ERAS®) Society recommendations. World J Surg. 2012;37:285–305. doi:10.1007/s00268-012-1787-6.

5. Feldman LS, Baldini G, Lee L, et al. Enhanced recovery pathways: organization of evidence-based, fast-track perioperative care. In: Fink MP, editor. ACS surgery: principles and practice. New York: WebMD; 2013.

6. Weiss B. Health literacy: a manual for clinicians. Chicago, IL: American Medical Association and American Medical Association Foundation; 2003.

7. Nielsen-Bohlman L, Panzer A, Kindig D, editors. Health literacy: a prescription to end confusion. Washington, DC: The National Academies Press; 2004.

8. Bass L. Health literacy: implications for teaching the adult patient. J Infus Nurs. 2005;28:15–22.

9. Rootman I, Gordon-El-Bihbety D. A vision for a health literate Canada: report of the expert panel on health literacy. Ottawa, ON: Canadian Public Health Association; 2008. http://www.cpha.ca/en/portals/h-l/panel.aspx. Accessed 11 June 2009.

10. Wizowski L, Harper T, Hutchings T. Writing health information for patients and families: a guide to creating patient education materials that are easy to read, understand and use. 3rd ed. Hamilton: Hamilton Health Sciences; 2008.

11. Canadian Council on Learning. Health literacy in Canada: a healthy understanding. Ottawa, ON: Canadian Council on Learning; 2008. http://www.ccl-cca.ca/CCL/Reports/HealthLiteracy?Language=EN. Accessed 11 June 2009.

12. National Assessment of Adult Literacy. National Center for Education Statistics. USA: Department of Education; 2003.

13. Doyle G, Cafferkey K, Fullam J. The European Health Literacy Survey: results from Ireland. In: EU Health Literacy Survey. MSD/NALA Health Literacy Initiative. 2012. Available via healthliteracy.ie. http://www.healthliteracy.ie/wp-content/uploads/2010/11/EU-Health-Literacy-Survey-Full-Report.pdf. Accessed 28 Aug 2014.

14. Parikh N, Parker R, Nurss J, et al. Shame and health literacy: the unspoken connection. Patient Educ Couns. 1996;27:33–9.

15. Mayer G, Villaire M. Health literacy in primary care: a clinician's guide. New York: Springer; 2007.

16. Brown D, Ludwig R, Buck G, et al. Health literacy: universal precautions needed. J Allied Health. 2004;33:150–5.

17. Tamura-Lis W. Teach-back for quality education and patient safety. Urol Nurs. 2013;33(6):267–71. doi:10.7257/1053-816X.2013.33.6.267.

18. Zickuhr K. Generations online in 2010. Available from: http://pewinternet.org/Reports/2010/Generations-2010/Overview.aspx. Cited Nov 2010.

19. Caligtan CA, Carroll DL, Hurley AC, et al. Bedside information technology to support patient-centered care. Int J Med Inform. 2012;81:442–51.

20. Cornett S. The Ohio State University Health Literacy Distance Education. Module #7: guidelines for selecting and writing easy to read health materials. 2011. www.healthliteracy.osu.edu. Accessed 30 Nov 2011.

21. Osborne H. Health literacy from A to Z: practical ways to communicate your health message. Sudbury, MA: Jones and Bartlett; 2005.

22. Canadian Public Health Association. Plain Language Service. 2008. http://www.cpha.ca/en/pls/FAQ.aspx. Accessed 26 July 2009.
23. Rudd R. Literacy implications for health communications and for health. 2001. http://www.hsph.harvard.edu/healthliteracy/talk_rudd.html. Accessed 11 June 2009.
24. Doak C, Doak L, Root J. Teaching patients with low literacy skills. Philadelphia, PA: Lippincott; 1996.
25. Smith S, Trevena L, Nutbeam D, et al. Information needs and preferences of low and high literacy consumers for decisions about colorectal cancer screening: utilizing a linguistic model. Health Expect. 2008;11:123–36.
26. Macabasco-O'Connell A, Fry-Bowers EK. Knowledge and perceptions of health literacy among nursing professionals. J Health Commun. 2011;16 Suppl 3:295–307. doi :10.1080/10810730.2011.604389.
27. Houts PS, Doak CC, Doak LG, et al. The role of pictures in improving health communication: a review of research on attention, comprehension, recall, and adherence. Patient Educ Couns. 2006;61:173–90.

Key References

Weiss B. Health literacy: a manual for clinicians. Chicago, IL: American Medical Association and American Medical Association Foundation; 2003.
Wizowski L, Harper T, Hutchings T. Writing health information for patients and families: a guide to creating patient education materials that are easy to read, understand and use. 3rd ed. Hamilton: Hamilton Health Sciences; 2008.
Osborne H. Health literacy from A to Z: practical ways to communicate your health message. Sudbury, MA: Jones and Bartlett; 2005.
Houts PS, Doak CC, Doak LG, et al. The role of pictures in improving health communication: a review of research on attention, comprehension, recall, and adherence. Patient Educ Couns. 2006;61:173–90.

3. Medical Optimization and Prehabilitation

Thomas N. Robinson, Francesco Carli, and Celena Scheede-Bergdahl

Medical Optimization

Preoperative medical optimization goes beyond simple preoperative risk assessment and aims to improve surgical outcomes. A concept critical to successful preoperative medical optimization is to target patients with preexisting physiologic compromise in whom physiologic reserves can be improved to better withstand the planned surgical intervention. In contrast, a healthy non-compromised patient has relatively less to gain from preoperative medical optimization efforts. This chapter provides specific, practical recommendations to optimize postoperative outcomes by focusing on the optimizing pulmonary status, cardiac disease, medication management, glucose control, frailty, and prehabilitation (Table 3.1).

Pulmonary Interventions

Inspiratory Pulmonary Training

Inspiratory muscle training using incentive spirometry breathing exercises preoperatively reduces postoperative pulmonary complications. An example of a preoperative inspiratory muscle training regimen is training patients to perform 20 min daily of incentive spirometry breathing exercises for at least 2 weeks prior to an operation. Following cardiac operations, this protocol can reduce both serious pulmonary complications and pneumonia by 50 %.

L.S. Feldman et al. (eds.), *The SAGES / ERAS®*
Society Manual of Enhanced Recovery Programs for
Gastrointestinal Surgery, DOI 10.1007/978-3-319-20364-5_3,
© Springer International Publishing Switzerland 2015

Table 3.1. Preoperative medical optimization and prehabilitation—overview.

Pulmonary
• Inspiratory pulmonary training
• Smoking cessation
Medication management
• Anticoagulation
Cardiac
• Beta-blockers
Diabetes
• Glucose management
Geriatric assessment
• Assess frailty
Prehabilitation

Smoking Cessation

Stopping smoking can reduce postoperative complications. Numerous studies have found that smoking cessation can reduce postoperative complications, and particularly pulmonary complications, by more than 40 %. Evidence suggests that at least 4 weeks of no smoking is required to allow the postoperative benefits of smoking cessation; this fact may require delay in elective scheduling of an operation.

Cardiac Interventions

The literature regarding beta-blockade for reduction of postoperative myocardial ischemia is mixed and sometimes contradictory. The potential benefit of perioperative beta-blockade when used in high-risk patients is a reduction of postoperative ischemia, myocardial infarction, and cardiovascular death in high-risk patients. However, perioperative beta-blockade has been found in some studies to increase the risk of stroke and even death, particularly in beta-blocker naïve patients. Strong evidence exists both to continue beta-blockers in the perioperative period in patients who are chronically on beta-blockers and to prescribe beta-blockers for high-risk patients with coronary artery disease who are undergoing high-risk operations (e.g., major vascular operations).

Medication Management

Anticoagulation Management

Managing anticoagulants in the perioperative setting is becoming increasingly commonplace. The decision regarding anticoagulation around an elective operation balances the risk of thromboembolism against the risk of bleeding. In patients with a high risk of thromboembolism (e.g., mechanical heart valve, venous thromboembolism within 3 months, high-risk atrial fibrillation), bridging of oral warfarin anticoagulation with shorter lasting low-molecular-weight heparin injections is recommended. An evidence-based regimen for bridging therapy is described in Table 3.2. In patients with low risk of thromboembolism (e.g., bileaflet valve without risk factors, venous thromboembolism more than 12 months previously, low-risk atrial fibrillation), no bridging with low-molecular-weight heparin is recommended. In these low-risk cases, warfarin should be stopped 5 days prior to the planned operation and started 12–24 h postoperatively.

Target specific oral anticoagulants are a new class of oral anticoagulants. These medications are cleared by the kidneys. With normal renal function, the medications rivaroxaban and dabigatran should be stopped 24 h prior to a standard bleeding risk operation and 48–72 h prior to a high-risk bleeding operation.

Antiplatelet drugs represent a common dilemma in perioperative care. In general for low-bleeding-risk operations, antiplatelet therapy with aspirin and clopidogrel can be continued throughout the periopera-

Table 3.2. Bridging warfarin anticoagulation with low-molecular-weight heparin—an evidence-based approach.

Preoperative	
5 days pre-op	Stop warfarin 5 days
3 days pre-op	Begin subcutaneous low-molecular-weight heparin (enoxaparin 1 mg/kg Q12 h or dalteparin 200 IU/kg Q24 h)
24 h pre-op	Discontinue LMWH injections Administer approximately ½ total daily dose for the last dose
Postoperative	
Post-op LMWH resumption	Low-risk bleeding—24 h post-op High-risk bleeding—48–72 h post-op
12–24 h post-op	Resume warfarin
Lab testing	Check INR at 5–7 days

Acronyms: *LMWH* low-molecular-weight heparin

tive setting. For high-risk bleeding operations, aspirin should be stopped 5 days prior to the procedure for low-cardiovascular-risk patient and are recommended to be continued throughout the perioperative period in patients with high risk of an adverse cardiovascular event. And finally, clopidogrel should be stopped 5 days prior to major operations. If patient are at high risk of an adverse cardiovascular event, bridging therapy with short-acting GPIIb/IIIa antagonists may be considered.

Glucose Management

Patients with diabetes are at higher risk for postoperative morbidity and mortality. For diabetics, operations should be scheduled early in the morning to avoid prolonged periods of starvation. Additionally, patients with poorly controlled glucose or end-organ dysfunction related to diabetes should be recognized as high risk and optimal glucose control should be achieved preoperatively. While hyperglycemia is associated with development of complications, it is not yet clear which level of glycemia should be targeted to improve postoperative outcomes.

Frailty Evaluation

Older adults have increased surgical risk due to globally reduced physiologic reserves, a phenomenon termed frailty. Frailty by definition confers increased risk of adverse healthcare events including disability. The presence of frailty independently predicts adverse surgical outcomes including complications, need for discharge institutionalization, and mortality.

The measurement of frailty is completed by simple clinical tests that quantify the various domains, or characteristics, which make up the frail older adult. Frailty characteristics include impaired cognition, functional dependence, poor mobility, undernutrition, high comorbidity burden, and geriatric syndromes. A person is determined to be frail by summing the number of abnormal frailty characteristics present preoperatively. Frail older adults will have an accumulation of a higher number of abnormal frailty characteristics than the non-frail older adult. Clinical characteristics of frailty and simple clinical tools to measure these characteristics can be found in Table 3.3. Finding frailty in an older adult prior to an operation may be an indication for interventions such as prehabilitation.

Table 3.3. Characteristics of the frail older adult.

Frailty characteristic	Clinical measurement tool (abnormal score)
Impaired cognition	Mini-Cog Test (≤ 3) Mini-Mental Status Exam (≤ 24)
Functional dependence	Katz Activity of Daily Living Test (one or more dependent ADLs) Instrumental Activity of Daily Living Test (one or more dependent iADLs)
Poor mobility	Time Up-and-Go Test (≥ 15 s) 5 m walking speed (≥ 6 s)
Undernutrition	≥ 10 lb weight loss in past year Hypoalbuminemia (<3.4 g/dL)
High comorbidity burden	Charlson Index (≥ 3) Cumulative Illness Rating Score (≥ 3)
Geriatric syndromes	Unintentional fall in past 6-months (≥ 1 fall) Presence of a pressure ulcer

Prehabilitation

Impact of Surgery on Physical and Emotional Functions

Despite advances in surgical techniques, anesthetic pharmacology, and perioperative care, which have made even major operations safe and accessible to a variety of patients potentially at risk, there remains a group of patients who have suboptimal recovery. Almost 30 % of patients undergoing major abdominal surgery have postoperative complications, and, even in the absence of morbid events, major surgery is associated with 40 % reduction in functional capacity. Patients experience physical fatigue, disturbed sleep, and a decreased capacity to mentally concentrate for up to 9 weeks once they return home from surgery. Long periods of physical inactivity induce loss of muscle mass, deconditioning, pulmonary complications, and decubitus. Preoperative health status, functional capacity and muscle strength, and anxiety and depression correlate with postoperative fatigue, medical complications, and postoperative cognitive disturbances, and this is particularly true in the elderly, persons with cancer, and persons with limited physiological and mental reserve who are the most susceptible to the negative effects of surgery.

Traditionally efforts have been made to improve the recovery process by intervening in the postoperative period. However, the postoperative period may not be the most opportune time as any of these surgical patients are tired, depressed, and anxious. These patients may be awaiting extra treatment for the tumor and are therefore unwilling to be engaged in any rehabilitative process. Instead, the preoperative period may be a more appropriate time to engage the patients in building up physical reserve, and with the understanding that these activities would help them to overcome the stress of surgery.

What Is Surgical Prehabilitation?

The process of enhancing functional capacity of the individual to enable him or her to withstand an incoming stressor has been termed *prehabilitation*. Conventionally, patients are prepared for the stresses of surgery through education and positive reinforcement; however, the use of an exercise program prior to surgery is not routinely practiced.

The benefits of exercise have been demonstrated for the prevention/management of many chronic conditions, and in medicine, regular exercise has been shown to decrease the incidence of ischemic heart disease, hypertension, diabetes, stroke, and fractures in the elderly, related to improved balance and strength. With regular physical activity, there is increase in aerobic capacity, a decrease in sympathetic over-reactivity, an improvement of insulin sensitivity, and increased ratio of lean body mass to body fat. Exercise training, particularly in sports medicine, has been used as a method of preventing a specific injury or facilitating recuperation. Evidence seems to suggest that, by increasing the aerobic and muscle strength capacity of the patient by means of increased physical activity prior to surgery, physiological reserve increases and postoperative recuperation is facilitated.

The first published systematic review included 12 studies and concluded that preoperative exercise therapy was effective for reducing postoperative complication rates and accelerating the hospital discharge of patients undergoing cardiac and abdominal surgery. All four studies on cardiac and abdominal surgery reported the beneficial effect of inspiratory muscle training as a primary intervention. The risk of developing postoperative pulmonary complications was significantly higher in the group that did not receive training. Unfortunately, little information regarding the type of exercise, frequency, duration, and intensity was provided. Conversely, the outcome after joint arthroplasty was not significantly affected by preoperative exercise therapy. In the orthopedic groups, the prehabilitation program lasted for up to 6 weeks, while in the cardiac and abdominal group the average was 3–4 weeks. Whether these inconsistencies were due to variations in the physical status of the patients or the different muscle groups targeted was not established. More recently, another systematic review of eight studies demonstrated that exercise confers some physiologic improvement, however with limited clinical benefit not always translated into better clinical outcome.

An initial randomized trial conducted by our group in patients undergoing colorectal surgery comparing a 4-week home-based intense (aerobic and resistance) exercise program with a "sham" intervention consisting of a daily walk and breathing exercises before surgery showed a deterioration in postoperative functional capacity in the intense exercise group. Full adherence with the exercise program was very low. Predictors of poor surgical outcome included functional deterioration while waiting for surgery, age over 75 years, high anxiety, and lack of social support. These results suggest that an intervention based on intense exercise alone was not sufficient to enhance functional capacity if factors such as nutrition, anxiety, and other perioperative care elements (e.g., smoking and alcohol cessation, glycemic control, standardized intraoperative and early postoperative surgical and anesthetic care) were not taken into consideration during the program. This highlights the point that while physical activity undoubtedly has several benefits in restoring physiological reserve in preparation for abdominal surgery, one cannot exclude the important role played by other modalities such as pharmacological optimization, nutritional supplementation, cognitive enhancement, psychosocial support, and caregiver involvement.

Based on these findings, we designed a multimodal prehabilitation program consisting of moderate-intensity physical exercise, complemented by nutritional counseling/supplementation and anxiety reduction strategies. The benefits of this approach were supported by a recent pilot study, followed by a subsequent RCT comparing initiation of the program prior to colorectal cancer surgery or afterwards. In the prehabilitation program, over 80 % of patients recovered to their baseline functional walking capacity by 8 weeks, compared to only 40 % of patients in the control group (Fig. 3.1).

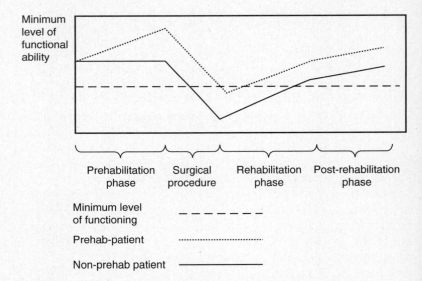

Fig. 3.1. Trajectory of functional capacity throughout the surgical process. Representation of trajectory of functional capacity demonstrates an abrupt decline postoperatively, followed by a slow return ("recovery") to baseline. A prehabilitation intervention, by increasing functional reserve preoperatively, results in less of a drop in capacity and faster return to baseline levels (from Carli F, Zavorsky GS. Optimizing functional exercise capacity in an elderly surgical population. Curr Opin Nutr Metab Care 2005;8:23–32, with permission).

Physical Activity as an Essential Component of Prehabilitation

Both strength and aerobic training increase endurance capacity, play an important role in weight management, improve muscle strength, reduce the risk of fall, and increase the range of motion in a number of joints, particularly in the elderly.

Current recommendations for aerobic exercise for the elderly population include a combination of moderate-to-vigorous intensities, if deemed appropriate for the individual. These intensities, on a scale of 1–10 representing a rating of perceived exertion (RPE), should be approximately 5–6 for moderate and 7–8 for vigorous exercises (Fig. 3.2). In the case of this population, the exercise intensity should start conservatively at first, and progress depending on the physical

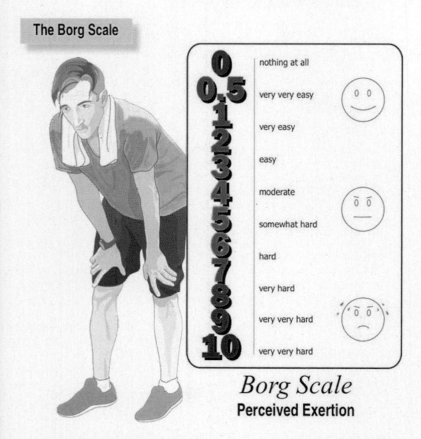

Fig. 3.2. Sample of the Rate of Perceived Exertion Scale (RPE, Borg). A scale such as this may be transferred onto a large poster board and mounted within view of the exercising patient. Often the RPE is *color* coded (from *green* or *blue* at rest to *red* at maximal efforts) or has cartoons representing effort. Key words represent exercise intensity (from Carli F, Scheede-Bergdahl C. Prehabilitation to enhance perioperative care. Anesthesiol Clin 2015;33:17–33, with permission).

status, abilities, and concurrent medical conditions of each individual. The intensity of exercise included in prehabilitation programs should introduce the activity at an intensity that is more than what the individual already partakes in, so that the body experiences the "stress" of additional work. It is, however, important to avoid prescribing exercise that is too intense, which may result in fatigue, injury, or—as in our previous experience—poor adherence. The modality of training may include activities such as walking, swimming, cycling, or other similar

Table 3.4. Key guidelines for older adults (2008 physical activity guidelines for Americans).

The following guidelines are the same for adults and older adults:
- All older adults should avoid inactivity. Some physical activity is better than none, and older adults who participate in any amount of physical activity gain some health benefits.
- For substantial health benefits, older adults should do at least 150 min (2 h and 30 min) a week of moderate-intensity or 75 min (1 h and 15 min) a week of vigorous-intensity aerobic physical activity, or an equivalent combination of moderate- and vigorous-intensity aerobic activity. Aerobic activity should be performed in episodes of at least 10 min, and preferably, it should be spread throughout the week.
- For additional and more extensive health benefits, older adults should increase their aerobic physical activity to 300 min (5 h) a week of moderate-intensity or 150 min a week of vigorous-intensity aerobic physical activity, or an equivalent combination of moderate- and vigorous-intensity activity. Additional health benefits are gained by engaging in physical activity beyond this amount.
- Older adults should also do muscle-strengthening activities that are of moderate or high intensity and involve all major muscle groups on 2 or more days a week, as these activities provide additional health benefits.

The following guidelines are just for older adults:
- When older adults cannot do 150 min of moderate-intensity aerobic activity a week because of chronic conditions, they should be as physically active as their abilities and conditions allow.
- Older adults should do exercises that maintain or improve balance if they are at risk of falling.
- Older adults should determine their level of effort for physical activity relative to their level of fitness.
- Older adults with chronic conditions should understand whether and how their conditions affect their ability to do regular physical activity safely.

Published by the United States Department of Health and Human Services (http://www.health.gov/paguidelines/guidelines/)

activity. Most importantly is that the patient enjoys the activity and is able to maintain the activity for at least 10 min per session. Physical activity guidelines for older adults are presented in Table 3.4.

As there is a decrease in skeletal muscle mass and muscle strength as a result of age and disease, the implementation of resistance training, which has been shown to reduce this rate of decline, is extremely important for prehabilitation. Such training has positive effects on functionality, health, and quality of life. Again, in order to achieve strength gains in untrained individuals, the patient should be able to perform 8–12 repetitions of each exercise, with the final one or two becoming "difficult to perform." These exercises should be progressed as the patient finds it "relatively easy" to perform the 12 repetitions. Resistance training exercises should be performed approximately 2–3 times a week on non-consecutive days, allowing for adequate recovery between sessions. Progressive prehabilitation strength-program guidelines for resistance training are recommended for elderly and frail people. A minimum of 8–10 different exercises involving the major, multi-jointed muscle groups (arms, shoulders, chest, abdomen, back, hips, and legs) are recommended. A sample training program has been included in Table 3.5.

Complementing Physical Activity with Nutrition

The nutritional status of patients scheduled for abdominal surgery is directly influenced by the presence of cancer or chronic disease which impacts on all aspects of intermediary (protein, carbohydrate, lipid, trace element, vitamin) metabolism. Thus, the primary goal of nutrition therapy during the prehabilitation period is to optimize nutrient stores preoperatively and provide adequate nutrition to compensate for the catabolic response of surgery postoperatively.

The benefits of integrating nutrition and physical exercise have been studied in elderly patients whereby it has been shown that a minimum of 140 g of carbohydrate taken 3 h before exercise increases liver and muscle glycogen and facilitates the completion of the exercise session. Also the time of ingesting a protein meal is of importance; elderly individuals who consume 10 g proteins immediately after weight training have their mean quadriceps fibre area increased by 24 % as well as their dynamic muscular strength.

With regard to the type of nutrients, a synergistic effect has been shown between arginine and fish oils with positive impact on postoperative morbidity. Whey protein is another nutritional component that has attracted the interest of exercise physiologists as it is a protein which is highly bioavailable, is rapidly digested, and contains all the indispensable amino acids. Whey protein is also associated with an increase in protein synthesis, and is found to score highest on the quality assessments used to assess protein quality, such as net protein utilization, biological value, and the protein digestibility. Finally, whey protein plays a role in oxidative stress defense, by increasing the content of intracellular stores of the antioxidant glutathione (GSH). GSH is a major intracellular antioxidant that neutralizes reactive oxygen species (ROS)

Table 3.5. Example of 4-week prehabilitation program including physical activity, nutrition, and relaxation exercises.

Aerobic exercise
- Start a slow walk in order to adequately warm up
- 30-min minimum of aerobic activity (walking/biking) three times per week at moderate intensity (4–6 on the Borg Scale). If the participant finds the activity to be easier (2–3 on the Borg Scale) then the walking pace or duration should be gradually increased. It is recommended not to surpass 7–8 on the Borg Scale. Example: Walk at a normal pace for 5 min and then walk at a quicker pace for 2 min and repeat for the duration of time

Resistance exercise
- All exercises are to be done starting with one set of about 10–12 repetitions. Number of sets and repetitions gradually increase to two sets, and 12–15 repetitions
  - Use of a Theraband/handheld weights and some body weight exercises
  - Body weight exercise involve the following:
  - Push-ups (wall, modified, or full)
  - Squats with the use of a chair
  - Hamstring curls
  - Calf raises
  - Abdominal crunches (chair or floor)
  - Theraband/handheld weight exercises involve the following:
  - Chest exercise
  - Deltoid lifts
  - Bicep curls
  - Triceps extension

Flexibility
- Flexibility exercises are given for the following muscles (each exercise should be performed twice and held for a minimum of 20 s):
  - Chest
  - Biceps
  - Triceps
  - Quadriceps
  - Hamstring
  - Calf

Breathing relaxation exercise
- Abdominal breathing (15 min twice daily)
- Use of relaxation CD (nature sounds and breathing instructions)

It is instructed to take protein within 30 min upon completion of the exercise regimen

---

by donating its sulfhydryl proton. Nutritional assessment and sufficient provision of proteins (1.5–2.0 g protein per kilogram body weight) are needed in patients with a history of weight loss, cancer, or chronic inflammatory diseases. In a recent prehabilitation nutrition RCT (no physical exercise) patients scheduled for colorectal resection for cancer received daily 2 g/kg body weight of protein for 4 weeks before surgery and their functional walking capacity (a measure of recovery, assessed by the 6-min walk test) increased by over 20 m in more than 50 % of the subjects. This was in contrast to patients who received 0.8 g/kg of proteins for 4 weeks as recommended, and their functional capacity decreased during the preoperative period.

Strategies to Attenuate the State of Anxiety and Depression Encountered Before Surgery

The physical burden of surgery is closely linked to the emotional one. Elevated levels of psychosocial distress seen in patients undergoing abdominal surgery are related to the diagnosis (cancer for example), the treatment (chemotherapy), and most often disability (stoma siting). Several studies have identified that anxiety and depression can impact on postoperative outcome; for example those who were more stressed on the third day after surgery stayed longer in hospital and those who were more optimistic were not often hospitalized. Depression was associated with more infection-related complication and poor wound healing.

In a recent prehabilitation study in patients who underwent colorectal resections, those who improved in functional capacity showed also positive changes in mental health and some aspects of the SF-36 subscale vitality. Anxiety at baseline was also associated with poorer recovery. The belief that fitness aided recovery was a strong predictor of improvement.

These observations indicate the need to incorporate mental strategies to interact with physical activity and enhance the effect of prehabilitation. Interventional studies that improve healing outcomes by reducing psychological stress provide further evidence of the impact of psychological and behavioral factors in wound repair, length of stay, less demand for analgesia postoperatively, and increased patient satisfaction. The use of information booklets and tailored messages on how to promote personal health help to empower patients in controlling their own health and becoming more involved in the healing process.

Who Would Benefit from Prehabilitation?

As people are living well in their late 70s, they are more likely to undergo surgery. Morbidity and mortality associated with surgery increase with advancing age once above 75 years of age. There is a large heterogeneity in this population with frail and cognitively impaired on one side and highly functional and robust from the other side. There has also been a shift in the comorbidity of this population with an increase in cancer, obesity, diabetes, cognitive impairment, and osteoarthritis. Comprehensive preoperative assessments which take into consideration functionality, comorbidity, cognition, social support, nutrition, and medical assessment could help at identifying those who are at risk of adverse events and formulating a treatment plan before surgery.

While there has been several studies emphasizing the benefit of long-term endurance training in patients with chronic heart failure and the positive effect of rehabilitation physical exercise after reconstructive surgery, few studies have focused on surgical prehabilitation in the elderly and patients with cancer with the intent to increase physiological reserve and enhance functional capacity in preparation of surgery. It is assumed that elderly, frail patients with medical comorbidities, with poor functional and social status, or at risk of malnutrition would need some attention.

The appropriate time for the development of a prehabilitation program would be during the preoperative assessment period for elective operations. At this time, the multidisciplinary team, which should include internal medicine, geriatrics, anesthesia, surgery, nutrition, kinesiologist/physiotherapist, and nursing, would devise a risk stratification model and identify the type and duration of prehabilitation needed in order to balance the potential benefit of such intervention versus the potential harms of delaying surgery.

Conclusions

Surgical prehabilitation is an emerging concept which derives from the realization that despite innovations in perisurgical care and technology some aspects of postoperative outcome have not significantly changed. This is probably due to other factors such as patients' health and functional status, which are modifiable. As the population gets older and surgical mortality decreases, patients are increasingly concerned with quality of life, community reintegration, and cognitive well-being. Innovative comprehensive preoperative risk evaluation and implementation of multidisciplinary prehabilitation programs need to be further developed and tested, particularly directed to patients at risk. The integrated role of physical exercise, adequate nutrition, and psychosocial balance, together with medical and pharmacological optimization, deserves to receive more attention.

Take-Home Messages

- Target preoperative medical optimization efforts on patients who have reduced physiologic reserves, not healthy individuals.
- Inspiratory muscle training with incentive spirometry and smoking cessation can reduce pulmonary complications.
- Measuring frailty in older adults includes quantification of characteristics including impaired cognition, functional dependence, poor mobility, undernutrition, high comorbidity burden, and the presence of a geriatric syndrome.
- Prehabilitation is a comprehensive preoperative program which aims to better prepare the patient to withstand the stress of surgery and promote faster recovery. This is critical for the most efficient implementation of subsequent treatment protocols.
- The program includes physical activity, adequate energy and protein intake, mental strategies to reduce psychological stress, and pharmacological optimization.

Suggested Reading

1. 2009 ACCF/AHA focused update on perioperative beta blockade—2009 writing group to review new evidence and update the 2007 guidelines on perioperative cardiovascular evaluation and care for noncardiac surgery. Circulation. 2009;120: 2123–51.
2. Robinson TN, Wallace JI, Wu DS, et al. Accumulated frailty characteristics predict postoperative discharge institutionalization in the geriatric patient. J Am Coll Surg. 2011; 213:37–42.
3. Carli F, Zavorsky G. Optimizing functional exercise capacity in the elderly surgical population. Curr Opin Clin Nutr Metab Care. 2005;8:23–32.
4. Silver JK, Baima J. Cancer prehabilitation. Am J Phys Med Rehabil. 2013;92:715–27.
5. Gillis C, Li C, Lee L, Awasthi R, Augustin B, Gamsa A, Liberman AS, Stein B, Charlebois P, Feldman L, Carli F. Prehabilitation vs rehabilitation, a randomized control trial in patients undergoing colorectal resection for cancer. Anesthesiology. 2014; 121(5):937–47.

4. Preoperative Fasting and Carbohydrate Treatment

Olle Ljungqvist

Preoperative Fasting

Preoperative fasting is a routine that aims to secure an empty stomach by the time of induction of anesthesia in order to reduce the risk of regurgitation of acid gastric content that may flow into the lungs and cause dangerous chemical pneumonia. Based on studies of gastric emptying of various foods and drinks, recent guidelines for elective surgery recommend that while solid food should not be taken within 6 h prior to induction of anesthesia, intake of clear liquids can be recommended to most patients until 2 h before anesthesia. Although this makes perfect sense to any health professional having studied the physiology of gastric emptying and/or fluid absorption and metabolism, this guideline is probably one of the most underused worldwide today. The reason for this is likely to be historic. But it may also relate to the reluctance of the medical community to change habits from traditional ways to evidence-based practice and the ease of sticking to a rule that is simple and well known.

The History of Overnight Fasting

The first surgery performed under general anesthesia was in Boston in 1846. Instead of operating on a patient intoxicated with alcohol, the most used "anesthetic" at that time, the introduction of ether resulted in a calm, pain-free patient. The introduction of ether anesthesia was a

L.S. Feldman et al. (eds.), *The SAGES / ERAS®*
Society Manual of Enhanced Recovery Programs for
Gastrointestinal Surgery, DOI 10.1007/978-3-319-20364-5_4,
© Springer International Publishing Switzerland 2015

sensation to say the least, and a major medical breakthrough that allowed for the development of modern surgery [1].

However, it only took 2 years until the first anesthesia death occurred. An unfortunate young woman died from suspected aspiration after a toenail extraction in Newcastle, UK. The operation had gone well, but afterwards the patient was not fully responsive and was given water and brandy by her doctor. She never recovered and very quickly died. Upon autopsy a full stomach was found as well as congested lungs and although the exact cause of death was never established, this was believed to be the result of aspiration [2]. The first certain case of death from aspiration was reported in 1862 [1]. Still, Lord Lister proposed in 1883 that while solids should be avoided before surgery, he proposed a cup of beef tea 2 h before the administration of chloroform [3]. A report on aspirations in women undergoing caesarean section in the USA in the 1940s also recommended a prolonged fasting period to reduce the risk [4]. In this report, none of the patients died. Nevertheless, based on no scientific testing, it was proposed in a textbook in 1964 for the first time that all patients should be fasting from midnight to the day of elective surgery to secure an empty stomach. Since then subsequent textbooks in anesthesia and surgery have stated the same rule. This is probably the best known medical "rule" in the world today, and it is still widely applied despite ample science showing that it has no data in its support.

The Science Behind Current Fasting Guidelines

Eventually, investigators started to challenge these routines. The pioneering work came from Canada and led by Dr. Roger Maltby [5] showing that intake of 150 ml of water fluids 2 h before surgery instead of overnight fasting actually resulted in a lower volume of fluids in the stomach at the time of surgery. Several follow-up randomized trials confirmed that intake of different types of clear fluids resulted in similar or lower gastric volumes at the time of anesthesia compared with those found after an overnight fast. Other large-scale studies of national data reported that aspirations were very rare events in elective surgery [6]. The majority of the aspirations occurred in emergency patients and often during nighttime. Fatal outcomes following aspirations were mainly found in patients with severe comorbidities. It was also found that fasting overnight was no a guarantee that the stomach was empty the next morning. Other factors apart from the period of fasting determine the volume in the stomach at any given time, such as gastric motility, fluid balance, and the type of food consumed.

Table 4.1. European Society of Anesthesiology (2011) selected items.

Item	Evidence	Recommendation
Clear fluids encouraged until 2 h before elective surgery	1++	A
Solids food prohibited for 6 h before elective surgery	1+	A
Is it safe to use specific carbohydrate-rich drinks 2 h before surgery? (*But not all carbohydrate drinks are necessarily safe*)	1++	A
Carbohydrate-rich drinks before surgery improve subjective well-being, reduce thirst and hunger and postoperative insulin resistance (*in 2011 little clear evidence to show reductions in length of stay or mortality*)	1++	A

From Smith I et al. Perioperative fasting in adults and children: guidelines from the European Society of Anaesthesiology. Eur J Anaesthesiol. 2011;28(8): 556–69; with permission

While the rule of nothing to eat or drink after midnight is simple and potentially easy to follow, it also results in some of the most disturbing and common complaints that the patients have before surgery. Thirst ranks amongst the most common complaints alongside hunger, anxiety, and difficulty to sleep [7], and thirst (and hunger to some extent) can be reduced by allowing free intake of clear fluids. Another complaint is headache from lack of caffeine in coffee drinkers, which can also be overcome by a simple change of practice.

With the growing evidence that allowing oral intake of fluids up until 2–3 h before an operation was safe and had patient benefits in terms of well-being, gradually national guidelines began to change. Guidelines from Canada and Norway were the first to change [8, 9] followed by several European countries and the USA. The recent European Society of Anesthesiology guidelines are also consistent with these recommendations [10] (Table 4.1).

Preoperative Carbohydrates

The Conceptual Idea

The idea behind the addition of carbohydrates to the oral drink stems from animal studies of severe stress such as near-fatal hemorrhage or endotoxemia. These studies showed that even a short period of fasting depleting or reducing liver glycogen before such stress was associated with more catabolic metabolic reactions and in its extreme also mortality (for review see [11]). These observations led to the idea that the metabolic state of the patient—fed or overnight fasted—may impact the metabolic response to elective surgery and potentially postoperative recovery.

The first studies addressing this in patients were done using a highly concentrated i.v. glucose infusion (20 % glucose infused at 5 mg/kg/min) given in a large vein overnight [12, 13]. The studies revealed a marked difference in metabolic response to surgery, with the infusion of a high load of glucose resulting in less protein loss and a 50 % reduction in postoperative insulin resistance. Because of the high osmolality of the solution however some patients suffered from irritation and even some mild pain near the infusion site, despite the use of a large peripheral vein. To simplify the treatment, a carbohydrate-rich drink was developed, tailored for preoperative use, and further studies on its potential impact were performed.

The main objective of preoperative carbohydrate treatment is to change the overnight fasted state to a fed state through the activation of insulin to the levels seen after a normal meal (about 5–6 times basal fasting levels). In addition, the administered carbohydrates should ensure that glycogen stores were filled. At the same time it was necessary that the drink would be emptied quickly enough to be safe for use in clinical practice within the then newly formed modernized fasting guidelines. This was achieved by using complex carbohydrates as the main source of the carbohydrates, allowing the drink to be hypo-osmolar, which had been shown to be important for faster gastric emptying. The drink that was developed and tested contains 12.5 % carbohydrates and has an osmolality of approximately 265 mosm/kg. Most trials used an evening dose of 800 ml (100 g of carbohydrate) the night before surgery and a morning dose of 400 ml (50 g) given approximately 2 h before the induction of anesthesia. Intake of the morning dose of the carbohydrate drink was shown to empty from the stomach in 90 min, only slightly slower than a similar amount of water [14], while evoking the desired insulin response.

Preoperative Carbohydrates and Postoperative Metabolism

Preoperative carbohydrates alter the metabolic state before the onset of surgery from the fasted to the fed state. This not only affects glucose metabolism, but also protein and fat metabolism. Normal ingestion of carbohydrates and nutrients in general results in activation of several key signaling systems in the muscle such as tyrosine kinase and phosphatidyl-inositol 3-kinase (PI3K) that govern the anabolic actions of insulin in muscle [15, 16]. Preoperative carbohydrate treatment results in higher activity of these signals after surgery. Other studies have shown that the main insulin-activated glucose transporter GLUT4 is less disturbed after surgery in patients given carbohydrates compared to those in a fasted state. These findings in muscle cells help explain the reports of less insulin resistance in patients given carbohydrates before the onset of surgery.

Several studies showed that both intravenous glucose and oral carbohydrates could reduce insulin resistance by about 50 % the day after surgery. Consistent findings were seen when the gold standard method for studying postoperative insulin resistance was used, namely the hyperinsulinemic normoglycemic clamp method. This is a somewhat cumbersome and relatively expensive method in which i.v. insulin is infused at levels similar to those seen after a meal, with a simultaneous infusion of glucose with variable rates; the lower the glucose infusion rate needed to maintain normoglycemia, the greater the degree of insulin resistance. Determining insulin sensitivity before and after an operation allows changes in insulin resistance to be calculated. In elective surgical patients, the degree of insulin resistance is related to the magnitude of the operation [17], while the level of insulin sensitivity before the operation, BMI, and gender have no influence on these changes. A higher degree of insulin resistance is a recognized risk factor for the development of postoperative complications [18]. Due to the relatively expensive investment for the clamp, many researchers have opted to use another method, homeostatic model assessment (HOMA). This method calculates an index based on the basal glucose and insulin levels. Thus, the measurements are made in a situation of fasting when insulin is not physiologically active. As such, HOMA measurement is unable to capture the main defect in postoperative insulin resistance, namely insulin-stimulated glucose uptake in muscle. This explains the lack of agreement between results obtained by the two methods [19]. For the purposes of answering if insulin resistance is present or not after surgery, only data based on the clamp method should be used.

The intracellular changes described above may help explain the mechanisms for how carbohydrate loading may result in improved protein metabolism and muscle function. One of the earliest studies of preoperative carbohydrates using intravenous infusion showed reduced postoperative protein losses. Later studies found better preservation of lean body mass with preoperative carbohydrate loading, with less than half the loss of mid-arm circumference after major abdominal surgery compared to placebo [20]. Yet another study reported that preoperative carbohydrates resulted in better preservation of quadriceps muscle strength 1 month after surgery, again compared to patients fasted before the operation [21].

Preoperative Carbohydrates and Clinical Outcomes

While physiological data supports the concept of preoperative carbohydrates, there is a need for further studies investigating the clinical impact. Studies support that preoperative carbohydrates improve patient well-being compared to fasting or placebo by reducing thirst, hunger, anxiety, and preoperative nausea. The effect on postoperative well-being was not as clear.

Regarding clinical data such as length of stay, an early meta-analysis indicated that preoperative carbohydrate may reduce postoperative stay by about 1 day after major abdominal surgery, while no beneficial effect was seen in studies with short length of stay to begin with (laparoscopic surgery with an estimated stay of 1–2 days) or with smaller data samples (orthopedics) [22]. The studies pooled for analysis were not of highest quality. A recent Cochrane analysis came to similar conclusions, but when studies were pooled comparing patients undergoing major abdominal surgery given carbohydrate treatment with patients in the fasted state or given placebo, length of stay was reduced by 1.66 days [23]. However, the authors point to heterogeneity and differences in study quality as affecting confidence in these conclusions. Studies investigating the impact of individual elements of enhanced recovery protocols are inconsistent, with some showing no effect of carbohydrates, while others concluding that this treatment has a significant positive effect on outcomes in multivariant analyses of length of stay and complications [24].

Can Any Carbohydrate Drink Be Used?

A problem facing many clinicians wanting to use preoperative carbohydrates is to find a drink that is suitable. There are a few commercial drinks available for this specific purpose. However, most studies investigated the Nutricia preOp formula. There are other preoperative carbohydrate drinks available but these have limited or even no testing behind them. There are numerous ways of mixing carbohydrates and depending on the way this is done very different physiological effects will be achieved. Hence not every carbohydrate drink will be useful, and some may even be potentially dangerous in surgery. A preoperative carbohydrate-rich drink must have certain properties: the drink should result in a marked elevation of insulin to secure a change in metabolism before the onset of the operation; it should pass the stomach sufficiently fast to be safe and fit with the prevailing fasting guidelines; it should achieve a metabolic reaction or have a measurable clinically significant effect on well-being before or after surgery or affect outcomes postoperatively.

There are several carbohydrate-containing drinks that have been tried that will predictably not be achieving these effects. For example, sports drinks purposefully contain a concentration of carbohydrates of around 6 %. A sports drink is designed to give fluids, salts, and some carbohydrates while not eliciting a marked insulin release. An elevation in insulin will block the release of free fatty acids that is a main fuel for working muscle. An elevation of insulin would counteract the desired effect of supporting the working muscle. Many nutritional supplements will yield a sufficient elevation of insulin, but they may not pass the stomach fast enough to be safe. The same is true for formulas with high osmolar content and/or fat-containing drinks. Apple and other juices (without pulp) are sometimes also used, but again there are many brands available, all of them different. While it is likely that many of them can serve the purpose, they have not been specifically tested and therefore more studies are needed for preoperative carbohydrate loading.

Take-Home Messages

- Overnight fasting for elective surgery is obsolete.
- Modern fasting guidelines should be employed.
- Intake of clear fluids until 2 h and solids until 6 h before anesthesia is safe.
- Preoperative carbohydrates improve well-being and postoperative insulin resistance and may reduce hospital stay.
- The effect of preoperative carbohydrates on postoperative complications is unclear.

References

1. Maltby JRYP. Fasting from midnight—the history behind the dogma. Best Pract Res Clin Anaesthesiol. 2006;20(3):363–78.
2. Simpson JY. Remarks on the alleged case of death from the action of chloroform. Lancet. 1848;1:175–6.
3. Lister J. On anaesthestics. In: Holmes T, editor. Holmes system of surgery. London: Lingmans Green and Co.; 1883.
4. Mendelson C. The aspiration of stomach contents into the lungs during obstetric anaesthesia. Am J Obstet Gynecol. 1946;52:191–205.
5. Maltby JR, et al. Preoperative oral fluids: is a five-hour fast justified prior to elective surgery? Anesth Analg. 1986;65(11):1112–6.
6. Olsson GL, Hallen B, Hambraeus-Jonzon K. Aspiration during anaesthesia: a computer-aided study of 185,358 anaesthetics. Acta Anaesthesiol Scand. 1986;30(1): 84–92.
7. Madsen M, Brosnan J, Nagy VT. Perioperative thirst: a patient perspective. J Perianesth Nurs. 1998;13(4):225–8.
8. Goresky GV, Maltby JR. Fasting guidelines for elective surgical patients. Can J Anaesth. 1990;37(5):493–5.
9. Soreide E, Fasting S, Raeder J. New preoperative fasting guidelines in Norway. Acta Anaesthesiol Scand. 1997;41(6):799.
10. Smith I, et al. Perioperative fasting in adults and children: guidelines from the European Society of Anaesthesiology. Eur J Anaesthesiol. 2011;28(8):556–69.
11. Ljungqvist O. Modulating postoperative insulin resistance by preoperative carbohydrate loading. Best Pract Res Clin Anaesthesiol. 2009;23:401–9.
12. Ljungqvist O, et al. Glucose infusion instead of preoperative fasting reduces postoperative insulin resistance. J Am Coll Surg. 1994;178(4):329–36.
13. Crowe PJ, Dennison A, Royle GT. The effect of pre-operative glucose loading on postoperative nitrogen metabolism. Br J Surg. 1984;71(8):635–7.
14. Nygren J, et al. Preoperative gastric emptying. Effects of anxiety and oral carbohydrate administration. Ann Surg. 1995;222(6):728–34.
15. Witasp A, et al. Increased expression of inflammatory pathway genes in skeletal muscle during surgery. Clin Nutr. 2009;28(3):291–8.
16. Gjessing PF et al. Preoperative carbohydrate supplementation attenuates post-surgery insulin resistance via reduced inflammatory inhibition of the insulin-mediated restraint on muscle pyruvate dehydrogenase kinase 4 expression. Clin Nutr. 2014 Dec 11. pii: S0261-5614(14)00302-1.
17. Thorell A, Nygren J, Ljungqvist O. Insulin resistance: a marker of surgical stress. Curr Opin Clin Nutr Metab Care. 1999;2(1):69–78.
18. Sato H, et al. The association of preoperative glycemic control, intraoperative insulin sensitivity, and outcomes after cardiac surgery. J Clin Endocrinol Metabol. 2010; 95(9):4338–44.
19. Baban B, et al. Determination of insulin resistance in surgery: the choice of method is crucial. Clin Nutr. 2015;34(1):123–8.

20. Yuill KA, et al. The administration of an oral carbohydrate-containing fluid prior to major elective upper-gastrointestinal surgery preserves skeletal muscle mass postoperatively—a randomised clinical trial. Clin Nutr. 2005;24(1):32–7.
21. Henriksen MG, et al. Preoperative feeding might improve postoperative voluntary muscle function. Clin Nutr. 1999;18 Suppl 1:82.
22. Awad S, et al. A meta-analysis of randomised controlled trials on preoperative oral carbohydrate treatment in elective surgery. Clin Nutr. 2013;32(1):34–44.
23. Smith MD, et al. Preoperative carbohydrate treatment for enhancing recovery after surgery. Cochrane Database Syst. 2014;8, CD009161. doi:10.1002/14651858.CD009161.pub2.
24. Gustafsson UO, et al. Adherence to the enhanced recovery after surgery protocol and outcomes after colorectal cancer surgery. Arch Surg. 2011;146(5):571–7.

5. Bowel Preparation: Always, Sometimes, Never?

J.C. Slieker and D. Hahnloser

Bowel preparation is used to empty the intestinal tube before an intervention, which can be for surgical reasons, or prior to a colonoscopy. The main goal when applied prior to colonoscopy seems evident: the colon must be empty in order for pathologic lesions to be detected. The main reason why it is prescribed prior to surgery is to provide a completely clean bowel to minimize the risk of intraoperative faecal spillage. Other reasons described are to diminish the volume of the bowel for better intraoperative handling, or to facilitate the possibility to palpate small intraluminal masses.

Different Ways to Prep the Bowel for Surgery

The ideal bowel preparation reliably empties the intestine of all faecal material, with no histologic alteration of the colonic mucosa, and with as little discomfort and side-effects as possible for the patient. Non-invasive possibilities of bowel preparation, which consist of oral liquid diet or minimal residue diet, combined with laxatives, give suboptimal results and must be started days before the planned intervention. The most commonly prescribed preoperative bowel preparations are polyethylene glycol (PEG) and sodium phosphate. Historically these prescribed solutions are called *mechanical bowel preparation* in the surgical literature; however, this nomenclature seems outdated since there is no actual "mechanical" aspect to these drugs. In this chapter we have chosen to speak of *bowel preparation*, as is done in the field of gastroenterology.

L.S. Feldman et al. (eds.), *The SAGES / ERAS®*
Society Manual of Enhanced Recovery Programs for
Gastrointestinal Surgery, DOI 10.1007/978-3-319-20364-5_5,
© Springer International Publishing Switzerland 2015

Polyethylene glycol (*PEG*) is iso-osmotic, non-absorbable and acts by retaining fluid in the colon. Four litres are required. It is generally well tolerated; however, up to 15 % of patients do not complete the preparation due to poor taste and/or the large volume. PEG can safely be given to patients with comorbidities such as electrolyte disturbances, renal failure, heart failure, and liver insufficiency. Reduced volume options are available in a 2-l formulation, combined with stimulant agents such as bisacodyl or prokinetic agents such as metoclopramide. They have been associated with an equivalent level of cleansing and better patient tolerance.

Sodium phosphate is hyperosmotic and therefore acts by drawing fluid into the colon. Smaller quantities (90 ml) are required. Both PEG and sodium phosphate are successful (>90 %); however, sodium phosphate has a higher patient compliance, less adverse gastrointestinal symptoms and greater willingness of patients to reuse. Nevertheless, significant fluid and electrolyte disbalances can occur in patient with comorbidities and in older patients (>65 years), the use of sodium sulphate is associated with a higher risk of hyponatremia necessitating a hospitalization.

Like sodium phosphate, *magnesium citrate* is a hyperosmotic agent that promotes bowel cleansing by increasing intraluminal fluid volume. Since magnesium is eliminated solely by the kidney, it should be used with extreme caution in patients with renal insufficiency or renal failure.

A *rectal enema* (0.5–1 l of a laxative substance into the rectum through the anus) can achieve a bowel preparation of the descending colon and rectum, but cannot extend further to the right colon.

Bowel preparation with *oral drugs* exists in the form of NaP tablets. The dosage consists of 32–40 tablets, combined with 250 ml of clear fluid per tablet. One study compared NaP tablets to 4 l of PEG, finding equal colon cleansing with fewer side effects.

No Bowel Preparation for Surgery

Several histological studies have shown that bowel preparation is associated with bowel wall alterations consisting of loss of superficial mucus and epithelial cells, as well as inflammatory changes such as lymphocyte and polymorphonuclear cell infiltration. In addition, bowel preparation can be associated with a higher rate of bowel contents spillage, because liquid contents cause higher rates of spillage. This showed a trend toward more infectious complications; however, this increase was not statistically significant. The degree of inadequate bowel preparation is described between 20 and 40 % in literature.

For all the above mentioned pathophysiological and patient-related reasons, the use of bowel preparation has been questioned in recent years. Patients in general do not like it, so do we really need it? Does it facilitate surgery? Are infectious and non-infectious complications decreased with bowel preparation? Does it facilitate the possibility to palpate small intraluminal masses intraoperatively? All these questions led to many prospective randomized trials and Cochrane reviews (Table 5.1). When we look at the evidence regarding infectious post-operative complications, we can subdivide the results for colon and rectum resections.

No Bowel Preparation for Colon Resections!

For colon resection all different meta-analyses performed in the past years uniformly conclude that there is no advantage of bowel preparation prior to surgery. Rates of anastomotic leakage and septic complications in patients without bowel preparation compared to patients with preoperative bowel preparation were equal or even lower. The latest Cochrane meta-analysis dating from 2011 combined 18 studies, comparing 2906 and 2899 patients in each group. No significant difference was found in the incidence of anastomotic leakage, wound infection, extra-abdominal infectious complication, peritonitis, reoperation, and mortality. A separate study on oncologic outcome between patients having received bowel preparation preoperatively versus a control group has shown no difference on long term survival between groups.

The evidence is sufficient to conclude that bowel cleansing can be safely omitted and induces no lower complication rate in colonic surgery. There is no statistically significant evidence that patients benefit from bowel preparation. Therefore, for right-sided resections no action is required. For left-sided resections many surgeons prescribe an enema the day before or the day of surgery to clean out the rectum and facilitate transanal stapled anastomosing of the bowel. Theoretically this can be also done through wash-out during surgery. However, this approach is not very frequently used and we recommend an enema (500 ml to 1 l) the day or morning before surgery.

Table 5.1. Overview of the available Cochrane meta-analyses on bowel preparation

Year Cochrane	RCTs included	Prep/no prep N=	% Leak Colon	% Leak Rectum	Bowel prep...	Bowel prep should be...
2003	6	576/583	1.2 % vs. 0.6 % (ns)	12.5 % vs. 12 % (ns)	...not reduce leak	...questioned
2005	9	789/803	2.9 % vs. 1.6 % (ns)	9.8 % vs. 7.5 % (ns)	...not reduce leak	...reconsidered
2009	13	2390/2387	2.9 % vs. 2.5 % (ns)	10 % vs. 6.6 % (ns)	...no benefit	...questioned
2011	18	2906/2899	3.0 % vs. 3.5 % (ns)	8.8 % vs. 10.3 % (ns)	...no benefit	Colon: omitted Rectum: selectively

No Bowel Preparation for Rectal Resections?

The possible benefit of a complete bowel preparation has also been studied in Cochrane meta-analyses. In 2011, it included seven studies, comparing 415 and 431 patients with regard to anastomotic leakage, infectious and non-infectious complications. The conclusion was identical to colon resections: no evidence of bowel preparation prior to surgery can be proven. However, one of the largest randomized controlled trials (Bretagnol 2010) showed more infectious complications in the group without any bowel preparation. There was a clear trend towards more anastomotic leakage (19 %) compared to the group with bowel preparation (10 %). The study was criticized for using absolutely no bowel cleaning in the control group, which seems to make transanal stapling difficulty, not to say "dirty".

A lavage of the rectum during the operation or a preoperative transanal enema is a possible solution. A rectum enema would be sufficient to clear the area of its faeces where the stapled anastomosis is made. On the other hand, rectal enema will not clean the entire colon and it is argued that if the rectal resections will be covered with a temporary ostomy then the entire colon distally to the ostomy should be emptied preoperatively, in order to limit the stool spillage in case of anastomotic leakage. One case-controlled study compared full bowel preparation to rectal enema only and found no increased infectious complications including anastomotic leakage in the latter group. However, the study was small (50 patients in each group) and not prospectively randomized. Therefore, many surgeons agree that some sort (e.g. enema, mechanical bowel preparation) of bowel preparation is still necessary for rectal resections with anastomosis, even though no significant effect was found. Further studies are required.

Oral Antibiotics and Bowel Preparation

Several recent studies have found that bowel preparation combined with the administration of oral antibiotics results in reduced surgical site infection. The hypothesis is that bowel preparation permits washout of the faeces, permitting the oral antibiotic to reduce the bacterial concentration of the colonic mucosa. However, this evidence is based on observational studies, and confirmation through randomized studies is needed. Furthermore, strict documentation of infectious complications and possible development of resistance should be included in these studies.

Bowel Preparation and Survival After Cancer Surgery

A recent analysis of a Swedish randomized study on mechanical bowel preparation 1995–1999 found significantly fewer recurrences and better cancer-specific and overall survival in the bowel preparation group. However, this study is a secondary analysis and is underpowered for the survival endpoints. In addition, it was unknown whether patients received adjuvant therapy, which could have influenced the oncological results.

Considerations for Laparoscopic Surgery

Many of the randomized studies and meta-analyses have not exclusively included laparoscopic resections, and therefore conclusions cannot be extrapolated to laparoscopic surgery. Logically, one does not expect the effect of bowel preparation on anastomotic leakage and other septic complications to be different between patients with a laparoscopic or open approach. However, the effect of bowel preparation on the volume of the bowel, and thus on exposure, could play an important role in the course of the laparoscopic intervention itself, perhaps especially in the area of single port laparoscopic surgery.

In a pig study a gain of 500 ml CO_2 pneumoperitoneum independently of the pressure was seen in the group receiving bowel preparation. Consequently, with preoperative bowel preparation the same volume of pneumoperitoneum could be obtained at lower intra-abdominal pressures. This could represent more space in technically challenging laparoscopic surgery. Two randomized studies in gynaecologic laparoscopy seem to conclude that there is no amelioration of surgical field exposure with bowel preparation. The difficulty of these studies is the outcome measure, which is the evaluation of the surgical field using a surgeon questionnaire. The surgeon's evaluation of the working space may be too subjective to detect significant differences in outcome.

In addition, it seems logical that a bowel full of stool requires a larger incision at the extraction site than an empty bowel. However, we do not know if this is really a relevant factor, especially in obese patients with fatty mesenteries.

Special Situations

Special considerations should be kept in mind for certain categories of interventions. With SILS (single incision laparoscopic surgery) or the future ileostomy as the extraction site, it may be impossible to extract a colon full of faeces, and bowel preparation should be prescribed preoperatively. When performing a combined endoscopic–laparoscopic resection, obviously full bowel preparation is needed. The construction of a neovagina deserves full attention considering infectious prevention, reason why full bowel preparation should be considered. In case of a colonic stent placed as a bridge to surgery, we recommend bowel preparation as stool can stay impacted in front of the stent.

However, despite the lack of evidence in favour of bowel preparation for standard colorectal surgery, different surveys amongst colorectal surgeons reveal bowel preparation is still prescribed preoperatively. Table 5.2 illustrates the gap between the evidence on bowel preparation and surgeon practices, showing that surgeons are not at ease to completely abandon bowel preparation. The reasons for this reluctance would be interesting to investigate.

Table 5.2. Results of published surveys among colorectal surgeons on practice regarding full bowel preparation

	Colon	Rectum
Switzerland (2008)	53 %	83 %
New Zealand and Australia (2010)	28 %	63 %
GB and Ireland (2010)	Right—17 % Left—43 %	72 %
Germany 2010		91 %
Austria 2010		79 %
Spain 2006/2007	Right—59 % Left—90 %	98 %

Conclusions

In conclusion, thorough mechanical cleansing of the bowel has long been considered essential prior to colorectal operations. One believed an empty bowel would diminish the risk of anastomotic leakage and septic complications. However, during the last decade several studies have uniformly concluded that there is no advantage of bowel preparation prior to colonic resections, finding equal or lower rates of anastomotic leakage and septic complications in patients without bowel preparation compared to patients with preoperative bowel preparation. There is some evidence that this conclusion is also valid in the field of rectum surgery, however more studies are needed. In most enhanced recovery protocols in Europe, full bowel preparation is omitted for colon surgeries including end-colostomies. For rectal cancer surgery some sort of bowel preparation (enema or full mechanical bowel preparation) is still performed.

Take Home Messages

- Bowel preparation leads to bowel wall alterations and inflammatory changes.
- PEG and sodium phosphate act differently, but are both equally effective in cleaning the bowel.
- Bowel preparation can safely be omitted in elective colon resections.
- For rectal resections the available evidence shows no benefit of bowel preparation; however, more studies are needed, especially for low rectal resections with protective temporary ileostomies.
- Despite the lack of evidence in favour of no bowel preparation it is still largely prescribed preoperatively, presumably for surgeon preference.

Suggested Readings

1. Güenaga KF, Matos D, Wille-Jørgensen P. Mechanical bowel preparation for elective colorectal surgery. Cochrane Database Syst Rev. 2011 Sep 7;(9):CD001544.
2. Bretagnol F, Panis Y, Rullier E. Rectal cancer surgery with or without bowel preparation: the French GRECCAR III multicenter single-blinded randomized trial. Ann Surg. 2010;252(5):863–8.

3. Wexner SD, Beck DE, Baron TH. A consensus document on bowel preparation before colonoscopy: prepared by a Task Force from the American Society of Colon and Rectal Surgeons (ASCRS), the American Society for Gastrointestinal Endoscopy (ASGE), and the Society of American Gastrointestinal and Endoscopic Surgeons (SAGES). Surg Endosc. 2006;20(7):1161.
4. Bucher P, Gervaz P, Egger JF. Morphologic alterations associated with mechanical bowel preparation before elective colorectal surgery: a randomized trial. Dis Colon Rectum. 2006;49(1):109–12.
5. Vlot J, Slieker JC, Wijnen R. Optimizing working-space in laparoscopy: measuring the effect of mechanical bowel preparation in a porcine model. Surg Endosc. 2013; 27(6):1980–5.

6. The Role of the Anesthesiologist in Reducing Surgical Stress and Improving Recovery

Francesco Carli

Although there have been major advances in surgical technology and anesthesia techniques, the relatively high rate of postoperative complications continues to have an impact on health care. Thanks to closer collaboration between different medical disciplines, a great deal of attention has been focused on how to improve the quality of surgical care, reduce perioperative morbidity, accelerate the recovery process and better utilize health resources. With this in mind, great effort has been pursued in the development and implementation of Enhanced Recovery After Surgery programs (ERP) with the intention to understand and identify the factors that keep patients in hospital longer than necessary and delay their return to baseline. The chapter elucidates the physiological mechanisms characteristic of the response to surgical stress and proposes a role of the anesthesiologist as a perioperative physician in addressing the strategies which can modify this response and facilitate recovery.

The Surgical Stress Response and the Development of Insulin Resistance

The cascade of events that are initiated with surgery are commonly referred to as the stress response which is characterized by a release in neuroendocrine hormones, and production of various inflammatory products (Fig. 6.1). The combination of both the systemic inflammatory response and hypothalamic-sympathetic stimulation acts on target organs including the brain, heart, muscle, and liver leading to release of

L.S. Feldman et al. (eds.), *The SAGES / ERAS®*
Society Manual of Enhanced Recovery Programs for
Gastrointestinal Surgery, DOI 10.1007/978-3-319-20364-5_6,
© Springer International Publishing Switzerland 2015

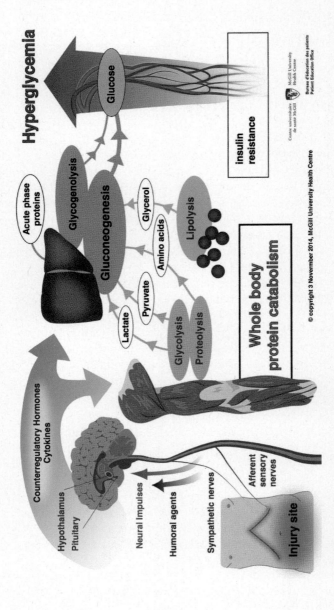

Fig. 6.1. Metabolic and inflammatory changes leading to a state of insulin resistance. (Courtesy of McGill University Health Centre Patient Education Office, Montreal, Quebec, Canada.).

anxiety, pain, tissue damage, ileus,
tachycardia, anorexia, hypoxia,
disruption of sleep patterns,
hypothermia, acidosis, hyperglycemia,
loss of body mass, impaired
homeostasis, altered fibrinolysis.

Fig. 6.2. Consequences of the stress response.

energy substrates (fat, carbohydrates, and protein) to use as fuel for vital organs such as brain, muscle, heart, and kidney. Negative consequences initiated by this response include anxiety, pain, tissue damage, ileus, tachycardia, anorexia, hypoxia, disruption of sleep patterns, hypothermia, acidosis, hyperglycemia, loss of body mass, impaired homeostasis, and altered fibrinolysis (Fig. 6.2). The magnitude of the inflammatory response is proportional to the degree of surgical insult. An obvious clinical example is the use of endoscopic surgical techniques when compared with open procedures, which are associated with an attenuated inflammatory response to surgery. The improved outcomes such as less pain and shorter hospitalization associated with laparoscopic techniques are generally well established.

The degree of the inflammatory response is variable and this might be related to genetic polymorphism. Patients with higher proinflammatory response were shown to be prone to a greater incidence of postoperative complications. Central to the physiological changes of the metabolic response to surgery, characterized by catecholamine release and hyperinflammation followed by immunosuppression, is the development of insulin resistance. A correlation has been demonstrated between high circulating values of CRP, a marker of the inflammatory response, and poor preoperative insulin sensitivity.

Insulin resistance can be defined as a condition wherein a normal concentration of insulin produces a subnormal biological response. In the context of the surgical stress response, the actions of insulin as a key anabolic hormone are reduced in order to rapidly mobilize energy substrate. This has been termed "the diabetes of injury." A significant correlation has been demonstrated between the degree of the patient's insulin sensitivity on the first postoperative day and length of hospital stay. Also a significant association has been reported between the

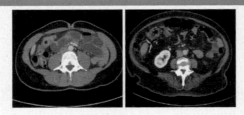

Core muscle size assessed by perioperative CT scan is related to mortality, postoperative complications, and hospitalization after major abdominal surgery

Langenbecks Arch Surg 399: 287-295 (2014)

Fig. 6.3. Poor preoperative physical status can lead to high morbidity and mortality. (From Hasselager R, Gogenur I. Core muscle size assessed by perioperative abdominal CT scan is related to mortality, postoperative complications, and hospitalization after major abdominal surgery: a systematic review. Langenbecks Arch Surg 2014; 399:287–95, with permission.).

magnitude of insulin resistance and complications. For every decrease in intraoperative insulin sensitivity by 20 %, the risk of serious complications was more than doubled after open heart surgery.

Insulin controls glucose, fat and protein metabolism, and with the presence of surgical injury, glucose and protein metabolism are altered. Hyperglycemia and protein breakdown represent the two main metabolic consequences of the surgical stress. The loss of muscle mass following major abdominal surgery amounts to approximately 50–70 g of protein per day (Fig. 6.3).

Preoperative conditions such as cancer, morbid obesity and metabolic syndrome, and perioperative elements such as fasting and starvation, pain, bed rest, and fatigue, have each been identified as contributing to the establishment of the postoperative insulin resistance state.

ERP and the Modulation of Stress Response

With the understanding that the pathophysiology of the stress response is multifactorial, therapeutic strategies should target those elements contributing to the development of insulin resistance as well as others with different physiological mechanisms. The modulation of the stress response would result in normalizing insulin action and the main components of metabolism, preserving protein stores. Many of these elements will be dealt in depth in the different chapters of this manual.

Getting the Patient Ready for Surgery

Elderly patients represent a great portion of surgical practice and although age per se does not preclude surgery, the presence of coexisting diseases such as hypertension, stroke, ischemic heart disease, hypercholesterolemia, and diabetes has a greater impact on postoperative morbidity and mortality than age alone. Other stressors such as obesity, frailty, malnutrition resulting from cancer also need also to be considered. Smoking, alcohol, anemia, poor nutritional status, and poor glycemic control can further impact on postoperative infection rate, immune function, and tissue healing. Preoperative anxiety, emotional distress, and depression have been shown to be associated with higher complication rates, greater postoperative pain, cognitive disturbances, and delayed convalescence.

The role of the preoperative clinic is to identify with sufficient time those patients who present a serious surgical and anesthetic risk and to attempt to optimize them from the physical, metabolic, nutritional, and mental point of view. Preparing the frail and deconditioned patient with a prehabilitation program aimed at increasing the functional reserve is a strategy which could be recommended if sufficient time (3–4 weeks) is available. It makes sense that the anesthesiologist, being knowledgeable in both surgical and medical disciplines, leads the preoperative program, in conjunction with internists, geriatricians, hematologists, nurses, physiotherapists and kinesiologists, nutritionists, and possibly psychologists. Besides these interventions, patients and caregivers need to be educated about the surgical process and empowered.

Arriving to the Operating Room in the Fed State

Although all societies of anesthesia recommend ingestion of clear fluids up to 2 h before surgery, the clinical practice in many hospitals still follows the old dogma of keeping the patient fasting from midnight.

Fasting has been shown to cause a decrease in insulin sensitivity, and to accentuate the development of postoperative insulin resistance. Research has shown that animals sustain trauma better in the fed rather than fasted state. The administration of preoperative oral carbohydrates raises insulin sensitivity by 50 %, and the impact on postoperative metabolic function is characterized by 50 % less postoperative insulin resistance, less risk of hyperglycemia and improved retention of protein and preservation of lean body mass.

Choosing Anesthesia Drugs to Facilitate Recovery

The choice of anesthetic drugs is based on the understanding that the physiologic and metabolic response to surgery has to be minimized and the prolongation of the effect of the anesthetic drugs on recovery has to be avoided. With this in mind, long acting anxiolytics (e.g., lorazepam) must be avoided and short acting anesthetic agents should be used. Bispectral index (BIS) can be used to monitor the depth of anesthesia and avoid deep sedation. Deep muscle relaxation is necessary for laparoscopic procedures in order to facilitate surgical exposure and avoid high intraperitoneal pressure which can lead to impaired hemodynamics and increased visceral pain. Adjuvant anesthetic drugs such as ketamine, dexmedetomidine, lidocaine, dexamethasone can be used for their opioid sparing effects. Nausea and vomiting prophylaxis (dexamethasone, droperidol, odansetron) is strongly advised.

The Role of Regional Anesthesia

As the central and peripheral nervous systems are identified as part of the pathway leading to the metabolic changes following surgery, it would make sense to block the afferent and efferent nociceptive stimuli in anticipation of the injury. There is sufficient evidence that epidural and spinal, and to some extent peripheral nerve blocks, play a major role in decreasing the development of postoperative insulin resistance, thus minimizing the catabolic response, and provide excellent pain relief while also sparing opioid side effects. This is particularly evident with open abdominal surgery, but not when laparoscopic approach is used. A possible side effect of epidural analgesia is hypotension which might impact on recovery. When epidural blockade is contraindicated alternative solutions are available such as intravenous lidocaine, abdominal field blocks, or pre-peritoneal catheter with continuous infusion of local anesthetics. When possible the surgeon should infiltrate the wound with local anesthetics.

Maintaining Homeostasis During Surgery

Hypothermia, fluid overload, hyperglycemia, exaggerated cardiovascular responses such as tachycardia, hypertension, hypotension, arrhythmias, and respiratory disturbances such as hypercapnia, elevated airway resistance, and hypoxia all need to be avoided during surgery. All these elements represent important stressors that can enhance the metabolic changes and have an impact on postoperative outcome.

Multimodal Analgesia to Facilitate Recovery

In view of the multifactorial nature and complexity of postoperative pain pathways, analgesia must be achieved with different classes of medications acting on multiple sites. Multimodal analgesic strategies aim not only to improve postoperative pain control but also to attenuate the multi-organ dysfunction induced by unrelieved pain but also reduce opioid side-effects such as nausea and vomiting and ileus, thus facilitating early resumption of oral diet and early mobilization.

Future Directions

The knowledge of surgical metabolism helps us to better understand the changes occurring when a series of therapeutic modalities is implemented; however, the connection between the physiological and the clinical outcome is not always evident. Many aspects of the inflammatory response to surgery such as postoperative fatigue, ileus, sympathetic activation, visceral pain, sleep disorders are still to be elucidated. The anesthesiologist is rightly positioned to work together with the perioperative team to address these aspects of surgical pathophysiology and facilitate the transfer of knowledge to clinical practice.

Take Home Messages

- The surgical stress response, if not controlled, can lead to physiologic and metabolic consequences and impact on patient recovery.
- The anesthesiologist can intervene starting from the preoperative optimization and continuing during the perioperative period to maintain homeostasis, and providing adequate analgesia, thus minimizing the untoward effects of surgical stress.
- This can only be achieved if closer collaboration is in place between the anesthesiologist and the surgeon and in conjunction with different specialties such as geriatrics, internal medicine, hematology, physiotherapy, nutrition.

Suggested Readings

1. Feldman L, Baldini G, Lee L, Carli F. Basic Surgical and Perioperative Consideraton. Enhanced Recovery Pathways: Organization of Evidence-Based, Fast-Track Perioperative Care. In: *Scientific American Surgery*. 2013;1–29.
2. Ljungqvist O. Insulin resistance and enhanced recovery after surgery. J Parenter Enteral Nutr. 2012;36:389–98.
3. White PF, Kehlet H, Neal JM, Schricker T, Carr DB, Carli F. The role of the anesthesiologist in fast-track surgery: from multimodal analgesia to perioperative medical care. Anesth Analg. 2007;104:1380–96.

7. Prevention of Hypothermia

Timothy E. Miller

Mild perioperative hypothermia, defined as a core body temperature between 34 and 36 °C, is common and preventable [1]. Without active interventions approximately 70 % of patient undergoing operations lasting 2 h or longer will become hypothermic [2]. This is of concern as mild perioperative hypothermia has been associated with adverse outcomes [1, 3]. This chapter will explore the causes of perioperative hypothermia, the potential adverse consequences for patients, and techniques and recommendations for avoiding inadvertent perioperative hypothermia.

Causes of Perioperative Hypothermia

Patients are frequently cool peripherally when they arrive in the operating theater (OR), wearing a thin gown with the body exposed to the cool hospital environment. General anesthesia then profoundly impairs our normal thermoregulatory responses [1]. Induction of anesthesia causes direct peripheral vasodilation, and decreases the threshold for shivering and vasoconstriction by 2–3 °C resulting in vasodilation and a distribution of heat from the core to the periphery (usually 2–4 °C cooler) which, without intervention, will decrease core temperature by 1–1.5 °C after 1 h of anesthesia [4]. This mechanism is accentuated when the periphery is already cool, with vasoconstriction constraining heat in the core and increasing the core-to-periphery gradient.

This initial redistribution, without intervention, is followed by a slower decrease in core temperature over the next few hours as heat loss exceeds heat production, with the rate depending on the size of the patient [4]. The addition of neuraxial anesthesia (spinal, epidural) will

L.S. Feldman et al. (eds.), *The SAGES / ERAS®*
Society Manual of Enhanced Recovery Programs for
Gastrointestinal Surgery, DOI 10.1007/978-3-319-20364-5_7,
© Springer International Publishing Switzerland 2015

exaggerate these responses by further inhibiting vasoconstriction, so that active thermal management is especially important in patients with combined general and regional anesthesia [5].

Adverse Consequences of Perioperative Hypothermia

Even mild perioperative hypothermia (34–36 °C) has been shown in large randomized controlled trials (RCTs) to be associated with adverse outcomes. Most importantly for major gastrointestinal surgery mild hypothermia triples the risk of surgical site infection (SSI) by directly impairing immunity, and by causing vasoconstriction, which decreases oxygen delivery to the wound [3]. In animal models mild hypothermia also impairs resistance to bacterial infection.

Mild hypothermia also significantly increases blood loss and the relative risk of transfusion by about 20 % for each 1 °C drop in core temperature, which is substantial and clinically significant [6]. The mechanism is multifactorial: hypothermia impairs platelet function, primarily by impairing release of thromboxane A_2 which is needed to form the initial platelet plug, as well as the function of enzymes in the clotting cascade [7]. This impairment in coagulation will not be apparent during routine coagulation screening as these tests are performed at 37 °C [8].

Prospective randomized controlled trials also show that mild hypothermia can cause other complications such as shivering (which increases oxygen consumption) [9], a threefold increase in adverse cardiac events [10, 11], and prolonged hospital stay [3]. Hypothermia also prolongs the duration of action of anesthetic and neuromuscular blocking agents that can result in delayed recovery [12]. Finally and importantly hypothermia is very unpleasant for patients, can persist for several hours, and is often remembered as one of the worst aspects of their perioperative experience [13]. This discomfort is also stressful for patients and elevates blood pressure, heart rate, and plasma catecholamine levels [14]. These factors, along with shivering, presumably contribute to the significant and serious increase cardiac events.

Temperature Monitoring

The patient's temperature should be monitored perioperatively to help prevent inadvertent hypothermia, and also to enable warming to be adjusted to avoid hyperpyrexia which can occur in prolonged procedures with active warming, or if the patient develops a systemic inflammatory response syndrome (SIRS).

Core body temperature should be measured in patients undergoing general anesthesia for longer than 30 min. Core temperature can be reliably monitored at the tympanic membrane, pulmonary artery (with a pulmonary artery catheter), distal esophagus, or nasopharynx. Bladder, rectal, oral, and forehead skin temperatures can be measured clinically but may not reliably reflect core temperature.

Recommendations for Perioperative Care

Prevention of hypothermia mainly requires attention to detail and the adoption of a few simple measures during the patient's perioperative journey.

Preoperative

Preoperative assessment is clinically important to help identify patients at risk of inadvertent perioperative hypothermia, and can help anesthesia providers prepare suitable warming methods. Patients at high risk have a high severity of illness on admission, low body mass index (BMI), age >65 years, and anemia, and are planned to undergo combined general and regional anesthesia, or major surgery [2, 15]. It is also important for anesthesia providers to be aware of the patient's planned position during surgery, and the area available for warming devices; for instance the lithotomy position or "prepping in a leg" for a possible skin graft can significantly alter the options available for intraoperative patient warming.

The initial redistribution of heat from the central thermal compartment to cooler peripheral tissues is difficult to treat, but it can be reduced. Preoperatively, patients should be encouraged to be active if possible (e.g., walk to the operating department), which generates body heat. They should also be encouraged to verbalize when they feel cold.

Patients should be nursed in a warm environment to minimize peripheral cooling. There is some evidence that pre-emptive skin surface warming for 1–2 h preoperatively is effective in reducing the initial redistribution of heat that occurs after induction of anesthesia [16]. The most important site is the legs, which is the largest contributor to the peripheral thermal compartment. If the patient's preoperative temperature is below 36 °C, then it is advisable to start forced-air warming preoperatively.

Intraoperative

The most important factor in determining intraoperative heat loss is operating room temperature. Room temperatures above 23 °C in adults (up to 26 °C in infants) will help to maintain normothermia, but will be uncomfortable for the operating room staff. Therefore it is recommended that ambient temperature is maintained at 21 °C or above, especially during induction of anesthesia or when the patient is exposed; if normothermia is maintained, this may be reduced once active warming is established [17].

Airway Heating and Humidification

Approximately 10 % of metabolic heat production is lost via the respiratory tract, from both the heating and humidification of inspiratory gases. This can be reduced by routine humidification of airway gases, although the overall effect on core temperature is minimal [18].

Intravenous Fluid Warming

Administration of 1 l of intravenous (IV) fluid at room temperature (21 °C) or one unit of refrigerated blood decreases the core body temperature by approximately 0.25 °C. Therefore whilst patients cannot be warmed by using fluid warmers (fluid given cannot substantially exceed body temperature), heat loss can be prevented, especially when large amounts of fluid are given. Administration of warmed IV fluid has been shown to decrease the incidence of hypothermia in gynecologic, abdominal, and orthopedic surgery [19]. Their use has been recommended for all intraoperative IV infusions >500 ml in adults [17]. At low flow rates, there are no clinically important differences between any of the available fluid warmers. At higher flow rates the Hotline countercurrent water heat exchanger (Level 1 Technologies Inc, Rockland, MA, USA) consistently delivers the warmest fluid outlet temperatures [19]. During massive transfusion or whenever very high flow rates are needed, high volume systems with powerful heaters are recommended to deliver large amounts of warm fluid quickly (e.g., level 1 infusor, Belmont).

Cutaneous Warming Devices

The simplest way to decrease cutaneous heat loss is to apply a cotton blanket, or surgical drape to the skin to trap a layer of still air below the covering and act as a passive insulator. A single layer will reduce heat loss by approximately 30 %, with additional layers only adding marginal benefit [20]. Warming the blanket may increase patient satisfaction but has little benefit, and the benefit is short-lived [20]. Therefore passive warming can help to reduce heat loss but usually insufficient to prevent mild hypothermia.

The most common intraoperative warming systems are forced-air convective warming systems or forced-air warmers, which distribute heated air generated by a power unit through a specially designed blanket. About 90 % of metabolic heat is lost via the skin surface, and forced-air warmers have a dual benefit of almost completely eliminating this loss where they are sited, and transferring heat to the body. Heat transfer per unit area is relatively low, but as long as a large surface area is available for heating forced-air warmers are generally very effective and maintain normothermia even during major procedures [18, 21]. They are superior to passive insulation both in preventing hypothermia and rewarming already hypothermic patients [19]. Forced-air warming is also inexpensive and remarkably safe, and has therefore become the routine method of warming surgical patients. It is preferable to cover most of the exposed area when possible in order to counteract the heat loss coming from large abdominal incisions.

By comparison, circulating water mattresses are generally less effective [22]. Little heat is lost from the back, and therefore water mattresses do not effectively reduce heat loss. All of the trials comparing circulating water mattresses with forced-air warmers have favored forced-air warming [19]. However when forced-air warming cannot be used for practical reasons, they should be considered in patients at low to medium risk of inadvertent hypothermia. The cost is comparable with forced-air warming devices.

In high-risk patients newer alternative warming devices are now available that use adhesive circulating water garments and "energy transfer pads" to improve local heat transfer efficiency. An example is the Kimberley Clark Patient Warming System (Kimberley Clark, Roswell, GA), which uses adhesive pads with microchannels for circulating water that can be applied to the back, legs, or chest. The use of temperature management systems incorporating energy transfer pads warms healthy volunteers twice as fast as forced-air warming [23]. Intraoperatively they have also been shown to be more effective than forced-air warming, as well as offering more flexibility in warming sites [24, 25]. They are however considerably more expensive than other warming methods and are therefore probably best reserved for operations in which forced-air warming may be inadequate for maintaining normothermia. Examples include major abdominal surgery in the lithotomy position, major vascular surgery, or polytrauma; where both a large amount of the body is exposed (with considerable heat loss), and there is a restricted area available for warming.

Alternatively in high-risk patients combinations of devices can be used. The combination of two forced-air warming devices (upper and lower body covers) and a posterior water mattress has been shown to be equivalent to water garments, and considerable cheaper, although less practical [26].

Other warming methods include heating or humidifying the carbon dioxide gas used for insufflation in laparoscopic procedures. However in a Cochrane review this method did not improve the patient's temperature or pain scores after surgery [27].

Warmed fluids should be used by the surgical team when irrigation of the abdominal cavity is needed since the large surface area of the peritoneum, exposed to ambient temperature, can contribute to significant loss of heat.

Postoperative

Active warming should be continued into the postoperative period until the patient's temperature is greater than 36 °C, and they are comfortably warm [17]. As there is no limitation on the available surface area for warming postoperatively, this is usually achieved, if needed, with forced-air warming.

Conclusion

Every patient should have a perioperative warming management plan. This plan should include not only choosing the appropriate body warming device for the patient and surgery but also limiting preoperative cooling and exposed body surfaces, ensuring the room temperature is above 21 °C, and using warmed IV fluids appropriately.

During major surgery or in high-risk cases, a single warming device may not eliminate the risk of inadvertent hypothermia, and therefore combinations of warming modalities or newer more expensive circulating water garments may be appropriate.

Take Home Messages

- Mild perioperative hypothermia, defined as a core body temperature between 34 and 36 °C, is common and preventable.
- Mild hypothermia can cause a variety of adverse events such as increased risk of surgical wound infection, adverse myocardial events, coagulopathy, shivering, and prolonged post-anesthetic recovery.
- The most important factor in determining intraoperative heat loss is operating room temperature. It is recommended that ambient temperature is maintained at 21 °C or above.
- Intravenous fluid warmers should be used for all intraoperative IV infusions >500 ml in adults.
- Forced-air warming is inexpensive, effective, and remarkably safe, and has therefore become the routine method of warming surgical patients.
- In high-risk cases circulating water garments or combinations of warming may be appropriate.

References

1. Sessler DI. Complications and treatment of mild hypothermia. Anesthesiology. 2001;95:531–43.
2. Bernard H. Patient warming in surgery and the enhanced recovery. Br J Nurs. 2013;22:319–20.
3. Kurz A, Sessler DI, Lenhardt R. Perioperative normothermia to reduce the incidence of surgical-wound infection and shorten hospitalization. Study of Wound Infection and Temperature Group. N Engl J Med. 1996;334:1209–15.

4. Sessler DI. Perioperative heat balance. Anesthesiology. 2000;92:578–96.

5. Joris J, Ozaki M, Sessler DI, Hardy AF, Lamy M, McGuire J, Blanchard D, Schroeder M, Moayeri A. Epidural anesthesia impairs both central and peripheral thermoregulatory control during general anesthesia. Anesthesiology. 1994;80:268–77.

6. Rajagopalan S, Mascha E, Na J, Sessler DI. The effects of mild perioperative hypothermia on blood loss and transfusion requirement. Anesthesiology. 2008;108:71–7.

7. Valeri CR, Feingold H, Cassidy G, Ragno G, Khuri S, Altschule MD. Hypothermia-induced reversible platelet dysfunction. Ann Surg. 1987;205:175–81.

8. Staab DB, Sorensen VJ, Fath JJ, Raman SB, Horst HM, Obeid FN. Coagulation defects resulting from ambient temperature-induced hypothermia. J Trauma. 1994; 36:634–8.

9. Sharkey A, Lipton JM, Murphy MT, Giesecke AH. Inhibition of postanesthetic shivering with radiant heat. Anesthesiology. 1987;66:249–52.

10. Frank SM, Fleisher LA, Breslow MJ, Higgins MS, Olson KF, Kelly S, Beattie C. Perioperative maintenance of normothermia reduces the incidence of morbid cardiac events. A randomized clinical trial. JAMA. 1997;277:1127–34.

11. Nesher N, Zisman E, Wolf T, Sharony R, Bolotin G, David M, Uretzky G, Pizov R. Strict thermoregulation attenuates myocardial injury during coronary artery bypass graft surgery as reflected by reduced levels of cardiac-specific troponin I. Anesth Analg. 2003;96:328–35. Table of contents.

12. Lenhardt R, Marker E, Goll V, Tschernich H, Kurz A, Sessler DI, Narzt E, Lackner F. Mild intraoperative hypothermia prolongs postanesthetic recovery. Anesthesiology. 1997;87:1318–23.

13. Kumar S, Wong PF, Melling AC, Leaper DJ. Effects of perioperative hypothermia and warming in surgical practice. Int Wound J. 2005;2:193–204.

14. Frank SM, Higgins MS, Breslow MJ, Fleisher LA, Gorman RB, Sitzmann JV, Raff H, Beattie C. The catecholamine, cortisol, and hemodynamic responses to mild perioperative hypothermia. A randomized clinical trial. Anesthesiology. 1995;82:83–93.

15. Billeter AT, Hohmann SF, Druen D, Cannon R, Polk Jr HC. Unintentional perioperative hypothermia is associated with severe complications and high mortality in elective operations. Surgery. 2014;156(5):1245–52.

16. Just B, Trevien V, Delva E, Lienhart A. Prevention of intraoperative hypothermia by preoperative skin-surface warming. Anesthesiology. 1993;79:214–8.

17. NICE National Institute for Health and Care Excellence. CG65 Clinical practice guideline. The management of inadvertent perioperative hypothermia in adults. 2008. http://pathways.nice.org.uk/pathways/inadvertent-perioperative-hypothermia?fno=1.

18. Hynson JM, Sessler DI. Intraoperative warming therapies: a comparison of three devices. J Clin Anesth. 1992;4:194–9.

19. John M, Ford J, Harper M. Peri-operative warming devices: performance and clinical application. Anaesthesia. 2014;69:623–38.

20. Sessler DI, Schroeder M. Heat loss in humans covered with cotton hospital blankets. Anesth Analg. 1993;77:73–7.

21. Giesbrecht GG, Ducharme MB, McGuire JP. Comparison of forced-air patient warming systems for perioperative use. Anesthesiology. 1994;80:671–9.

22. Kurz A, Kurz M, Poeschl G, Faryniak B, Redl G, Hackl W. Forced-air warming maintains intraoperative normothermia better than circulating-water mattresses. Anesth Analg. 1993;77:89–95.

23. Wadhwa A, Komatsu R, Orhan-Sungur M, Barnes P, In J, Sessler DI, Lenhardt R. New circulating-water devices warm more quickly than forced-air in volunteers. Anesth Analg. 2007;105:1681–7.

24. Grocott HP, Mathew JP, Carver EH, Phillips-Bute B, Landolfo KP, Newman MF, Duke Heart Center Neurologic Outcome Research Group. A randomized controlled trial of the Arctic Sun Temperature Management System versus conventional methods for preventing hypothermia during off-pump cardiac surgery. Anesth Analg. 2004;98:298–302. Table of contents.

25. Galvao CM, Liang Y, Clark AM. Effectiveness of cutaneous warming systems on temperature control: meta-analysis. J Adv Nurs. 2010;66:1196–206.

26. Perez-Protto S, Sessler DI, Reynolds LF, Bakri MH, Mascha E, Cywinski J, Parker B, Argalious M. Circulating-water garment or the combination of a circulating-water mattress and forced-air cover to maintain core temperature during major upper-abdominal surgery. Br J Anaesth. 2010;105:466–70.

27. Birch DW, Manouchehri N, Shi X, Hadi G, Karmali S. Heated $CO(2)$ with or without humidification for minimally invasive abdominal surgery. Cochrane Database Syst Rev. 2011:CD007821.

8. Prevention of Postoperative Nausea and Vomiting

Robert Owen and Tong Joo Gan

Postoperative nausea and vomiting (PONV) are common and unpleasant complications of anesthesia and surgery. The overall incidence rate of PONV for all surgical patients is estimated to be 25–30 %, while the rate of PONV in high-risk patients can be as high as 80 % [1–4]. An estimated 0.18 % of patients experience intractable PONV, which may result in prolonged postanesthesia care unit (PACU) stay, unanticipated hospital readmission, and increased health care costs [5–7]. PONV represents one of the most common reasons for poor patient satisfaction scores in the postoperative period [8]. One survey found that patients would be willing to pay up to $100, at their own expense, for complete and effective antiemetic treatment [9].

The aim of this chapter will be to summarize the evidence for the implementation of PONV protocols within an enhanced recovery after surgery program (ERP). Literature used for these recommendations come from randomized control trials, meta-analyses, and consensus guidelines. We will address the following: identifying high-risk patients, minimizing risks, administering appropriate prophylactic antiemetic and rescue treatment, and recommending a treatment algorithm for use in an ERP protocol.

Identifying High-Risk Patients

There are several factors that have been associated with increased risk of PONV, but to effectively stratify risk, one should focus on those factors that independently predict PONV. These factors include female sex, history of PONV or motion sickness, nonsmoking status, younger

L.S. Feldman et al. (eds.), *The SAGES / ERAS®*
Society Manual of Enhanced Recovery Programs for
Gastrointestinal Surgery, DOI 10.1007/978-3-319-20364-5_8,

age, general versus regional anesthesia, use of volatile anesthetics and nitrous oxide, postoperative opioids, duration of surgery, and type of surgery (cholecystectomy, laparoscopic, gynecological) [10]. The increased incidence of PONV with laparoscopic surgeries and cholecystectomies is particularly relevant when considering ERP protocols for gastrointestinal surgery [11]. To ease the task in risk stratification, Apfel et al. [1] developed a simplified risk score, based on four predictors: female gender, history of motion sickness or PONV, nonsmoking status, and the use of opioids for postoperative analgesia. The incidence of PONV in patients with 0, 1, 2, 3, or 4 of these risk factors was 10, 21, 39, 61, and 79 % respectively (Fig. 8.1) [1]. The use of this simplified risk score to guide therapeutic interventions has been shown to dramatically reduce institutional rates of PONV [12–14] (Fig. 8.2).

Reducing Baseline Risks

There are several strategies that can be used to reduce the baseline risk of PONV: Avoiding general anesthesia by the use of regional anesthesia; Using propofol, an antiemetic in its own right, for induction and maintenance of anesthesia; Avoiding nitrous oxide; Avoiding volatile anesthetics; Minimizing intraoperative and postoperative opioids; and adequate hydration [10]. The complete avoidance of general anesthesia is not generally practical for gastrointestinal surgery; however, the use of transversus abdominis plane (TAP) blocks as part of the analgesic regimen reduced incidence of PONV in colonic surgery patients [15]. This same effect has not been shown for epidural analgesia [16, 17]. This could be related to the amount of opioid used. Similarly, propofol for induction and maintenance of anesthesia (total IV anesthesia [TIVA]) has been shown to reduce the risk of PONV by approximately 25 % [14]. Additionally, two meta-analyses have shown that omitting nitrous oxide reduced both early and late PONV, except when baseline risks were already low [18, 19]. Early PONV, specifically, may be reduced by avoiding volatile anesthetics, as they have been identified as the primary cause of early PONV [20].

Another primary cause of PONV can be avoided by reducing or minimizing postoperative opioids [1, 19–24]. To achieve adequate analgesia without opioids, one can utilize several modalities including regional or neuraxial analgesia, opioid adjuncts such as nonsteroidal anti-inflammatory drugs (NSAIDs), cyclooxygenase-2 (COX-2) inhibitors, acetaminophen, calcium antagonists (gabapentin, pregabalin),

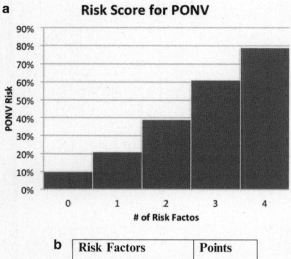

Fig. 8.1. (a) Risk score for PONV. (b) Risk factors contribute to simplified risk score from Apfel et al. These can be used to predict a patient's risk for PONV. (A, From Apfel, C.C., et al., *A Simplified Risk Score for Predicting Postoperative Nausea and Vomiting: Conclusions from Cross-validations between Two Centers.* Anesthesiology, 1999. 91(3): p. 693, with permission).

and NMDA receptor antagonists (ketamine). NSAIDs and COX-2 inhibitors have been shown, in randomized controlled trials and meta-analyses, to have a morphine-sparing effect in the postoperative period [25–27]. To a lesser degree, ketamine may offer a similar morphine-sparing effect [28].

The volume and type of fluid administered in the perioperative period can influence the incidence of PONV and bowel function. Optimal fluid management in an ERP protocol involves judicious administration of

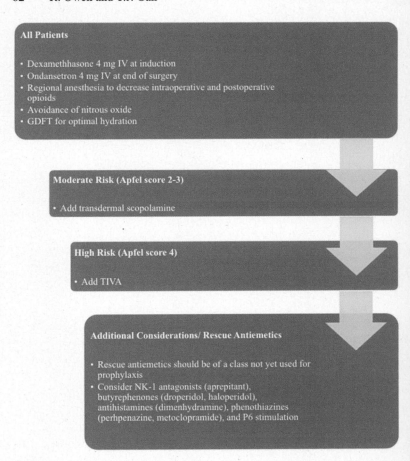

Fig. 8.2. Treatment algorithm for preventing PONV for patients in an ERP protocol.

background crystalloids, while optimizing hemodynamics with colloids as part of a goal-directed fluid therapy (GDFT) [29]. A meta-analysis shows that GDFT, aimed at maximizing flow-related hemodynamic values, reduces PONV, as well as hospital stay, complications, and ileus [30]. Meanwhile, Gustafsson et al. [31] showed that fluid overload can increase complications, particularly cardiovascular complications, in colorectal patients. This same study also showed that preoperative carbohydrate drinks, as part of an ERP protocol, can significantly reduce PONV [31]. It is therefore recommended that to minimize PONV in an

ERP protocol, excessive crystalloids administration should be avoided. GDFT strategy based on hemodynamic variables should be available in patients undergoing major or high-risk surgery.

PONV Prophylaxis

Prophylactic treatment with antiemetics is a key aspect of PONV prevention. Several classes of antiemetics exist for this purpose and each will be discussed in turn; the benefits and side effects of these classes are listed in Table 8.1. Recommended doses and times of administration for specific antiemetics are listed in Table 8.2.

Table 8.1. Benefits and side effects of the main classes of PONV prophylactic antiemetics and alternative treatment strategy.

Antiemetic class	Benefits	Side effects
5-HT$_3$ receptor antagonists (e.g., ondansetron, dolasetron, granisetron, tropisetron)	Specific for PONV Do not have sedative side effects	Headache, constipation, elevated liver enzymes, risk of QT prolongation
NK-1 receptor antagonists (e.g., aprepitant, casopitant, rolapitant)	Long duration of action Improved efficacy against vomiting Do not have sedative side effects	Headache, constipation
Corticosteroids (e.g., dexamethasone, methylprednisolone)	Do not have sedative side effects Long duration of action	Hyperglycemia in obese and diabetic patients, may increase risk of wound infection
Butyrophenones (e.g., droperidol, haloperidol)	Improved prophylaxis against nausea	Sedation with high doses, hypotension, extrapyramidal side effects, neuroleptic malignant syndrome, droperidol has an FDA "black box" warning regarding QTc prolongation. However the risk is considered minimal with antiemetic doses

(continued)

Table 8.1. (continued)

Antiemetic class	Benefits	Side effects
Antihistamines (e.g., dimenhydrinate, meclizine)	Effective against motion sickness Meclizine has longer duration of action	Sedation, dry mouth, restlessness
Anticholinergics (e.g., scopolamine)	Effective against motion sickness Transdermal preparation has long duration of action and can be applied the night before surgery	Sedation, visual disturbances, dry mouth, dizziness, restlessness, central cholinergic syndrome
Phenothiazines (e.g., perphenazine)	Long duration of action	Extrapyramidal side effects, hypotension, restlessness, anticholinergic syndrome, may cause sedation
Acupuncture (P6 stimulation)	Improved efficacy against nausea	None reported when used for PONV prophylaxis
TIVA with Propofol	Effective against early PONV Reduces the incidences of PDNV	Increased risk of awareness

Adapted from Habib, A.S.G., Gan, T.J., *What is the Best Strategy for Prevention of Postoperative Nausea and Vomiting.* Evidence-Based Practice of Anesthesiology. 3rd ed. Philadelphia, PA: Elsevier/Saunders, 2013. p. 294–300, with permission

5-HT$_3$ Receptor Antagonists

The 5-HT$_3$ antagonists are a unique group of drugs that were developed specifically for the management of nausea and vomiting. In general, their antiemetic (anti-vomiting) effects are stronger than their anti-nausea effects [32]. Most of the available research on this class of drugs focuses on ondansetron. A dose of 4 mg ondansetron has a number needed to treat (NNT) of approximately 6 for prevention of vomiting (0–24 h) and approximately 7 for prevention of nausea [32]. The 8 mg oral disintegrating tablet (ODT) is equally effective to the 4 mg IV dose [33]. Other 5-HT$_3$ antagonists which have been shown to be effective in preventing PONV include: granisetron 0.35–3 mg IV [34], tropisetron 2 mg IV [35], ramosetron 0.3 mg IV [36, 37], and palonosetron 0.075 mg

Table 8.2. Antiemetic doses and timing for prevention of PONV.

Drug	Dose	Timing
Aprepitant	40 mg per os	At induction
Casopitant	150 mg per os	At induction
Dexamethasone	4–5 mg IV	At induction
Dimenhydrinate	1 mg/kg IV	
Droperidol[a]	0.625–1.25 mg IV	End of surgery
Granisetron	0.35–3 mg IV	End of surgery
Haloperidol	0.5–<2 mg IM/IV	
Methylprednisolone	40 mg IV	
Ondansetron	4 mg IV, 8 mg ODT	End of surgery
Palonosetron	0.075 mg IV	At induction
Perphenazine	5 mg IV	
Ramosetron	0.3 mg IV	End of surgery
Rolapitant	70–200 mg per os	At induction
Scopolamine	Transdermal patch	Prior evening or 2 h before surgery
Tropisetron	2 mg IV	End of surgery

Adapted from Gan, T.J., et al., *Consensus guidelines for the management of postoperative nausea and vomiting.* Anesth Analg, 2014. 118(1): p. 85–113, with permission

[a]See FDA black box warning

IV [38, 39]. Of these, tropisetron and ramosetron are not available in the United States.

One reason 5-HT_3 antagonists are widely used for the prevention of PONV is their favorable side effect profile. All, except palonosetron, have been shown to prolong the QTc interval [10]. For ondansetron specifically, the U.S. FDA recommends that the dose should not exceed 16 mg in a single dose because of the risks to the QTc interval. The number-needed-to-harm (NNH) for a single dose of ondansetron is 36 for headache, 31 for elevated liver enzymes, and 23 for constipation [19]. All 5-HT_3 antagonists are considered to be equally safe.

Corticosteroids

Dexamethasone 4–5 mg IV has widely been used prophylactically to prevent PONV. It has been shown to be especially effective against late PONV [40]. A recent meta-analysis showed that the NNT for TIVA over 24 h was 3.7 (95 % CI, 3.0–4.7) [41]. There is also the added benefit that dexamethasone 0.1 mg/kg has been shown to be an effective adjunct in multimodal strategies to reduce postoperative pain and opioid consumption [42]. Recently, an increasing number of studies have used a higher dose of dexamethasone 8 mg IV. One such study found that preoperative dexamethasone 8 mg enhances the postdischarge quality of recovery in addition to reducing nausea, pain, and fatigue [43]. However, a recent meta-analysis showed no clinical advantage of higher dose 8–10 mg IV dexamethasone compared with 4–5 mg IV [41].

There is conflicting data concerning the safety of dexamethasone. Most studies show that a single dose of perioperative dexamethasone does not appear to increase the risk of wound infection [40, 42]. However, dexamethasone has been shown to cause significant increases in blood glucose levels that occur 6–12 h postoperatively in normal subjects [44, 45], those with impaired glucose tolerance [45], type 2 diabetics [46], and obese patients [45]. Additionally, one recent retrospective case-control study showed that patients who developed a postoperative wound infection were significantly more likely to have received a single perioperative dose of dexamethasone 4–8 mg IV, and thus concluded that dexamethasone may increase the postoperative risk of wound infection [47]. However, these patients were also less likely ($p = 0.001$) to have received a prophylactic antibiotics. Based on the totality of evidence, a single dose of 4–8 mg dexamethasone is not associated with an increased risk and hence is recommended [48, 49]. The increase in blood sugar is predictable, and should be monitored in labile diabetics. Methylprednisolone 40 mg IV is also effective for the prevention of late PONV, as it has a similarly long half-life [50, 51]. There is no evidence to suggest that methylprednisolone differs from dexamethasone in terms of adverse effects.

Butyrophenones

Droperidol and haloperidol are two butyrophenones that have been shown to be effective for the prophylactic prevention of PONV. An effective dose of droperidol for preventing PONV is 0.625–1.25 mg IV [52–54]. It has been shown to have similar efficacy to ondansetron, with an NNT of approximately 5 for the prevention of PONV within 24 h [54]. However, in 2001, the FDA issued a black box restriction on the use of droperidol over concerns of QTc prolongation. Despite this, studies have shown that droperidol has equal effects on the QTc interval as ondansetron [55, 56]. Furthermore, the combination of droperidol and ondansetron, while being more effective than either drug alone for the prevention of PONV, had no greater effect on the QTc interval than either drug alone [57]. It is believed, therefore, that at dosing levels appropriate for the prevention of PONV, droperidol can be safely used without significant cardiovascular events.

At low doses, 0.5–2 mg IM or IV, haloperidol effectively reduced the risk of PONV with an NNT between 4 and 6 [58]. Haloperidol carries a warning of QTc prolongation on its label; however at these low doses cardiac arrhythmias have not been reported. Nonetheless, haloperidol is not regarded as a first antiemetic of choice, as it also carries risk of extrapyramidal symptoms. The use of haloperidol for PONV and the IV route of administration is not an FDA-approved indication.

Antihistamines

Antihistamines are older drugs with antiemetic effects. The antihistamine dimenhydrinate can be used as an antiemetic in doses of 1 mg/kg IV, where it has shown to have similar efficacy to the $5\text{-}HT_3$ receptor antagonists, dexamethasone, and droperidol [59, 60]. Despite this, there are too few direct comparisons with other antiemetics; furthermore, there is not enough data to determine optimal administration timing, dose response, or side effect profile [10].

Anticholinergics

Transdermal scopolamine (TDS) has the added benefit that it can be applied the evening before surgery or 2–4 h before the start of anesthesia because of its 2- to 4-h onset of effect [61, 62]. TDS has been shown to have equal effectiveness in single drug therapy studies comparing it to ondansetron and droperidol [63]. TDS prevented nausea and vomiting up to 24 h after surgery with an NNT of 6 [64]. The most common adverse effects include visual disturbances (NNH=5.6), dry mouth (NNH=13), and dizziness (NNH=50) [64].

Phenothiazines

Perphenazine and metoclopramide are two phenothiazines that have been used for the management of PONV. A review of 6 RCTs showed a relative risk reduction (RRR) of 0.5 (95 % CI, 0.37–0.67) for PONV when using 5 mg IV perphenazine [65]. This same review showed no significant increase in sedation or drowsiness when compared with a placebo [65]. Metoclopramide is not effective at 10 mg dose. However, efficacy has been demonstrated at higher doses. The NNT for metoclopramide 10, 25, and 50 mg for PONV at 24 h is 30, 16, and 11, respectively [66]. The NNH for extrapyramidal symptoms with 25 or 50 mg metoclopramide is 140 [66].

NK-1 Receptor Antagonists

The most widely studied of the neurokinin-1 (NK-1) receptor antagonists and the only one currently available is aprepitant. Compared with ondansetron, aprepitant has a longer duration of action, with a half-life of 9–13 h [67]. While it was shown to be similar to ondansetron in achieving complete response (no vomiting and no use of rescue antiemetic) for 24 h after surgery, it was shown to be more effective than ondansetron at preventing vomiting at 24 and 48 h after surgery and in reducing nausea severity during the first 48 h after surgery [68, 69]. The side effect profile of aprepitant is similar to that of ondansetron [69]. The role of aprepitant as a routine prophylactic agent has not yet been established due to limited clinical experience and higher costs [70]. Casopitant and rolapitant are similar long-acting NK-1 antagonists which have shown comparable efficacy, but have not yet been approved for use [10].

Other Techniques

The use of propofol as part of TIVA has been shown to decrease the incidence of early PONV, with an NNT of 5 [70, 71]. The use of TIVA reduces the risk of PONV by approximately 25 % [14]. A systematic review of 58 studies has shown that TIVA is also useful for the prevention of postdischarge nausea and vomiting (PDNV) [72]. TIVA with propofol is, therefore, a useful alternative for those at increased risk for PONV and PDNV.

Acustimulation at P6 has also been shown to decrease the need for rescue antiemetics with a similar effectiveness of prophylactic ondansetron, droperidol, metoclopramide, cyclizine, and prochlorperazine [73, 74].

Stimulation can be achieved before or after surgery by experienced acupuncturists or noninvasive stimulation devices. Prevention of nausea was more effective than prevention of vomiting [73]. This represents a useful alternative for patients wary of pharmaceutical prophylaxis.

Combination Therapy and Rescue Antiemesis

When considering a multimodal approach to PONV prophylaxis, a combination of antiemetics of different classes should be used [10]. Many studies have shown that the combination of 5-HT$_3$ antagonists and either dexamethasone or droperidol is more effective in preventing PONV than monotherapy with any of the drugs [75, 76].

Similarly, treatment of patients for which prophylactic treatment is insufficient should consist of an antiemetic of a different class than those used for prophylaxis [10]. Repeating medication that was given for PONV prophylaxis within the first 6 h after initial dose provided no additional benefit [77].

PONV Management Algorithm

When evaluating treatment strategies for the prevention of PONV, it is important to reduce baseline risks and identify high-risk patients. Studies have shown, however, that purely risk-based treatment guidelines have been poorly implemented [78]. Considering this, multimodal baseline prevention strategies augmented for high-risk patients are the best strategy for preventing PONV in the ERP setting. A treatment algorithm for preventing PONV is outlined in Fig. 8.2. Risk reduction methods should be used for all patients by avoiding nitrous oxide and reducing need for intraoperative and postoperative opioids by using regional and neuraxial techniques. Additionally, prophylactic treatment with ondansetron and dexamethasone should be used for all patients unless they are specifically contraindicated. For patients with an increased risk, TDS should also be added. High-risk patients should receive ondansetron, dexamethasone, TDS, and TIVA using propofol. Rescue antiemetics should include a class of drug not used for prophylaxis.

Conclusions

PONV remains a common cause of patient discomfort and dissatisfaction of significant importance to patients. Extensive resources exist to prevent this unpleasant side effect. Here, we have evaluated the available evidence, outlined the various resources, and proposed an effective treatment algorithm that can be implemented by perioperative care teams in an ERP protocol, even at busy institutions. A summary of take home messages is provided below.

Take Home Messages

- Evaluate all patients for risk of PONV.
- Minimize risk of PONV by avoiding nitrous oxide, reducing the doses of intraoperative and postoperative opioids.
- Avoidance of hypovolemia and hypervolemia.
- Appropriate use of antiemetic prophylaxis, with combination therapy in patients at high risk of PONV.
- Use different class of antiemetic for rescue therapy when prophylactic therapy fails.

References

1. Apfel CC, et al. A simplified risk score for predicting postoperative nausea and vomiting: conclusions from cross-validations between two centers. Anesthesiology. 1999; 91(3):693.
2. Kovac A. Prevention and treatment of postoperative nausea and vomiting. Drugs. 2000;59(2):213–43.
3. Koivuranta M, et al. A survey of postoperative nausea and vomiting. Anaesthesia. 1997;52(5):443–9.
4. Sinclair DR, Chung F, Mezei G. Can postoperative nausea and vomiting be predicted? Anesthesiology. 1999;91(1):109–18.
5. Fortier J, Chung F, Su J. Unanticipated admission after ambulatory surgery – a prospective study. Can J Anaesth. 1998;45(7):612–9.
6. Gold BS, et al. Unanticipated admission to the hospital following ambulatory surgery. JAMA. 1989;262(21):3008–10.
7. Hill RP, et al. Cost-effectiveness of prophylactic antiemetic therapy with ondansetron, droperidol, or placebo. Anesthesiology. 2000;92(4):958–67.
8. Myles PS, et al. Patient satisfaction after anaesthesia and surgery: results of a prospective survey of 10,811 patients. Br J Anaesth. 2000;84(1):6–10.

9. Gan T, et al. How much are patients willing to pay to avoid postoperative nausea and vomiting? Anesth Analg. 2001;92(2):393–400.

10. Gan TJ, et al. Consensus guidelines for the management of postoperative nausea and vomiting. Anesth Analg. 2014;118(1):85–113.

11. Apfel CC, et al. Evidence-based analysis of risk factors for postoperative nausea and vomiting. Br J Anaesth. 2012;109(5):742–53.

12. Pierre S, Benais H, Pouymayou J. Apfel's simplified score may favourably predict the risk of postoperative nausea and vomiting. Can J Anaesth. 2002;49(3):237–42.

13. Pierre S, et al. A risk score-dependent antiemetic approach effectively reduces postoperative nausea and vomiting – a continuous quality improvement initiative. Can J Anaesth. 2004;51(4):320–5.

14. Apfel CC, et al. A factorial trial of six interventions for the prevention of postoperative nausea and vomiting. N Engl J Med. 2004;350(24):2441–51.

15. McDonnell JG, et al. The analgesic efficacy of transversus abdominis plane block after abdominal surgery: a prospective randomized controlled trial. Anesth Analg. 2007;104(1):193–7. doi:10.1213/01.ane.0000250223.49963.0f.

16. Jorgensen H, et al. Epidural local anaesthetics versus opioid-based analgesic regimens on postoperative gastrointestinal paralysis. PONV and pain after abdominal surgery. Cochrane Database Syst Rev. 2000;4:CD001893.

17. Marret E, Remy C, Bonnet F. Meta-analysis of epidural analgesia versus parenteral opioid analgesia after colorectal surgery. Br J Surg. 2007;94(6):665–73.

18. Tramer M, Moore A, McQuay H. Omitting nitrous oxide in general anaesthesia: meta-analysis of intraoperative awareness and postoperative emesis in randomized controlled trials. Br J Anaesth. 1996;76(2):186–93.

19. Tramer M, Moore A, McQuay H. Meta-analytic comparison of prophylactic antiemetic efficacy for postoperative nausea and vomiting: propofol anaesthesia vs omitting nitrous oxide vs total i.v. anaesthesia with propofol. Br J Anaesth. 1997;78(3):256–9.

20. Apfel CC, et al. Volatile anaesthetics may be the main cause of early but not delayed postoperative vomiting: a randomized controlled trial of factorial design. Br J Anaesth. 2002;88(5):659–68.

21. Roberts GW, et al. Postoperative nausea and vomiting are strongly influenced by postoperative opioid use in a dose-related manner. Anesth Analg. 2005;101(5):1343–8.

22. Moiniche S, et al. Nonsteroidal antiinflammatory drugs and the risk of operative site bleeding after tonsillectomy: a quantitative systematic review. Anesth Analg. 2003;96(1):68–77. table of contents.

23. Polati E, et al. Ondansetron versus metoclopramide in the treatment of postoperative nausea and vomiting. Anesth Analg. 1997;85(2):395–9.

24. Sukhani R, et al. Recovery after propofol with and without intraoperative fentanyl in patients undergoing ambulatory gynecologic laparoscopy. Anesth Analg. 1996;83(5):975–81.

25. Marret E, et al. Effects of nonsteroidal antiinflammatory drugs on patient-controlled analgesia morphine side effects: meta-analysis of randomized controlled trials. Anesthesiology. 2005;102(6):1249–60.

26. Elia N, Lysakowski C, Tramer MR. Does multimodal analgesia with acetaminophen, nonsteroidal antiinflammatory drugs, or selective cyclooxygenase-2 inhibitors and patient-controlled analgesia morphine offer advantages over morphine alone? Meta-analyses of randomized trials. Anesthesiology. 2005;103(6):1296–304.

27. Gan TJ, et al. Presurgical intravenous parecoxib sodium and follow-up oral valdecoxib for pain management after laparoscopic cholecystectomy surgery reduces opioid requirements and opioid-related adverse effects. Acta Anaesthesiol Scand. 2004;48(9):1194–207.

28. Elia N, Tramer MR. Ketamine and postoperative pain – a quantitative systematic review of randomised trials. Pain. 2005;113(1-2):61–70.

29. Miller TE, et al. Reduced length of hospital stay in colorectal surgery after implementation of an enhanced recovery protocol. Anesth Analg. 2014;118(5):1052–61.

30. Bundgaard-Nielsen M, et al. Monitoring of peri-operative fluid administration by individualized goal-directed therapy. Acta Anaesthesiol Scand. 2007;51(3):331–40.

31. Habib ASG, Gan TJ. What is the best strategy for prevention of postoperative nausea and vomiting. Evidence-based practice of anesthesiology. 3rd ed. Philadelphia, PA: Elsevier/Saunders, 2013. p. 294–300.

32. Tramer MR, et al. Efficacy, dose-response, and safety of ondansetron in prevention of postoperative nausea and vomiting: a quantitative systematic review of randomized placebo-controlled trials. Anesthesiology. 1997;87(6):1277–89.

33. Grover VK, Mathew PJ, Hegde H. Efficacy of orally disintegrating ondansetron in preventing postoperative nausea and vomiting after laparoscopic cholecystectomy: a randomised, double-blind placebo controlled study. Anaesthesia. 2009;64(6): 595–600.

34. Erhan Y, et al. Ondansetron, granisetron, and dexamethasone compared for the prevention of postoperative nausea and vomiting in patients undergoing laparoscopic cholecystectomy : A randomized placebo-controlled study. Surg Endosc. 2008;22(6): 1487–92.

35. Kranke P, et al. Tropisetron for prevention of postoperative nausea and vomiting: a quantitative systematic review. Anaesthesist. 2002;51(10):805–14.

36. Lee HJ, et al. Preoperatively administered ramosetron oral disintegrating tablets for preventing nausea and vomiting associated with patient-controlled analgesia in breast cancer patients. Eur J Anaesthesiol. 2008;25(9):756–62.

37. Choi YS, et al. Effect of ramosetron on patient-controlled analgesia related nausea and vomiting after spine surgery in highly susceptible patients: comparison with ondansetron. Spine (Phila Pa 1976). 2008;33(17):E602–6.

38. Kovac AL, et al. A randomized, double-blind study to evaluate the efficacy and safety of three different doses of palonosetron versus placebo in preventing postoperative nausea and vomiting over a 72-hour period. Anesth Analg. 2008;107(2):439–44.

39. Candiotti KA, et al. A randomized, double-blind study to evaluate the efficacy and safety of three different doses of palonosetron versus placebo for preventing postoperative nausea and vomiting. Anesth Analg. 2008;107(2):445–51.

40. Henzi I, Walder B, Tramer MR. Dexamethasone for the prevention of postoperative nausea and vomiting: a quantitative systematic review. Anesth Analg. 2000;90(1): 186–94.

41. De Oliveira Jr GS, et al. Dexamethasone to prevent postoperative nausea and vomiting: an updated meta-analysis of randomized controlled trials. Anesth Analg. 2013;116(1):58–74.

42. De Oliveira Jr GS, et al. Perioperative single dose systemic dexamethasone for postoperative pain: a meta-analysis of randomized controlled trials. Anesthesiology. 2011;115(3):575–88.

43. Murphy GS, et al. Preoperative dexamethasone enhances quality of recovery after laparoscopic cholecystectomy: effect on in-hospital and postdischarge recovery outcomes. Anesthesiology. 2011;114(4):882–90.

44. Eberhart LH, et al. Randomised controlled trial of the effect of oral premedication with dexamethasone on hyperglycaemic response to abdominal hysterectomy. Eur J Anaesthesiol. 2011;28(3):195–201.

45. Nazar CE, et al. Dexamethasone for postoperative nausea and vomiting prophylaxis: effect on glycaemia in obese patients with impaired glucose tolerance. Eur J Anaesthesiol. 2009;26(4):318–21.

46. Hans P, et al. Blood glucose concentration profile after 10 mg dexamethasone in non-diabetic and type 2 diabetic patients undergoing abdominal surgery. Br J Anaesth. 2006;97(2):164–70.

47. Percival VG, Riddell J, Corcoran TB. Single dose dexamethasone for postoperative nausea and vomiting – a matched case-control study of postoperative infection risk. Anaesth Intensive Care. 2010;38(4):661–6.

48. Ali Khan S, McDonagh DL, Gan TJ. Wound complications with dexamethasone for postoperative nausea and vomiting prophylaxis: a moot point? Anesth Analg. 2013;116(5):966–8.

49. Colin B, Gan TJ. Cancer recurrence and hyperglycemia with dexamethasone for postoperative nausea and vomiting prophylaxis: more moot points? Anesth Analg. 2014;118(6):1154–6.

50. Miyagawa Y, et al. Methylprednisolone reduces postoperative nausea in total knee and hip arthroplasty. J Clin Pharm Ther. 2010;35(6):679–84.

51. Weren M, Demeere JL. Methylprednisolone vs. dexamethasone in the prevention of postoperative nausea and vomiting: a prospective, randomised, double-blind, placebo-controlled trial. Acta Anaesthesiol Belg. 2008;59(1):1–5.

52. Domino KB, et al. Comparative efficacy and safety of ondansetron, droperidol, and metoclopramide for preventing postoperative nausea and vomiting: a meta-analysis. Anesth Analg. 1999;88(6):1370–9.

53. Fortney JT, et al. A comparison of the efficacy, safety, and patient satisfaction of ondansetron versus droperidol as antiemetics for elective outpatient surgical procedures. S3A-409 and S3A-410 Study Groups. Anesth Analg. 1998;86(4):731–8.

54. Henzi I, Sonderegger J, Tramer MR. Efficacy, dose-response, and adverse effects of droperidol for prevention of postoperative nausea and vomiting. Can J Anaesth. 2000; 47(6):537–51.

55. Charbit B, et al. Prolongation of QTc interval after postoperative nausea and vomiting treatment by droperidol or ondansetron. Anesthesiology. 2005;102(6):1094–100.

56. White PF, et al. Effect of low-dose droperidol on the QT interval during and after general anesthesia: a placebo-controlled study. Anesthesiology. 2005;102(6):1101–5.

57. Chan MT, et al. The additive interactions between ondansetron and droperidol for preventing postoperative nausea and vomiting. Anesth Analg. 2006;103(5):1155–62.
58. Buttner M, et al. Is low-dose haloperidol a useful antiemetic?: A meta-analysis of published and unpublished randomized trials. Anesthesiology. 2004;101(6):1454–63.
59. Kothari SN, et al. Antiemetic efficacy of prophylactic dimenhydrinate (Dramamine) vs ondansetron (Zofran): a randomized, prospective trial inpatients undergoing laparoscopic cholecystectomy. Surg Endosc. 2000;14(10):926–9.
60. Kranke P, et al. Dimenhydrinate for prophylaxis of postoperative nausea and vomiting: a meta-analysis of randomized controlled trials. Acta Anaesthesiol Scand. 2002; 46(3):238–44.
61. Apfel CC, et al. Transdermal scopolamine for the prevention of postoperative nausea and vomiting: a systematic review and meta-analysis. Clin Ther. 2010;32(12): 1987–2002.
62. Bailey PL, et al. Transdermal scopolamine reduces nausea and vomiting after outpatient laparoscopy. Anesthesiology. 1990;72(6):977–80.
63. White PF, et al. Transdermal scopolamine: an alternative to ondansetron and droperidol for the prevention of postoperative and postdischarge emetic symptoms. Anesth Analg. 2007;104(1):92–6.
64. Kranke P, et al. The efficacy and safety of transdermal scopolamine for the prevention of postoperative nausea and vomiting: a quantitative systematic review. Anesth Analg. 2002;95(1):133–43. doi:10.1097/00000539-200207000-00024.
65. Schnabel A, et al. Efficacy of perphenazine to prevent postoperative nausea and vomiting: a quantitative systematic review. Eur J Anaesthesiol. 2010;27(12):1044–51.
66. Wallenborn J, et al. Prevention of postoperative nausea and vomiting by metoclopramide combined with dexamethasone: randomised double blind multicentre trial. BMJ. 2006;333(7563):324.
67. Dando T, Perry C. Aprepitant. Drugs. 2004;64(7):777–94.
68. Diemunsch P, et al. Single-dose aprepitant vs ondansetron for the prevention of postoperative nausea and vomiting: a randomized, double-blind phase III trial in patients undergoing open abdominal surgery. Br J Anaesth. 2007;99(2):202–11.
69. Gan TJ, et al. A randomized, double-blind comparison of the NK1 antagonist, aprepitant, versus ondansetron for the prevention of postoperative nausea and vomiting. Anesth Analg. 2007;104(5):1082–9. Tables of contents.
70. Scuderi PE, White PF. Novel therapies for postoperative nausea and vomiting: statistically significant versus clinically meaningful outcomes. Anesth Analg. 2011;112(4): 750–2.
71. Visser K, et al. Randomized controlled trial of total intravenous anesthesia with propofol versus inhalation anesthesia with isoflurane-nitrous oxide: postoperative nausea with vomiting and economic analysis. Anesthesiology. 2001;95(3):616–26.
72. Gupta A, et al. Comparison of recovery profile after ambulatory anesthesia with propofol, isoflurane, sevoflurane and desflurane: a systematic review. Anesth Analg. 2004;98(3):632–41. table of contents.
73. Frey UH, et al. Effect of P6 acustimulation on post-operative nausea and vomiting in patients undergoing a laparoscopic cholecystectomy. Acta Anaesthesiol Scand. 2009;53(10):1341–7.

74. Frey UH, et al. P6 acustimulation effectively decreases postoperative nausea and vomiting in high-risk patients. Br J Anaesth. 2009;102(5):620–5.
75. Eberhart LH, et al. Droperidol and 5-HT3-receptor antagonists, alone or in combination, for prophylaxis of postoperative nausea and vomiting. A meta-analysis of randomised controlled trials. Acta Anaesthesiol Scand. 2000;44(10):1252–7.
76. Habib AS, El-Moalem HE, Gan TJ. The efficacy of the 5-HT3 receptor antagonists combined with droperidol for PONV prophylaxis is similar to their combination with dexamethasone. A meta-analysis of randomized controlled trials. Can J Anaesth. 2004;51(4):311–9.
77. Kovac AL, et al. Efficacy of repeat intravenous dosing of ondansetron in controlling postoperative nausea and vomiting: a randomized, double-blind, placebo-controlled multicenter trial. J Clin Anesth. 1999;11(6):453–9.
78. Franck M, et al. Adherence to treatment guidelines for postoperative nausea and vomiting. How well does knowledge transfer result in improved clinical care? Anaesthesist. 2010;59(6):524–8.

9. Thromboprophylaxis

David Bergqvist

Postoperative venous thromboembolism (VTE) is a well-known and sometimes lethal complication, and prophylactic measures to decrease the risk have been documented in a vast number of publications. Today this is reflected in several guidelines [1], and although there are some different views among surgeons, the majority of high-risk patients receive some form of prophylaxis today. When new surgical methods are introduced or old ones are modified, it would seem important to define the risk for various complications, VTE being one, and whether or not thromboprophylaxis should be used. A potential problem is to extrapolate routines without having data supporting the evidence. It is only a little more than a decade the principles of ERPs (enhanced or early recovery after surgery, also called fast-track programs or early recovery programs) were pioneered by Henrik Kehlet in Denmark. Since then these principles have been adopted in many types of surgery and nowadays, the patients are mobilized and sent home rapidly also after rather major surgical treatments. Intuitively this would decrease the risk for VTE. The aim of this chapter is to analyze the risk of VTE after ERAS and the evidence on when and how to use thromboprophylaxis. In Table 9.1 factors are listed, which may reduce the risk of VTE in ERP patients.

Methodology

A literature search has been undertaken using the various terms for ERP given above combined with various terms for VTE and VTE prophylaxis. Most studies on ERP have not been made to analyze postoperative VTE, and there are therefore several problems related to the focus of this article (Table 9.2). As recently pointed out by Neville et al. [2] and Nicholson et al. [3], the large literature on ERP is skewed by

L.S. Feldman et al. (eds.), *The SAGES / ERAS®*
Society Manual of Enhanced Recovery Programs for
Gastrointestinal Surgery, DOI 10.1007/978-3-319-20364-5_9,
© Springer International Publishing Switzerland 2015

Table 9.1. Factors potentially reducing the risk
of VTE in ERP patients.

- Less trauma/minimal invasive techniques
- Less surgical stress
- Intraoperative goal-directed fluid therapy
- Less postoperative complications
- Early mobilization
- Short hospital stay

Table 9.2. Problem concerning ERP and VTE when analyzing the
literature.

- Few studies with direct focus on VTE
- Various diagnoses and definitions
- Few (if any) RCTs on VTE
- Too small sample sizes in RCTs to study VTE
- Historical controls, center comparisons
- Pulmonary and respiratory complications not always defined (PE?)
- Autopsy rate
- Thromboprophylaxis not mentioned or "up to the surgeon"
- Time for follow-up varies

poor study design and quality. When these authors performed systematic
searches only between 1 and 2 % of the identified papers could be
included for qualitative synthesis.

Results

The frequency of VTE after ERP without prophylaxis is virtually
unknown, especially as the use of prophylaxis is often not reported or
used in an unsystematic way, i.e., at the discretion of the surgeon in
charge. In a review on laparoscopic cholecystectomy, Lindberg et al. [4]
identified 60 publications with 153,832 patients without or with various
prophylactic measures. The incidence of clinically diagnosed deep vein
thrombosis (DVT) was 0.03 %, the incidence of pulmonary embolism
(PE) 0.06 %, the incidence of fatal pulmonary embolism (FPE) 0.02 %,
and the mortality 0.08 %. These results have recently been updated and
verified [5]. In a Cochrane review [6], analyzing the short-term benefit
of laparoscopic colorectal resection, 25 studies were identified, in six of
which DVT was registered. The frequency was 0.6 % in 545

laparoscopically treated patients compared with 1.1 % in 535 with conventional open surgery.

Until spring 2014 there were 17 studies with a total of 13,783 patients (18–4718) concerning ERP and with VTE mentioned, none of them being a randomized trial (RCT) and in 9 there was no information on thromboprophylaxis. In the remaining eight studies acetyl salicylic acid, low molecular weight heparin (LMWH), unfractionated heparin, rivaroxaban, or leg compression were used in "high-risk" patients, high risk only rarely being defined. The surgical procedures were colorectal (8), arthroplasty (4), cystectomy (2), liver surgery (2), and esophageal surgery (1). From these studies it is hardly possible to draw any conclusions on the use of prophylaxis.

Husted et al. [7] analyzed 1977 consecutive patients operated on with knee or hip joint arthroplasty (2004–2008). Thromboprophylaxis with LMWH started postoperatively and continued until discharge. The length of stay decreased from 7.3 days to 3.1 days during this period and simultaneously VTE and death decreased. The authors concluded that the risk of clinical VTE with the fast-track regimen and short duration of thromboprophylaxis compared favorably with extended prophylaxis after conventional surgery (up to 4 weeks). These findings were further verified in a recent prospective cohort study (4924 patients) on fast-track hip and knee arthroplasty, where prophylaxis (LMWH or factor Xa inhibition) was used during hospitalization when length of stay was shorter than 5 days [8]. Again the incidence of VTE was very low and there was only one FPE (0.02 %). In another large observational study (with historical control), there was no difference in VTE between conventional surgery and ERP after hip and knee replacement, but thromboprophylaxis also changed between the two periods (from mechanical/aspirin to extended tinzaparin) [9], again showing the difficulty drawing conclusions from non-RCT with several potential biases.

In a similar but small registry study on fast-track laparoscopic resection for rectal cancer (102 patients), thromboprophylaxis was given as a combination of preoperatively instituted tinzaparin and graded compression stockings [10]. No clinical VTE was seen, two patients developed pneumonia (differential diagnosis towards PE not clear), and three patients died, none of VTE.

Table 9.3 summarizes how recent guidelines deal with thromboprophylaxis. The use of prophylaxis recommended in the guidelines is basically extrapolated from knowledge based on studies on conventional surgical procedures for a similar diagnosis.

Table 9.3. Recommendations in recent guidelines and consensus reviews on ERP and thromboprophylaxis.

- Rectal/pelvic surgery [14, 15]
    - Compression stockings and LMWH (4 weeks when increased risk)
- Pancreaticoduodenectomy [16]
    - LMWH for 4 weeks. Mechanical measures added in high-risk patients
- Cystectomy for bladder cancer [17, 18]
    - Compression stockings and LMWH (4 weeks in patients at high risk)
- ACCP and NICE guidelines do not distinguish ERP from conventional surgery [1, 19]

Discussion

There are several problems worth mentioning in the context of VTE and ERP. The main ones are summarized in Table 9.1. There are data from various types of studies that the risk of VTE is probably low or very low. There could be several reasons why the incidence of DVT postoperatively is decreasing, the explanation probably being complex and not fully understood. So the proportion of DVT after total knee replacement decreased significantly between 1993 and 2005, warfarin being used throughout [11]. An important factor, common to all surgeries, is early mobilization, the importance of which clearly shown after knee arthroplasty [12]. Mobilizing patients less than 24 h postoperatively versus on the second postoperative day reduced the incidence of DVT from 27.6 to 1.0 %!

One problem, when contemplating on trials of thromboprophylaxis in ERP patients, is which diagnostic method to use. Most prospective studies on conventional surgery have used venography, fibrinogen uptake test or, recently, ultrasonography. Although discussions have sometimes been rather lively on the clinical relevance of detecting asymptomatic DVT in surveillance programs, there are data supporting a correlation between asymptomatic DVT and FPE. A trend in recent thromboprophylactic studies is more to use clinically overt VTE, often combined with proximal venographic DVT, and not to look for distal asymptomatic DVT.

Regarding thromboprophylaxis in fast-track surgery, there would seem to be a major need for RCTs. An example of the problem performing historical comparisons is illustrated in the paper by McDonald et al. [13], where 0.9 % VTE was seen in the ERP group versus 0.4 % in the historical control group. There could be several explanations but the result is totally contradictory to common sense and knowledge. Whichever diagnostic method used, with the low risk of VTE such studies would, however, need large patient populations, and it is not reasonable to believe in industrial support for such trials, despite pharmacological substances being evaluated. Another way to go would be using well-designed prospective population-based registries. It would seem important that surgeons dealing with ERP include patients in such studies, which need to be multicentric to obtain conclusive results within a reasonable time.

Until we have more firm data we have to extrapolate from present-day knowledge and use known risk factors to motivate prophylaxis in individual patients such as genetic prothrombotic predisposition, presence of malignant disease, presence of varicose veins, previous VTE, previous major orthopedic event, duration of immobilization, and type of anesthesia used (general versus epidural).

In this chapter focus has been on abdominal/pelvic and orthopedic operations, where most data exist. Recently, the ERP concept has also been extended to other types of surgery, for instance coronary bypass, aortic aneurysm repair, lung resection, bariatric surgery, esophageal surgery, and vaginal hysterectomy. Some of these are high-risk procedures and systematic studies are needed and should be stimulated.

Concluding Remarks

The risk of VTE in ERPs seems to be low but few studies focus on this problem specifically, and there are no RCTs. Fast-track programs, however, do not increase mortality compared with conventional regimens. The risk groups in need of thromboprophylaxis are unknown. Multicenter studies with noncommercial support should be stimulated. Guidelines on VTE need reconsiderations and in these risk factor categorizations should include ERP. Until further data are available, thromboprophylaxis (with LMWH or one of the new oral IIa or Xa inhibitors) should be used after individual risk factor assessment. This must include time for mobilization as well as the risk of hemorrhagic complications.

Take Home Messages

- The risk of VTE in ERPs seems to be low but few studies focus on this problem specifically, and there are no RCTs.
- Guidelines on VTE need reconsiderations and in risk factor categorization should include ERP.

- Until further data are available, thromboprophylaxis (with LMWH or one of the new oral IIa or Xa inhibitors) should be used after individual risk factor assessment including time for mobilization as well as the risk of hemorrhagic complications.

References

1. Guyatt GH, Akl EA, Crowther M, Gutterman DD, Schuunemann HJ, American College of Chest Physicians Antithrombotic T et al. Executive summary: antithrombotic therapy and prevention of thrombosis. 9th ed. American College of Chest Physicians Evidence-Based Clinical Practice Guidelines. Chest. 2012;141 (2 Suppl):7S–47S. PubMed Central PMCID: 3278060.
2. Neville A, Lee L, Antonescu I, Mayo NE, Vassiliou MC, Fried GM, et al. Systematic review of outcomes used to evaluate enhanced recovery after surgery. Br J Surg. 2014;101(3):159–70. PubMed.
3. Nicholson A, Lowe MC, Parker J, Lewis SR, Alderson P, Smith AF. Systematic review and meta-analysis of enhanced recovery programmes in surgical patients. Br J Surg. 2014;101(3):172–88. PubMed.
4. Lindberg F, Bergqvist D, Rasmussen I. Incidence of thromboembolic complications after laparoscopic cholecystectomy: review of the literature. Surg Laparosc Endosc. 1997;7(4):324–31.
5. Rondelli F, Manina G, Agnelli G, Becattini C. Venous thromboembolism after laparoscopic cholecystectomy: clinical burden and prevention. Surg Endosc. 2013;27(6): 1860–4. PubMed.
6. Schwenk W, Bohm B, Fugener A, Muller JM. Intermittent pneumatic sequential compression (ISC) of the lower extremities prevents venous stasis during laparoscopic cholecystectomy. A prospective randomized study. Surg Endosc. 1998;12(1):7–11.
7. Husted H, Otte KS, Kristensen BB, Orsnes T, Wong C, Kehlet H. Low risk of thromboembolic complications after fast-track hip and knee arthroplasty. Acta Orthop. 2010;81(5):599–605. PubMed Central PMCID: 3214750.
8. Jorgensen CC, Jacobsen MK, Soeballe K, Hansen TB, Husted H, Kjaersgaard-Andersen P, et al. Thromboprophylaxis only during hospitalisation in fast-track hip and knee arthroplasty, a prospective cohort study. BMJ Open. 2013;3(12):e003965. PubMed Central PMCID: 3863129.
9. Malviya A, Martin K, Harper I, Muller SD, Emmerson KP, Partington PF, et al. Enhanced recovery program for hip and knee replacement reduces death rate. Acta Orthop. 2011;82(5):577–81. PubMed Central PMCID: 3242954.
10. Stottmeier S, Harling H, Wille-Jorgensen P, Balleby L, Kehlet H. Pathogenesis of morbidity after fast-track laparoscopic colonic cancer surgery. Colorectal Dis. 2011; 13(5):500–5. PubMed.
11. Xing KH, Morrison G, Lim W, Douketis J, Odueyungbo A, Crowther M. Has the incidence of deep vein thrombosis in patients undergoing total hip/knee arthroplasty

changed over time? A systematic review of randomized controlled trials. Thromb Res. 2008;123(1):24–34. PubMed.

12. Pearse EO, Caldwell BF, Lockwood RJ, Hollard J. Early mobilisation after conventional knee replacement may reduce the risk of postoperative venous thromboembolism. J Bone Joint Surg Br. 2007;89(3):316–22. PubMed.

13. McDonald DA, Siegmeth R, Deakin AH, Kinninmonth AW, Scott NB. An enhanced recovery programme for primary total knee arthroplasty in the United Kingdom – follow up at one year. Knee. 2012;19(5):525–9. PubMed.

14. Lassen K, Soop M, Nygren J, Cox PB, Hendry PO, Spies C, et al. Consensus review of optimal perioperative care in colorectal surgery: Enhanced Recovery After Surgery (ERAS) Group recommendations. Arch Surg. 2009;144(10):961–9. PubMed.

15. Nygren J, Thacker J, Carli F, Fearon KC, Norderval S, Lobo DN, et al. Guidelines for perioperative care in elective rectal/pelvic surgery: Enhanced Recovery After Surgery (ERAS((R))) Society recommendations. World J Surg. 2013;37(2):285–305. PubMed.

16. Lassen K, Coolsen MM, Slim K, Carli F, de Aguilar-Nascimento JE, Schafer M, et al. Guidelines for perioperative care for pancreaticoduodenectomy: Enhanced Recovery After Surgery (ERAS(R)) Society recommendations. World J Surg. 2013;37(2):240–58. PubMed.

17. Cerantola Y, Valerio M, Persson B, Jichlinski P, Ljungqvist O, Hubner M, et al. Guidelines for perioperative care after radical cystectomy for bladder cancer: Enhanced Recovery After Surgery (ERAS((R))) society recommendations. Clin Nutr. 2013;32(6):879–87. PubMed.

18. Patel HR, Cerantola Y, Valerio M, Persson B, Jichlinski P, Ljungqvist O, et al. Enhanced recovery after surgery: are we ready, and can we afford not to implement these pathways for patients undergoing radical cystectomy? Eur Urol. 2014;65(2):263–6. PubMed.

19. Hill J, Treasure T, Guideline Development Group. Reducing the risk of venous thromboembolism (deep vein thrombosis and pulmonary embolism) in patients admitted to hospital: summary of the NICE guideline. Heart. 2010;96(11):879–82. PubMed.

10. Surgical Site Infection Prevention

Elizabeth C. Wick and Jonathan E. Efron

Surgical site infections (SSI) are the leading surgical complication with rates varying based on procedure, ranging from <1 % to upwards of 20 %. It is estimated that SSI cost an estimated $1 billion annually [1–3]. SSI are associated with increased morbidity and are a leading risk factor for readmission during the 30-day period after hospital discharge [4]. In addition to patient harm, SSI are associated with increased health care use, such as increased length of hospital stay, doctor visits, use of wound care supplies, and home care. Increasingly, SSI and readmission are being used as a quality metric in surgical care by the Centers for Medicare and Medicaid Services and other payers with mandatory reporting of SSI rates after colon and hysterectomy surgery being mandated in January 2013 with anticipated impact on reimbursement in 2015.

SSI prevention has been a challenge with the complexity of surgical patients and the perioperative care arena. There continues to be a need for well-designed randomized controlled trials to evaluate best practices for SSI prevention. Emerging evidence does support the implementation of bundled interventions to reduce SSI risk. Bundle elements vary slightly depending on the procedure, but core elements to consider including are: skin preparation; bowel preparation with oral antibiotics; pre- and intraoperative antibiotic use; use of wound protectors; laparoscopy; glucose control; fluid restriction; and temperature management. The evidence to support these interventions is elaborated on in this chapter.

L.S. Feldman et al. (eds.), *The SAGES / ERAS®*
Society Manual of Enhanced Recovery Programs for
Gastrointestinal Surgery, DOI 10.1007/978-3-319-20364-5_10,
© Springer International Publishing Switzerland 2015

Regulatory Requirements for SSI Prevention

Surgical Care Improvement Project (SCIP)

In the United States, the Surgical Care Improvement Project (SCIP) was an initiative led by stakeholder organizations with the common goal of significantly reducing surgical morbidity and mortality. The original intent of SCIP was to improve hospital compliance with the use of prophylactic antibiotics for elective surgery and later extended to broader SSI prevention measures as well as other surgical harm. Hospital-level compliance is publically reported on the hospitalcompare.gov website and tied to value based purchasing. SCIP measures related to SSI prevention include:

- Prophylactic antibiotics received within 1 h prior to surgical incision.
- Appropriate prophylactic antibiotic selection.
- Prophylactic antibiotics discontinued within 24 h of surgery.
- Cardiac surgery patients with controlled 6 am postsurgery blood glucose.
- Active warming or the maintenance of normothermia for colon surgery.

Although level 1 evidence supports each measure, hospital compliance has failed to translate into reduced SSI rates [5–7]. As of January 1, 2015, in the United States, the SCIP measures are no longer part of the Medicare value based purchasing program.

Emerging Evidence for SSI Prevention

Antibiotic Redosing

Redosing of antimicrobial surgical prophylaxis during procedures is an important strategy to prevent surgical site infection (SSI). Intraoperative redosing is supported by clinical and pharmacological studies and recommended by the Therapeutic Guidelines on Antimicrobial Prophylaxis in Surgery—a consensus document developed by multiple specialty societies (http://www.ajhp.org/content/70/3/195.full. pdf+html). The goal is to achieve and maintain adequate serum and tissue levels of the antimicrobial agent for the entire period during which the wound is open [8]. Antimicrobial agents need to be redosed if the procedure time exceeds two half-lives of the antimicrobial agents or if there is excessive blood loss (>1500 ml) [8–12]. Intraoperative redosing may also be warranted if factors such as extensive burns shorten the half-life of the antimicrobial agent. Intraoperative redosing may NOT be warranted if factors such as renal failure prolong the half-life of the antimicrobial agent. Recommended intraoperative redosing intervals (from the initiation of the preoperative dose) of some commonly utilized agents are:

- Cefazolin: redose every 3-4 h.
- Cefotetan: redose every 6 h.
- Cefoxitin: redose every 2 h (very short half-life, consider using an alternative prophylaxis for colorectal surgery).
- Clindamycin: redose every 6 h.
- Vancomycin: redose every 12 h.

Certain agents do not require intraoperative redosing (e.g., ertapenem, gentamicin [5 mg/kg], metronidazole) due to their pharmacokinetic properties.

Weight-Based Dosing of Cephalosporins

Weight-based dosing of Cephalosporin preoperative antimicrobial prophylaxis for obese patients aims to achieve adequate serum and tissue levels to prevent SSI. This strategy is supported by clinical and pharmacological studies, recommended by the CDC in the HICPAC (Healthcare Infection Control Practices Advisory Committee) Guidelines for Prevention of Surgical Site Infection (2004) [8], and suggested in the latest version of the Therapeutic Guidelines on Antimicrobial Prophylaxis in Surgery. The preoperative antimicrobial prophylaxis dose of cefazolin should be increased from 1 to 2 g for patients with weight >80 kg and to 3 g for patients with weight >120 kg. Preoperative doses of 1 g cefazolin may not be sufficient to achieve serum and tissue concentrations greater than the MIC for common gram-negative and gram-positive pathogens [13, 14]. Whether to use ideal body weight or actual body weight for these dosing calculations remains to be determined. Doubling the normal dose of cephalosporins produces concentrations in obese patients similar to those achieved with normal doses in normal-weight patients [15]. For simplification, some hospitals have implemented a standardized preoperative prophylaxis dose of Cefazolin 2 g for all adult patients and 3 g for patients with weight >120 kg and administer Cefotetan and Cefoxitin antimicrobial prophylaxis (when indicated) at a dose of 2 g for all adult patients.

Skin Preparation

Careful skin preparation with the appropriate agent is a critical step for prevention of surgical site infections. The skin harbors approximately 10^{12} bacteria. Common skin organisms include Staphylococcus spp., Streptococcus spp., Propionibacterium acnes, Corynebacterium spp., and Acinetobacter spp. The goal of a surgical skin preparation is to reduce the burden of skin microorganisms prior to incision [16]. The most commonly used preparations are chlorhexidine, povidone-iodine, and/or alcohol. To optimize efficacy, either chlorhexidine or povidone-iodine should be combined with alcohol solution because alcohol is the most effective strategy to reduce skin bacteria, but without another agent the effect is not durable. Commercially available combination preps include Chloraprep [2 % chlorhexidine gluconate and 70 % isopropyl alcohol] and DuraPrep [iodine povacrylex and isopropyl alcohol] [17]. A randomized controlled study of patients undergoing clean-contaminated procedures compared chloraprep and povidone-iodine scrub and paint. The chloraprep group had a lower overall, superficial and deep space infection rates but there was no difference in organ space infections (overall 9.5 % vs. 16.1 %) [18]. Recommendations for the use of alcohol-based skin preparations:

- Preparation should be applied according to manufacturer's specifications (duration and amount of preparation).
- Preparation MUST be allowed to dry on the skin prior to incision.
- Preparation should NOT be washed off.
- Education about fire precautions is important prior to instituting an alcohol-based prep protocol.

  - Avoid pooling and dripping of solution.
  - Prep should be dry (approximately 3 min) prior to draping the patient.

Preoperative Chlorhexidine Bathing

Preoperative bathing with chlorhexidine (CHG) 4 % to prevent SSI is becoming more common. CHG bathing preoperatively as compared to soap significantly reduces the microbiological burden of the skin, but it has been challenging to demonstrate an associated reduction in SSI. Studies from Hayek et al. (cluster randomized controlled trial) and Wihlborg et al. (randomized controlled trial) totaling 3500 patients reported reductions in SSI with chlorhexidine bathing [19, 20] while all other studies, totaling 6900 patients, found no decrease in SSI. Despite the lack of evidence, adoption of CHG bathing is widespread, likely because it is a simple intervention to implement and relatively low cost—between 1 and 12 dollars per patient depending on the formulation selected. Most protocols recommend bathing with CHG the night before and morning of surgery with either packages of CHG soap or impregnated washcloths. Alternatively, to improve compliance, some hospitals have advocated CHG use only prior to surgery with supervised application in the preoperative area of the operating room. Providers should consider using CHG bathing if they note an increase in a significant number of wound infections associated with skin bacteria such as Staphylococcus spp. or Streptococcus spp. as is commonly seen in cardiac and orthopedic surgery and in some instances in gastrointestinal surgery.

Perioperative Glucose Control

Hyperglycemia in hospitalized patients is common. In a survey of patients admitted to a community teaching hospital, hyperglycemia was present in 38 % of medical and surgical admissions (26 % had a known history of diabetes and 12 % had no preoperative history). In cardiac surgery, degree of postoperative hyperglycemia correlates with SSI [21, 22]. Although tight glucose control has not been studied with the same rigor in the general surgery patient, case series and analyses of statewide surgical collaboratives have identified an association between hyperglycemia and postoperative complications. Diabetic patients undergoing colorectal surgery had a 15 % rate of SSI; on multivariate analysis, higher glucose levels were associated with increased risk of SSI. However, implementation of SSI prevention bundles including glucose control (<200 mg/dl (11.1 mmol/l) or <180 mg/dl (10 mmol/l)) has not demonstrated improvements in SSI [23–25]. A Cochrane review of the topic found that there was insufficient evidence to support perioperative strict glycemic control for SSI prevention [26]. Based on the draft version of the revised HICPAC guidelines, perioperative glycemic control should be aimed at maintaining glucose levels less than 200 mg/dl (<11.1 mmol/l) in diabetic and nondiabetic patients. To achieve this in the perioperative area, the Canadian program, Safer Health Care Now, recommends:

- Blood glucose levels on all patients in pre-op evaluation.
- Assign responsibility and accountability for blood glucose monitoring and control.
- Diabetics or anyone with blood glucose >180 mg/dl (>10 mml/l) should be flagged to have a repeat level the day of surgery and follow-up every 2 h.
- Surgeon and anesthesiologist should be notified of blood glucose >180 mg/dl (>10 mml/l).

There are also several interventions included in Enhanced Recovery programs that aim to preserve perioperative insulin sensitivity, such as preoperative carbohydrate drinks and avoidance of prolonged fasting, afferent neural blockade, and early resumption of oral intake.

Mechanical Bowel Preparation with Oral Antibiotics for Colorectal Surgery

The use of oral antibiotics to decontaminate the colon was one of the earliest strategies to reduce infectious complications in colorectal surgery patients. For the past 20 years, much of the surgical infection research has focused on the role of preoperative intravenous antibiotics to reduce SSI rates and based on well-designed randomized studies this has become standard of care in the perioperative period and included as a SCIP measure. The combination of preoperative intravenous antibiotics combined with oral antibiotics with or without mechanical bowel has not been studied with the same rigor.

The use of oral antibiotics for colon surgery was first described in the 1940s. Small follow-up reports with different combinations of oral antibiotics (varying amounts of aerobic and anaerobic bacteria coverage) demonstrated that this treatment resulted in marked decontamination of the colon and decreased SSI. Washington et al. conducted the first randomized trial comparing oral neomycin/tetracycline plus mechanical bowel preparation with placebo plus mechanical bowel preparation and demonstrated decreased infectious complications in group receiving oral antibiotics (43 % placebo, 41 % neomycin, 5 % neomycin and tetracycline) [27]. Subsequent work by Nichols, Condon, and Clark popularized the use of neomycin and erythromycin with mechanical bowel preparation [28, 29]. These studies were criticized because intravenous antibiotics were not administered. In 2002, Lewis et al., conducted a randomized controlled trial comparing oral neomycin and metronidazole plus systemic antibiotics to systemic antibiotics alone (17 % placebo and 5 % neomycin and metronidazole) [30]. Oral antibiotics were associated with a decreased SSI rate and this finding was corroborated by a meta-analysis of 13 other trials demonstrating that oral antibiotic use was associated with decreased SSI. Most recently, evaluation of the Michigan Surgical Quality Collaborative (MSQC) data (NSQIP methodology) using a propensity matched analysis found that patients who received oral antibiotics and mechanical bowel preparation as compared to those receiving mechanical bowel preparation alone had a lower rate of superficial and organ space infections [31]. Similar results were found with analysis of the Veterans Affairs Hospital data. A recent Cochrane review of perioperative antibiotic prophylaxis found that use of preoperative oral antibiotics was associated with reduction in SSI [32].

Although there are still unanswered questions about the optimal use of oral antibiotics and mechanical bowel preparation, the evidence supports the addition of oral antibiotics when mechanical bowel preparation is used. The consensus guidelines endorsed by the American Society of Hospital Pharmacists support their use in colorectal surgery. Mechanical bowel preparation without oral antimicrobials does not reduce the risk of SSI. A Cochrane review from 2011 comparing mechanical bowel preparation to no bowel preparation found no difference in SSI rates in the two groups for open colon surgery; however these studies did not include oral antibiotics with the mechanical preparations. Nonetheless, guidelines from the ERAS Society state that mechanical bowel preparation should not be used routinely for colonic surgery. There is less data available for rectal surgery, laparoscopic surgery, or when a diverting ileostomy is planned (see Chap. 3).

Judicious Management of Volume, Temperature, and Oxygenation in the Perioperative Patient

Historical inquiry into surgical site infections has suggested that these infections occur during a "decisive period" intraoperatively when soft tissue is directly exposed to skin and enteric flora while the tissue is concurrently stressed [33]. Improving wound edge tissue oxygenation, maintaining euvolemia, and preventing intraoperative hypothermia are suggested to reduce the physiologic stress of surgery.

Improving Wound Edge Tissue Oxygenation

Low levels of tissue oxygen tension have long been associated with impaired wound healing and postoperative infections [34–37]. One commonly employed means of addressing poor tissue oxygenation has been the administration of highly concentrated supplemental oxygen. A number of clinical trials have tested different time intervals and criteria for the administration of 80 % FiO_2 to reduce the risk of SSI. Unfortunately, these studies have been complicated by intermittently successful attainment of oxygen-rich wound edges [35] and the varied array of anesthesia modalities available. In general, the consensus supported by the draft HICPAC guidelines is that patients who have required endotracheal intubation benefit the most from high fraction oxygen inspiration and supplementation should be continued into the immediate postextubation period [38–41].

Maintaining Euvolemia

In addition to ensuring blood oxygen tension is adequate, a related intervention has been optimizing the delivery of inspired oxygen to the periphery. On one hand, hypovolemia contributes to vascular constriction and poor tissue perfusion. However, hypervolemia decreases the oxygen carrying capacity and immune response of more concentrated blood. Few studies have been designed to specifically identify an ideal level of fluid resuscitation to reduce SSI, but common practice has been to maintain euvolemia to avoid the drawbacks of either extreme [38–40].

Preventing Hypothermia

The relationship between physiologic stress and surgical site infections has also led many to question whether low body temperature during surgery may be unduly stressing the exposed tissues. A number of studies explore the relationship of tight temperature regulation and surgical site infection outcomes [36, 42, 43]. Although these studies vary widely in methodology and specific temperature targets, all of them support at least some minimal degree of temperature maintenance. The draft

HICPAC guideline incorporates these findings and gives a high quality recommendation for warming versus no warming while providing a moderate quality recommendation for intraoperative only warming versus a longer perioperative warming period (pre-, intra-, postoperative).

Wound Protectors and Laparoscopy

Small single institution studies as well as personal experiences support the use of wound protectors for SSI prevention. A recent meta-analysis of six randomized controlled studies demonstrated an almost 50 % reduction in SSI with the use of wound protectors in gastrointestinal surgery. Wound protectors are available from a variety of companies, some with two rings and some with one—no specific format has been demonstrated to be superior [44]. The laparoscopic approach is also associated with a lower SSI rate and should be considered when technically feasible [45].

Conclusions

SSI prevention continues to be a challenge. This is likely a reflection of both the weak evidence to support many commonplace SSI prevention interventions and the challenges of translating research into practice. But, as more care is transitioned to protocols and pathways, it is likely that the variability in surgical care will continue to decrease and implementation of many of the SSI prevention intervention will be more consistent. For optimal results, SSI prevention interventions should be incorporated into enhanced recovery protocols.

Take Home Messages

- Effective SSI prevention requires that perioperative teamwork is fostered and a culture of safety is developed with all care providers (surgeons, anesthesia providers, and nurses).
- Key enhanced recovery principles like nutrition, glucose management, and normothermia are also important for SSI prevention.

- If a bowel preparation is used, mechanical bowel preparation with oral antibiotics is superior to mechanical bowel preparation alone.
- Optimization of SSI prevention processes requires continuous review of compliance with key process indicators at the patient level and systems-level innovations to ensure high reliability.

References

1. de Lissovoy G, Fraeman K, Hutchins V, Murphy D, Song D, Vaughn BB. Surgical site infection: incidence and impact on hospital utilization and treatment costs. Am J Infect Control. 2009;37:387–97. doi:10.1016/j.ajic.2008.12.010.
2. Wick EC, Hirose K, Shore AD, Clark JM, Gearhart SL, Efron J, Makary MA. Surgical site infections and cost in obese patients undergoing colorectal surgery. Arch Surg. 2011;146:1068–72. doi:10.1001/archsurg.2011.117.
3. Smith RL, Bohl JK, McElearney ST, Friel CM, Barclay MM, Sawyer RG, Foley EF. Wound infection after elective colorectal resection. Ann Surg. 2004;239:599–605. discussion 605-7.
4. Wick EC, Shore AD, Hirose K, Ibrahim AM, Gearhart SL, Efron J, Weiner JP, Makary MA. Readmission rates and cost following colorectal surgery. Dis Colon Rectum. 2011;54:1475–9. doi:10.1097/DCR.0b013e31822ff8f0.
5. Hawn MT, Vick CC, Richman J, Holman W, Deierhoi RJ, Graham LA, Henderson WG, Itani KM. Surgical site infection prevention: time to move beyond the surgical care improvement program. Ann Surg. 2011;254:494–9. doi:10.1097/SLA.0b013e31822c6929. discussion 499–501.
6. Stulberg JJ, Delaney CP, Neuhauser DV, Aron DC, Fu P, Koroukian SM. Adherence to surgical care improvement project measures and the association with postoperative infections. JAMA. 2010;303:2479–85. doi:10.1001/jama.2010.841.
7. Ingraham AM, Cohen ME, Bilimoria KY, Dimick JB, Richards KE, Raval MV, Fleisher LA, Hall BL, Ko CY. Association of surgical care improvement project infection-related process measure compliance with risk-adjusted outcomes: implications for quality measurement. J Am Coll Surg. 2010;211:705–14. doi:10.1016/j.jamcollsurg.2010.09.006.
8. Bratzler DW, Houck PM, Surgical Infection Prevention Guidelines Writers Workgroup, American Academy of Orthopaedic Surgeons, American Association of Critical Care Nurses, American Association of Nurse Anesthetists, American College of Surgeons, American College of Osteopathic Surgeons, American Geriatrics Society, American Society of Anesthesiologists, American Society of Colon and Rectal Surgeons, American Society of Health-System Pharmacists, American Society of PeriAnesthesia Nurses, Ascension Health, Association of periOperative Registered Nurses, Association for Professionals in Infection Control and Epidemiology, Infectious Diseases Society of America, Medical Letter, Premier, Society for Healthcare

Epidemiology of America, Society of Thoracic Surgeons, Surgical Infection Society. Antimicrobial prophylaxis for surgery: an advisory statement from the National Surgical Infection Prevention Project. Clin Infect Dis. 2004;38:1706–15, DOI: 10.1086/421095.

9. Engelman R, Shahian D, Shemin R, Guy TS, Bratzler D, Edwards F, Jacobs M, Fernando H, Bridges C, Workforce on Evidence-Based Medicine, Society of Thoracic Surgeons. The Society of Thoracic Surgeons practice guideline series: antibiotic prophylaxis in cardiac surgery, part II: antibiotic choice. Ann Thorac Surg. 2007;83:1569–76. DOI: S0003-4975(06)01840-6 [pii].

10. Swoboda SM, Merz C, Kostuik J, Trentler B, Lipsett PA. Does intraoperative blood loss affect antibiotic serum and tissue concentrations? Arch Surg. 1996;131:1165–71. discussion 1171–2.

11. Markantonis SL, Kostopanagiotou G, Panidis D, Smirniotis V, Voros D. Effects of blood loss and fluid volume replacement on serum and tissue gentamicin concentrations during colorectal surgery. Clin Ther. 2004;26:271–81. DOI: S0149291804900252 [pii].

12. Morita S, Nishisho I, Nomura T, Fukushima Y, Morimoto T, Hiraoka N, Shibata N. The significance of the intraoperative repeated dosing of antimicrobials for preventing surgical wound infection in colorectal surgery. Surg Today. 2005;35:732–8. DOI: 10.1007/s00595-005-3026-3 [doi].

13. Edmiston CE, Krepel C, Kelly H, Larson J, Andris D, Hennen C, Nakeeb A, Wallace JR. Perioperative antibiotic prophylaxis in the gastric bypass patient: do we achieve therapeutic levels? Surgery. 2004;136:738–47. DOI: S003960600400412X [pii].

14. Conklin CM, Gray RJ, Neilson D, Wong P, Tomita DK, Matloff JM. Determinants of wound infection incidence after isolated coronary artery bypass surgery in patients randomized to receive prophylactic cefuroxime or cefazolin. Ann Thorac Surg. 1988;46:172–7.

15. Slama TG, Sklar SJ, Misinski J, Fess SW. Randomized comparison of cefamandole, cefazolin, and cefuroxime prophylaxis in open-heart surgery. Antimicrob Agents Chemother. 1986;29:744–7.

16. Mangram AJ, Horan TC, Pearson ML, Silver LC, Jarvis WR, Guideline for Prevention of Surgical Site Infection. Centers for Disease Control and Prevention (CDC) Hospital Infection Control Practices Advisory Committee. Am J Infect Control. 1999;27: 97–132. quiz 133–4; discussion 96.

17. Swenson BR, Hedrick TL, Metzger R, Bonatti H, Pruett TL, Sawyer RG. Effects of preoperative skin preparation on postoperative wound infection rates: a prospective study of 3 skin preparation protocols. Infect Control Hosp Epidemiol. 2009;30: 964–71. doi:10.1086/605926.

18. Darouiche RO, Wall Jr MJ, Itani KM, Otterson MF, Webb AL, Carrick MM, Miller HJ, Awad SS, Crosby CT, Mosier MC, Alsharif A, Berger DH. Chlorhexidine-alcohol versus povidone-iodine for surgical-site antisepsis. N Engl J Med. 2010;362:18–26. doi:10.1056/NEJMoa0810988.

19. Wihlborg O. The effect of washing with chlorhexidine soap on wound infection rate in general surgery. A controlled clinical study. Ann Chir Gynaecol. 1987;76:263–5.

20. Hayek LJ, Emerson JM. Preoperative whole body disinfection – a controlled clinical study. J Hosp Infect. 1988;11(Suppl B):15–9.

21. Latham R, Lancaster AD, Covington JF, Pirolo JS, Thomas Jr CS. The association of diabetes and glucose control with surgical-site infections among cardiothoracic surgery patients. Infect Control Hosp Epidemiol. 2001;22:607–12. doi:10.1086/501830.

22. Presutti E, Millo J. Controlling blood glucose levels to reduce infection. Crit Care Nurs Q. 2006;29:123–31.

23. Pastor C, Artinyan A, Varma MG, Kim E, Gibbs L, Garcia-Aguilar J. An increase in compliance with the Surgical Care Improvement Project measures does not prevent surgical site infection in colorectal surgery. Dis Colon Rectum. 2010;53:24–30. doi:10.1007/DCR.0b013e3181ba782a.

24. Forbes SS, Stephen WJ, Harper WL, Loeb M, Smith R, Christoffersen EP, McLean RF. Implementation of evidence-based practices for surgical site infection prophylaxis: results of a pre- and postintervention study. J Am Coll Surg. 2008;207:336–41. doi:10.1016/j.jamcollsurg.2008.03.014.

25. Liau KH, Aung KT, Chua N, Ho CK, Chan CY, Kow A, Earnest A, Chia SJ. Outcome of a strategy to reduce surgical site infection in a tertiary-care hospital. Surg Infect (Larchmt). 2010;11:151–9. doi:10.1089/sur.2008.081.

26. Kao LS, Meeks D, Moyer VA, Lally KP. Peri-operative glycaemic control regimens for preventing surgical site infections in adults. Cochrane Database Syst Rev. 2009;3:CD006806. doi:10.1002/14651858.CD006806.pub2.

27. Washington 2nd JA, Dearing WH, Judd ES, Elveback LR. Effect of preoperative antibiotic regimen on development of infection after intestinal surgery: prospective, randomized, double-blind study. Ann Surg. 1974;180:567–72.

28. Clarke JS, Condon RE, Bartlett JG, Gorbach SL, Nichols RL, Ochi S. Preoperative oral antibiotics reduce septic complications of colon operations: results of prospective, randomized, double-blind clinical study. Ann Surg. 1977;186:251–9.

29. Nichols RL, Broido P, Condon RE, Gorbach SL, Nyhus LM. Effect of preoperative neomycin-erythromycin intestinal preparation on the incidence of infectious complications following colon surgery. Ann Surg. 1973;178:453–62.

30. Lewis RT. Oral versus systemic antibiotic prophylaxis in elective colon surgery: a randomized study and meta-analysis send a message from the 1990s. Can J Surg. 2002;45:173–80.

31. Englesbe MJ, Brooks L, Kubus J, Luchtefeld M, Lynch J, Senagore A, Eggenberger JC, Velanovich V, Campbell Jr DA. A statewide assessment of surgical site infection following colectomy: the role of oral antibiotics. Ann Surg. 2010;252:514–9. doi:10.1097/SLA.0b013e3181f244f8. discussion 519–20.

32. Nelson RL, Glenny AM, Song F. Antimicrobial prophylaxis for colorectal surgery. Cochrane Database Syst Rev. 2009;1:CD001181. doi:10.1002/14651858.CD001181. pub3.

33. MILES AA, MILES EM, BURKE J. The value and duration of defence reactions of the skin to the primary lodgement of bacteria. Br J Exp Pathol. 1957;38:79–96.

34. Hopf HW, Hunt TK, West JM, Blomquist P, Goodson 3rd WH, Jensen JA, Jonsson K, Paty PB, Rabkin JM, Upton RA, von Smitten K, Whitney JD. Wound tissue oxygen

tension predicts the risk of wound infection in surgical patients. Arch Surg. 1997;132:997–1004. discussion 1005.

35. Jonsson K, Jensen JA, Goodson 3rd WH, Scheuenstuhl H, West J, Hopf HW, Hunt TK. Tissue oxygenation, anemia, and perfusion in relation to wound healing in surgical patients. Ann Surg. 1991;214:605–13.

36. Kurz A, Sessler DI, Lenhardt R. Perioperative normothermia to reduce the incidence of surgical-wound infection and shorten hospitalization. Study of Wound Infection and Temperature Group. N Engl J Med. 1996;334:1209–15. doi:10.1056/NEJM199605093341901.

37. Meyhoff CS, Wetterslev J, Jorgensen LN, Henneberg SW, Hogdall C, Lundvall L, Svendsen PE, Mollerup H, Lunn TH, Simonsen I, Martinsen KR, Pulawska T, Bundgaard L, Bugge L, Hansen EG, Riber C, Gocht-Jensen P, Walker LR, Bendtsen A, Johansson G, Skovgaard N, Helto K, Poukinski A, Korshin A, Walli A, Bulut M, Carlsson PS, Rodt SA, Lundbech LB, Rask H, Buch N, Perdawid SK, Reza J, Jensen KV, Carlsen CG, Jensen FS, Rasmussen LS, PROXI Trial Group. Effect of high perioperative oxygen fraction on surgical site infection and pulmonary complications after abdominal surgery: the PROXI randomized clinical trial. JAMA. 2009;302:1543–50. doi: 10.1001/jama.2009.1452 [doi].

38. Belda FJ, Aguilera L, Garcia de la Asuncion J, Alberti J, Vicente R, Ferrandiz L, Rodriguez R, Company R, Sessler DI, Aguilar G, Botello SG, Orti R, Spanish Reduccion de la Tasa de Infeccion Quirurgica Group. Supplemental perioperative oxygen and the risk of surgical wound infection: a randomized controlled trial. JAMA. 2005;294:2035–42. DOI: 294/16/2035 [pii].

39. Bickel A, Gurevits M, Vamos R, Ivry S, Eitan A. Perioperative hyperoxygenation and wound site infection following surgery for acute appendicitis: a randomized, prospective, controlled trial. Arch Surg. 2011;146:464–70. DOI: 10.1001/archsurg.2011.65 [doi].

40. Greif R, Akca O, Horn EP, Kurz A, Sessler DI, Outcomes Research Group. Supplemental perioperative oxygen to reduce the incidence of surgical-wound infection. N Engl J Med. 2000;342:161–7. DOI: 10.1056/NEJM200001203420303 [doi].

41. Pryor KO, Fahey 3rd TJ, Lien CA, Goldstein PA. Surgical site infection and the routine use of perioperative hyperoxia in a general surgical population: a randomized controlled trial. JAMA. 2004;291:79–87. DOI: 10.1001/jama.291.1.79 [doi].

42. Melling AC, Ali B, Scott EM, Leaper DJ. Effects of preoperative warming on the incidence of wound infection after clean surgery: a randomised controlled trial. Lancet. 2001;358:876–80. doi:10.1016/S0140-6736(01)06071-8.

43. Barone JE, Tucker JB, Cecere J, Yoon MY, Reinhard E, Blabey Jr RG, Lowenfels AB. Hypothermia does not result in more complications after colon surgery. Am Surg. 1999;65:356–9.

44. Edwards JP, Ho AL, Tee MC, Dixon E, Ball CG. Wound protectors reduce surgical site infection: a meta-analysis of randomized controlled trials. Ann Surg. 2012;256: 53–9. DOI: 10.1097/SLA.0b013e3182570372 [doi].

45. Kiran RP, El-Gazzaz GH, Vogel JD, Remzi FH. Laparoscopic approach significantly reduces surgical site infections after colorectal surgery: data from national surgical quality improvement program. J Am Coll Surg. 2010;211:232–8. doi:10.1016/j.jamcollsurg.2010.03.028.

Key References

Healthcare Infection Control Practices Advisory Committee Guidelines for the Prevention of SSI (DRAFT version). https://www.federalregister.gov/articles/2014/01/29/2014-01674/draft-guideline-centers-for-disease-control-and-prevention-draft-guideline-for-the-prevention-of.

Clinical Practice Guidelines for Antimicrobial Prophylaxis in Surgery. http://www.ajhp.org/content/70/3/195.full.pdf+html.

11. Fluid Management

Sherif Awad and Dileep N. Lobo

The past two decades have hosted a resurgence of research interest into perioperative fluid and electrolyte therapy. Numerous studies and subsequent systematic reviews/meta-analyses have examined the effects on outcomes of different *type* (crystalloids, colloids, balanced and unbalanced solutions) [1], *volume* (restricted *versus* liberal fluid regimens) [2] and technology to *guide* intraoperative fluid therapy (goal-directed therapy *versus* conventional therapy) [3]. Importantly, there are now ample data that clearly demonstrate the aforementioned factors to have a direct effect on surgical outcome (morbidity and mortality) [2, 4, 5]. Key aims of enhanced recovery after surgery protocols (ERP) [6] include amelioration of physiological and metabolic stress, maintenance and rapid recovery of physiological function, and finally, reduced postoperative morbidity, mortality and length of hospital stay (LOHS). As most patients undergoing elective surgery will require intravenous fluid and electrolyte therapy, the importance of optimal fluid and electrolyte management (within and outwith ERP protocols) to the success of such protocols becomes readily apparent. As extensive reviews on perioperative fluid and electrolyte therapy have been published elsewhere [7–9], the present chapter aims to serve as a practical guide to optimising fluid therapy in patients undergoing elective surgery.

Optimal Fluid and Electrolyte Management

The aim of the ideal perioperative fluid and electrolyte therapy regimen is maintenance of 'zero' fluid balance coupled with minimal weight gain or loss. Key to understanding the plethora of recent studies into

L.S. Feldman et al. (eds.), *The SAGES / ERAS®*
Society Manual of Enhanced Recovery Programs for
Gastrointestinal Surgery, DOI 10.1007/978-3-319-20364-5_11,
© Springer International Publishing Switzerland 2015

perioperative fluid therapy in major surgery is use of standard definitions and terminology. Terms commonly used in previous randomised controlled trials (RCTs) to refer to different fluid regimens included 'standard', 'restricted', 'overload', 'liberal' and 'balance'. These terms have led to confusion and difficulty in making inferences from pooled data from RCTs. This was clearly demonstrated by our group, in a meta-analysis of nine RCTs on crystalloid-based perioperative fluid therapy in over 800 patients undergoing elective open abdominal surgery [2]. No apparent differences in postoperative complications or LOHS were noted when 'restricted' [as per author definitions] fluid regimens were compared with 'standard or liberal' [as per author definitions] fluid regimens. However, when fluid regimens were reclassified and patients were grouped into those who were managed in a state of fluid 'balance' [between 1.75 and 2.75 L/day] or 'imbalance' [fluid overload or underhydration], the former group had significantly fewer complications (risk ratio 0.59 (95 % CI 0.44–0.81), $P = 0.0008$) and a shorter LOHS (WMD -3.44 (95 % CI -6.33 to -0.54) days, $P = 0.02$) [2]. These data highlight the importance of maintaining patients in a state of zero fluid balance and it would appear that worse outcomes occur in patients who gain more than 2.5 kg in weight as a result of salt and water overload. Thus, to achieve optimal postoperative outcomes (reduced complications and LOHS), surgical programmes should implement near-zero fluid balance directed pathways utilising minimal weight gain as a quality indicator. Yet it is not uncommon to see septic surgical patients gain up to 12.5 L in total body water (i.e. 12.5 kg weight gain) in the first 48 h following resuscitation with crystalloids [10]. As the body is unable to excrete excess salt with ease, it takes up to 3 weeks to lose this excess accumulated fluid. Although salt and water overload may sometimes be an inevitable consequence of resuscitation of the injured and critically ill, this scenario is often and unnecessarily encountered after elective surgery, thereby delaying recovery, increasing complications and prolonging hospital stay. This highlights the importance of appropriately identifying patients' fluid status and indications for perioperative fluid and electrolyte therapy prior to commencing it (Table 11.1). Indeed, numerous authors and bodies have called for fluid and electrolyte therapy to be accorded the same status as drug prescriptions. Another key component of optimal fluid and electrolyte management is choosing the appropriate intravenous fluid therapy regimen. A summary of constituents and indications for use of the various fluid regimens is given in Table 11.2.

Table 11.1. Indications for intravenous fluid.

Indication for parenteral fluid therapy	Definition	Situational example	Example of appropriate fluid prescription
Maintenance	Provide daily physiological fluid and electrolyte requirements	Patient unable to drink, with no ongoing fluid and electrolyte losses	25–35 mL/kg water, 1 mmol/kg Na^+ and K+ and 100 g dextrose per day
Replacement	Provide maintenance requirements and add like for like replacement for ongoing fluid and electrolyte losses	Vomiting, intestinal fistulae, diarrhoea	Daily maintenance requirement + like for like for what is being lost in fistula in terms of volume and electrolyte content (e.g. 0.9 % saline with added potassium for vomiting/high nasogastric tube aspirates)
Resuscitation	Administration of fluid and electrolytes to restore intravascular volume	Multisystem trauma, acute postoperative haemorrhage, sepsis	2 L bolus of balanced crystalloid (e.g. Hartmann's solution/ Plasmalyte/Ringer's Lactate 148). Further fluids dependent on response to initial bolus

From Lobo DN. Recent advances in perioperative fluid therapy. In Taylor I, Johnson CD (eds.) Recent Advances in Surgery 36. London, JP Medical Publishers, 2014, pp 1–14, with permission

Optimising Preoperative Hydration Status

Preoperative counselling and preparation is a key component of ERP protocols. Of equal importance is the preoperative identification of patients at risk of developing perioperative fluid and electrolyte imbalance. Use of the H.E.A.D pneumonic may aid this process:

- *H*istory, which should be focussed on identifying cardiac, respiratory, renal and gastrointestinal morbidity which could result in fluid imbalance.

Table 11.2. Properties of commonly prescribed crystalloids.

	Plasma[a]	0.9 % NaCl	Hartmann's	Ringer's lactate (USP)	Ringer's acetate	Plasma-Lyte 148	Sterofundin	0.18 % NaCl/4 % dextrose	Plasma-Lyte 56 Maintenance	0.45 % saline	5 % dextrose
Na^+ (mmol/L)	135–145	154	131	130	130	140	145	31	40	77	0
Cl^- (mmol/L)	95–105	154	111	109	112	98	127	31	40	77	0
$[Na^+]:[Cl^-]$ ratio	1.28–1.45:1	1:1	1.18:1	1.19:1	1.16:1	1.43:1	1.14:1	1:1	1:1	1:1	–
K^+ (mmol/L)	3.5–5.3	0	5	4	5	5	4	0	13	0	0
HCO_3^-/Bicarbonate precursor (mmol/L)	24–32	0	29 (Lactate)	28 (Lactate)	27 (Acetate)	27 (Acetate) 23 (gluconate)	24 (Acetate) 5 (malate)	0	16 (Acetate)	0	0
Ca^{2+} (mmol/L)	2.2–2.6	0	2	1.4	1	0	2.5	0	0	0	0
Mg^{2+} (mmol/L)	0.8–1.2	0	0	0	1	1.5	1	0	1.5	0	0
Glucose (mmol/L)	3.5–5.5	0	0	0	0	0	0	222.2 (40 g)	277.8 (50 g)	0	277.8 (50 g)
pH	7.35–7.45	4.5–7.0	5.0–7.0	6.0–7.5	6.0–8.0	4.0–8.0	5.1–5.9	4.5	3.5–6.0	4.5–7.0	3.5–5.5
Osmolality (mOsm/L)	275–295	308	278	273	276	295	309	284	389	154	278

From Lobo DN, Lewington AJP, Allison SP. Basic Concepts of Fluid and Electrolyte Balance. Bibliomed—Medizinische Verlagsgesellschaft mbH: Melsungen; 2013, with permission
[a]Normal laboratory range from Nottingham University Hospitals, Nottingham

- *E*xamination, paying particular attention to clinical evidence of dehydration and/or inappropriate distribution of fluid in body compartments (e.g. peripheral oedema or ascites). Clinical findings should be corroborated with laboratory indicators such as haemoglobin, urea and creatinine.
- *A*ppropriate medications should be commenced (e.g. beta-blockers), highlighted (e.g. beta-blockers, diuretics, nonsteroidal agents), or discontinued (e.g. aspirin, clopidogrel and nonsteroidals in certain circumstances).
- *D*eficits in fluid balance should be estimated and replaced like for like (Table 11.2) with the aim of achieving zero balance at arrival at the anaesthetic room.

There is level I evidence in support of shortened preoperative fasting protocols, and numerous national anaesthetic societies now permit solid food intake up to 6 h before and clear noncarbonated fluids up to 2 h before induction of anaesthesia. However, patients may not readily follow these guidelines and in clinical practice (even within the context of ERP protocols) alterations in theatre schedules mean it not uncommon to find patients fasted from food for longer periods (even up to 18 h). It is, therefore, of importance that patients are encouraged and provided the opportunity to maintain oral fluid intake (ideally carbohydrate containing drinks) up to 2 h preoperatively to avoid fluid depletion. Similarly, mechanical bowel preparation leads to losses of salt and water, and does not seem to decrease risk of infection when used without oral antibiotics, at least in open colon resection [11]. The routine use of mechanical bowel preparation is discouraged in ERP protocols [6]. If used, patients should receive supplemental intravenous fluid therapy to replace GI losses and ensure zero fluid balance. Induction of anaesthesia in patients with a fluid deficit further reduces the effective circulatory volume by decreasing sympathetic tone. Finally, use of premedication, hypnotics and long-acting sedatives reduce patients' ability to drink and mobilise postoperatively thereby hampering early recovery, which is a key aim of ERP protocols.

Intraoperative Individualised Goal-Directed Therapy (GDT)

Intraoperative assessment of fluid status is difficult, as a formal physical examination cannot always be conducted. Traditionally heart rate, blood pressure, and urine output have been used to guide intraoperative fluid therapy; however, volume deficits may not become apparent until they exceed 10 % of body weight. Other common intraoperative confounders such as activation of nociceptive pathways by surgical stimulation and changes in body temperature may distort interpretation of the patient's real-time volume status. Finally, the use of static measurements such as end-diastolic and central venous pressure to estimate volume responsiveness can be influenced by numerous factors including comorbid cardiovascular pathologies and CO_2 pneumoperitoneum during laparoscopic surgery. The latter affects cardiovascular parameters through effects on reduced preload, and hypercarbia-induced vasodilatation and myocardial depression. Goal-directed therapy (GDT) principally aims to guide intravenous fluid and vasopressor/inotropic therapy using measurements of cardiac output or other similar parameters to improve stroke volume, cardiac index and splanchnic perfusion. A number of devices such as the transesophageal Doppler (TOD), arterial pulse contour analysis, lithium dilution and transpulmonary thermodilution techniques can be used to monitor and direct GDT. Algorithms usually involve intraoperative measurement of stroke volume corrected flow time (FTc) in the descending aorta and administering a 200–250 mL fluid bolus over 5–10 min if FTc is <0.35 s. A stroke volume increase of more than 10 % or an FTc <0.35 s indicates intravascular hypovolemia. Conversely, if the stroke volume does not increase after the initial bolus or if the FTc is >0.4 s, a further bolus is not necessary and background continuous crystalloid infusion is continued. Such an individualised intraoperative algorithm improves splanchnic perfusion without causing excessive interstitial oedema. Previous meta-analyses comparing GDT with conventional therapy reported reduced incidence of postoperative and gastrointestinal complications, need for ICU stay and LOHS in patients undergoing major surgery [12, 13]. However, recent meta-analysis of 31 studies of 5292 patients did not demonstrate difference in mortality [5]. Furthermore, appraisal of these 'historical' GDT studies highlighted no data comparing GDT with patients receiving 'restrictive' fluid therapy (near-zero fluid balance). Two recent studies have demonstrated no differences between GDT and no GDT in patients managed with ERP protocols, with avoidance of postoperative fluid overload in occurrence of postoperative complications and LOHS [14, 15]. Thus, the value of GDT within the setting of ERP patients receiving zero-balance fluid therapy remains unclear. Moreover, the use of hydroxyethyl starch for GDT has been limited severely by the European Medicines Agency's cautions [16] on the use of starch in light of the recent randomised controlled trials [17–20] showing harm caused by starch when used for resuscitation. However, a recent study has suggested that either crystalloid or HES may be used with equal efficacy for flow-directed fluid therapy, but both groups of patients received in excess of 5 L of fluid on the day of surgery, which is far in excess of what most patients being managed with ERP protocols receive [21]. A number of hospitals have now moved to gelatins for GDT, but at present there is no evidence to suggest that gelatins are equivalent to starches for this indication. Surprisingly, there is little published data on the utility of goal-directed technologies (GDT) within the setting of laparoscopic (CO_2 pneumoperitoneum) major abdominal surgery. Furthermore, the specific effects of differing pressures of CO_2 pneumoperitoneum (low-pressure [e.g. 8–10 mmHg] vs. normal/high pressure [e.g. 12–15 mmHg]) and steep Trendelenburg/reverse Trendelenburg positioning on GDT parameters have not been studied. That said, however, preliminary data suggest haemodynamic consequences in fluid optimised patients with pneumoperitoneum include decreased stroke volume, cardiac output, and oxygen delivery, coupled with increased systemic vascular resistance [22]. A study in patients undergoing laparoscopic colorectal surgery within an enhanced recovery setting failed to demonstrate differences in intraoperative indexed oxygen delivery (DO_2I) between patients who received epidural versus spinal analgesia. Furthermore, this study identified patients with DO_2I <400 mL/min/m^2 had higher incidence of anastomotic leak (22 %) than patients with DO_2I >400 mL/min/m^2 (1.8 %) [22].

Optimal Postoperative Fluid Therapy

Despite clear data on the harmful effects of perioperative salt and water overload, perioperative fluid prescribing practices have changed little over the past two decades. Up to one in five surgical patients may suffer adverse events directly consequent from improper fluid prescribing [23]. Surgeons may fail to appreciate that there is little margin of error with fluid administration, in that a 2.5–3 L fluid overload is sufficient to increase morbidity. Within the context of an ERP protocol, failure to achieve and maintain zero balance has potential deleterious effects (Fig. 11.1) on respiratory (increased pneumonia), gastrointestinal (prolonged ileus, splanchnic oedema, lower anastomotic bursting pressures and increased leak), patient mobility (reduced due to peripheral oedema causing stiffness) and well-being (increased nausea and reduced mental ability to undertake complex tasks). Conversely, deleterious

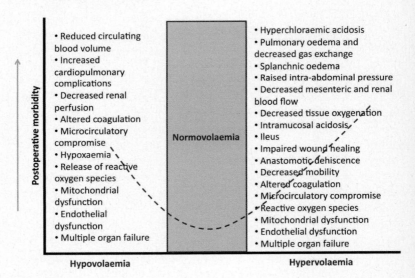

Fig. 11.1. Dose-response curve of fluid therapy demonstrating the adverse effects of fluid imbalance. (From Varadhan KK and Lobo DN. Perioperative fluid management in enhanced recovery. In: Francis N, et al. (eds.). Manual for Fast Track Recovery in Colorectal Surgery. London: Springer, 2012, with kind permission of Springer Science + Business Media).

effects may occur from perioperative underhydration which results in decreased venous return, cardiac output, diminished tissue perfusion and oxygen delivery. Furthermore, underhydration increases blood viscosity and pulmonary viscosity, resulting in plug formation and atelectasis.

A postoperative zero-balance schedule for fluid and electrolyte therapy should be clearly documented, individualised to patient needs and communicated to clinical teams. Changes in patient weight, which should be recorded daily if possible, are a sensitive means of gauging the quality of zero-balance fluid therapy and should alert the resident team to potential increased risk of morbidity. An appropriate time to agree and formulate such a schedule would be at the 'sign-out' moment of the WHO checklist [24] following major surgery considering the following factors:

- Intraoperative fluid administered and losses encountered.
- Maintenance fluids requirements (25–35 mL/kg water, 1 mmol/kg sodium and potassium, and 100 g dextrose per day).
- Replacement fluid requirements (expected ongoing losses from stomas, fistulae, drains and nasogastric tubes [if utilised], and open wounds).

- Minimal acceptable urine output (e.g. 0.5 mL/kg/h, averaged over 4 h), frequency of recordings and a protocol for managing reduced urine output postoperatively.

We have previously reviewed the history of 0.9 % sodium chloride solution ('normal saline') and how it came into routine clinical use [25]. It is now the most commonly utilised crystalloid in clinical practice with over 10 and 200 million litres being prescribed in the UK and the USA annually, respectively. With its content of 154 mmol/L sodium and 154 mmol/L of chloride being 10 and 50 % higher than that found in extracellular fluid, it is far from a physiological solution and often results in hyperchloraemia. In healthy volunteers, bolus infusions of 0.9 % saline are excreted slower than 5 % dextrose or balanced crystalloids (e.g. Hartmann's solution, Ringer's lactate or Plasma-Lyte 148) [26]. There have been numerous studies that support use of chloride-restrictive strategy perioperatively [4, 27, 28]. Analysis of a quality-assured database of outcomes of 2778 patients undergoing major open abdominal surgery demonstrated that use of 0.9 % saline on the day of surgery (compared with balanced crystalloids) was associated with higher in-hospital mortality (5.6 % vs. 2.9 %), complication rates (33.7 % vs. 23 %), greater requirement for blood transfusion and a near fivefold higher need for dialysis [4]. Another intensive care study demonstrated that patients who received chloride-restricted fluids (such as Hartmann's solution or Plasma-Lyte 148) had decreased incidence of acute kidney injury [odds ratio, OR, 0.59, $P < 0.001$] and need for renal replacement therapy [OR 0.52, $P = 0.004$] compared with those who received chloride-rich fluids, amongst which was 0.9 % saline [28]. Finally, in a study of 22,851 surgical patients, acute postoperative hyperchloraemia occurred in 22 % and was associated with increased risk of 30-day mortality, longer hospital stay and higher likelihood to having postoperative renal dysfunction [27]. Thus, it would appear that evidence on the harmful effects of routine use of 0.9 % saline is accumulating and it may be preferable to use balanced crystalloids perioperatively. Saline use should be restricted to patients with metabolic alkalosis, hypochloraemia due to persistent vomiting/high nasogastric aspirates or neurosurgical patients in whom the relative hypo-osmolarity of balanced crystalloids may be harmful.

ERP protocols recommend the use of mid-thoracic epidurals which work to effectively achieve analgesia, block stress hormone release, attenuate the reduction in postoperative insulin sensitivity, and prevent gut paralysis by blocking sympathetic outflow [6]. Epidural-induced

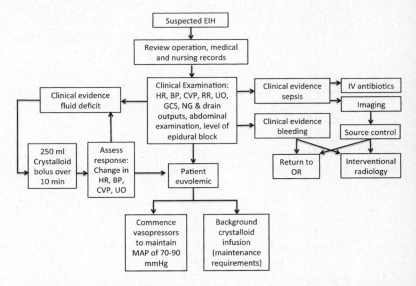

Fig. 11.2. Postoperative algorithm for the management of epidural-induced hypotension (EIH). *BP* blood pressure, *CVP* central venous pressure, *EIH* epidural-induced hypotension, *GCS* Glasgow coma scale, *HR* heart rate, *MAP* mean arterial pressure, *NG* nasogastric, *OR* operating room, *RR* respiratory rate, *UO* urine output.

hypotension is frequently encountered postoperatively. A zero-balance fluid therapy protocol should provide guidance on management of epidural-induced hypotension (Fig. 11.2), since not infrequently, the latter results in excessive infusion of fluids resulting in fluid imbalance. Epidural-induced hypotension in the adequately hydrated patient should be treated with vasopressors, although this usually requires ongoing haemodynamic monitoring, which may not be practical in some centres. If necessary a 250–500 mL bolus of balanced colloid rather than crystalloid should be used.

The optimal means of providing fluids after surgery is via the oral route, which along with early commencement of oral nutrition facilitates early return of bowel function and allows for early discontinuation of the intravenous drip, aiding mobility and faster recovery. Systematic reviews have established the safety of early oral nutrition which reduces postoperative morbidity without increasing risk of anastomotic leak [29]. Aggressive treatment of postoperative nausea and vomiting (PONV) facilitates early intake of oral fluids and feeding. Prophylaxis of PONV should occur in all patients, with individuals at moderate risk of PONV (>2 factors of: female gender, nonsmoking status, history of motion sickness or PONV and postoperative opioids) receiving additional prophylactic agents at induction of anaesthesia (see Chap. 8).

Fluid Management in Patients with Complications

In uncomplicated patients the early postoperative phase is associated with oliguria, salt and water retention. Average urine output over 4 h should be used in the assessment of oliguria. If there is associated hypotension, this should be treated with boluses (e.g. 250 mL) of crystalloids or colloids titrated to patient response, guided if possible by flow-based therapy. Furthermore, correction of any fluid deficits, electrolyte abnormalities, careful monitoring of continuing losses and daily weighing should guide clinicians to achieving zero balance and improved clinical outcomes. Hypovolaemia secondary to gastrointestinal losses from diarrhoea, ileus, small bowel fistulae and stomas should be replaced volume for volume with balanced crystalloids. Blood transfusions, if needed, should be provided in the ratio of 1:1:1 of whole blood: FFP: platelets as appropriate, especially if massive blood transfusion is required. Early timely identification and treatment of sepsis (in particular reversible abdominal causes such as collections and anastomotic dehiscence) in line with application of surviving sepsis guidelines [30], particularly early source control, go hand in hand with early resuscitative efforts using fluid and electrolyte therapy.

Future Directions

Although much progress has been made in the past two decades to understand the intricacies of perioperative fluid therapy, there is a paucity of data from zero-balance fluid therapy schedules utilised as part of ERP pathways. Furthermore, studies should examine whether the application of a zero-balance schedule individualised to patient needs improves and makes safer postoperative fluid and electrolyte therapy. Finally, there should be detailed studies of the effects of CO_2 pneumoperitoneum on haemodynamic and GDT parameters.

Conclusions

There are now clear data demonstrating inappropriate perioperative fluid and electrolyte therapy to increase surgical complications and LOHS. The margin of error is surprisingly small and weight gain of as little as 2.5 kg (i.e. a positive fluid balance of 2.5 L) may be sufficient to cause increased morbidity. Perioperative fluid therapy schedules should aim to achieve zero fluid balance, which in recent studies has been shown to lead to equivalent outcomes to GDT. In view of recent data on the adverse effects of using 0.9 % saline perioperatively, it is preferable to use balanced crystalloids.

Take Home Messages

- The optimal perioperative fluid and electrolyte therapy regimen is maintenance of 'near-zero' fluid balance coupled with minimal weight gain or loss.
- Within ERP protocols, importance should be afforded to the preoperative identification of patients at risk of developing perioperative fluid and electrolyte imbalance.
- Intraoperative assessment of volume status is difficult. Whilst devices facilitating goal-directed therapy help guide intravenous fluid and vasopressor/inotropic therapy to improve stroke volume, cardiac index and splanchnic perfusion, their utility in ERP protocols has been questioned.
- Routine use of 0.9 % sodium chloride should be discouraged due to the harmful effects of resultant hyperchloraemia.

References

1. Perel P, Roberts I, Ker K. Colloids versus crystalloids for fluid resuscitation in critically ill patients. Cochrane Database Syst Rev. 2013;2:CD000567.
2. Varadhan KK, Lobo DN. A meta-analysis of randomised controlled trials of intravenous fluid therapy in major elective open abdominal surgery: getting the balance right. Proc Nutr Soc. 2010;69(4):488–98.
3. Wilms H, Mittal A, Haydock MD, van den Heever M, Devaud M, Windsor JA. A systematic review of goal directed fluid therapy: rating of evidence for goals and monitoring methods. J Crit Care. 2014;29(2):204–9.

4. Shaw AD, Bagshaw SM, Goldstein SL, et al. Major complications, mortality, and resource utilization after open abdominal surgery: 0.9 % saline compared to Plasma-Lyte. Ann Surg. 2012;255(5):821–9.

5. Grocott MP, Dushianthan A, Hamilton MA, et al. Perioperative increase in global blood flow to explicit defined goals and outcomes after surgery: a Cochrane Systematic Review. Br J Anaesth. 2013;111(4):535–48.

6. Lassen K, Soop M, Nygren J, et al. Consensus review of optimal perioperative care in colorectal surgery: Enhanced Recovery After Surgery (ERAS) Group recommendations. Arch Surg. 2009;144(10):961–9.

7. Chowdhury AH, Lobo DN. Fluids and gastrointestinal function. Curr Opin Clin Nutr Metab Care. 2011;14(5):469–76.

8. Lobo DN, Awad S. Should chloride-rich crystalloids remain the mainstay of fluid resuscitation to prevent "pre-renal" acute kidney injury?: con. Kidney Int. 2014;86(6): 1096–105.

9. Mythen MG, Swart M, Acheson N, et al. Perioperative fluid management: consensus statement from the enhanced recovery partnership. Perioper Med (Lond). 2012;1:2.

10. Plank LD, Connolly AB, Hill GL. Sequential changes in the metabolic response in severely septic patients during the first 23 days after the onset of peritonitis. Ann Surg. 1998;228(2):146–58.

11. Slim K, Vicaut E, Launay-Savary MV, Contant C, Chipponi J. Updated systematic review and meta-analysis of randomized clinical trials on the role of mechanical bowel preparation before colorectal surgery. Ann Surg. 2009;249(2):203–9.

12. Abbas SM, Hill AG. Systematic review of the literature for the use of oesophageal Doppler monitor for fluid replacement in major abdominal surgery. Anaesthesia. 2008;63(1):44–51.

13. Giglio MT, Marucci M, Testini M, Brienza N. Goal-directed haemodynamic therapy and gastrointestinal complications in major surgery: a meta-analysis of randomized controlled trials. Br J Anaesth. 2009;103(5):637–46.

14. Brandstrup B, Svendsen PE, Rasmussen M, et al. Which goal for fluid therapy during colorectal surgery is followed by the best outcome: near-maximal stroke volume or zero fluid balance? Br J Anaesth. 2012;109(2):191–9.

15. Srinivasa S, Taylor MH, Singh PP, Yu TC, Soop M, Hill AG. Randomized clinical trial of goal-directed fluid therapy within an enhanced recovery protocol for elective colectomy. Br J Surg. 2013;100(1):66–74.

16. http://www.ema.europa.eu/docs/en_GB/document_library/Referrals_document/Solutions_for_infusion_containing_hydroxyethyl_starch/European_Commission_final_decision/WC500162361.pdf.

17. Brunkhorst FM, Engel C, Bloos F, et al. Intensive insulin therapy and pentastarch resuscitation in severe sepsis. N Engl J Med. 2008;358(2):125–39.

18. Myburgh JA, Finfer S, Bellomo R, et al. Hydroxyethyl starch or saline for fluid resuscitation in intensive care. N Engl J Med. 2012;367(20):1901–11.

19. Myburgh JA, Mythen MG. Resuscitation fluids. N Engl J Med. 2013;369(13): 1243–51.

20. Perner A, Haase N, Guttormsen AB, et al. Hydroxyethyl starch 130/0.42 versus Ringer's acetate in severe sepsis. N Engl J Med. 2012;367(2):124–34.

21. Yates DR, Davies SJ, Milner HE, Wilson RJ. Crystalloid or colloid for goal-directed fluid therapy in colorectal surgery. Br J Anaesth. 2014;112(2):281–9.

22. Levy BF, Fawcett WJ, Scott MJ, Rockall TA. Intra-operative oxygen delivery in infusion volume-optimized patients undergoing laparoscopic colorectal surgery within an enhanced recovery programme: the effect of different analgesic modalities. Colorectal Dis. 2012;14(7):887–92.

23. Walsh SR, Walsh CJ. Intravenous fluid-associated morbidity in postoperative patients. Ann R Coll Surg Engl. 2005;87(2):126–30.

24. Haynes AB, Weiser TG, Berry WR, et al. A surgical safety checklist to reduce morbidity and mortality in a global population. N Engl J Med. 2009;360(5):491–9.

25. Awad S, Allison SP, Lobo DN. The history of 0.9 % saline. Clin Nutr. 2008;27(2):179–88.

26. Chowdhury AH, Cox EF, Francis ST, Lobo DN. A randomized, controlled, double-blind crossover study on the effects of 2-L infusions of 0.9 % saline and plasma-lyte(R) 148 on renal blood flow velocity and renal cortical tissue perfusion in healthy volunteers. Ann Surg. 2012;256(1):18–24.

27. McCluskey SA, Karkouti K, Wijeysundera D, Minkovich L, Tait G, Beattie WS. Hyperchloremia after noncardiac surgery is independently associated with increased morbidity and mortality: a propensity-matched cohort study. Anesth Analg. 2013;117(2):412–21.

28. Yunos NM, Bellomo R, Hegarty C, Story D, Ho L, Bailey M. Association between a chloride-liberal vs chloride-restrictive intravenous fluid administration strategy and kidney injury in critically ill adults. JAMA. 2012;308(15):1566–72.

29. Lewis SJ, Andersen HK, Thomas S. Early enteral nutrition within 24 h of intestinal surgery versus later commencement of feeding: a systematic review and meta-analysis. J Gastrointest Surg. 2009;13(3):569–75.

30. Dellinger RP, Levy MM, Rhodes A, et al. Surviving sepsis campaign: international guidelines for management of severe sepsis and septic shock: 2012. Crit Care Med. 2013;41(2):580–637.

12. Postoperative Ileus: Prevention and Treatment

Martin Hübner, Michael Scott, and Bradley Champagne

Definition, Incidence, Risk Factors, Pathophysiology

Postoperative ileus (POI) is a transitory cessation of normal bowel activity. It is arguably the most frequent complication after digestive surgery; all the more surprising then to discover that the prevention and treatment of POI still pose many problems and not much progress has been made over the years in reducing its incidence and impact [1–4]. Besides the clinical impact, POI has a tremendous socioeconomic impact. It prolongs hospital stay by as much as 5 days and increases costs by about 8000 USD per patient [1, 4–6]. Furthermore POI appears to be the most frequent reasons for prolonged hospital stay and readmission after initial hospital stay [7, 8].

The problem begins with the lack of a standard definition of POI [9]. Vather et al. performed a systematic review of publications that included POI as primary endpoint. In a second step, an online survey informed opinion leaders of the variable definitions of POI identified in the review, in an attempt to come to standardized definitions [10]. The most important finding from the review was that definitions were extremely variable

---

The original version of this chapter was revised: A credit line has been added to the caption of Figure 12.1. The erratum to this chapter is available at: DOI 10.1007/978-3-319-20364-5_30

L.S. Feldman et al. (eds.), *The SAGES / ERAS®*
Society Manual of Enhanced Recovery Programs for
Gastrointestinal Surgery, DOI 10.1007/978-3-319-20364-5_12,
© Springer International Publishing Switzerland 2015

and sometimes contradictory. The author's suggested definitions were accepted by the expert panel with 80 % agreement and were as follows:

1. Postoperative ileus is the interval from surgery until both passage of flatus or stool AND tolerance of an oral diet. These two conditions are expected to be met before postoperative day (POD) 4.
2. Prolonged (pathological) POI is present if two of the following criteria are met on POD 4 without prior resolution of postoperative ileus: (1) nausea or vomiting; (2) food intolerance; (3) absence of flatus; (4) abdominal distension; (5) radiological confirmation.

Table 12.1. Postoperative ileus: risk factors, prevention, and treatment.

Risk factor	Prevention	Treatment
Patient		
Male gender	–	–
Comorbidities (pulmonary)	(Prehabilitation)	(Early mobilization, physiotherapy)
Procedure		
New ostomy	–	–
Surgical approach	(Minimally invasive surgery)	–
Emergency operation	–	–
Operation time	Consider pre-emptive conversion	–
Blood loss/transfusion	(Excellent surgical technique)	–
Perioperative care		
Fasting	No fasting	Early food intake
Fluid overload	Zero fluid balance Carbohydrates No bowel preparation	Early oral intake Early discontinuation of IV fluids
PONV	No nitrous oxide Short-acting anesthetics PONV prophylaxis	5HT3 antagonist
Opioid treatment	Opioid-sparing strategy	Opioid-sparing strategy
Immobilization	Prehabilitation Omission of drains, NG tubes Early removal/omission of urinary catheter	Early mobilization
Pharmacological agents		
Laxatives	?	+
Chewing gum	?	+
Opioid-sparing analgesia	+	–

(continued)

Table 12.1. (continued)

Risk factor	Prevention	Treatment
Lidocaine	+	−
Alvimopan	+	−
Neostigmine	−	?
WSCA	−	+

Risk factors for postoperative ileus are multifactorial and depend on the patient, the surgery, and the perioperative care pathway. Most of the patient- and surgery-related parameters are non-modifiable or can be corrected to a certain extent. In contrast, numerous preventive and therapeutic interventions are proven effective and are ideally combined within comprehensive perioperative care pathways in order to prevent ileus and to *enhance recovery*. Effective pharmacological interventions are acknowledged specifically

PONV postoperative nausea and vomiting, *NSAIDs* nonsteroidal anti-inflammatory drugs, *WSCA* water-soluble contrast agent

+ proven or probable effect

? potential effect but further studies required

Despite very different definitions, the incidence of POI has been reported to occur in about 15–25 % of patients undergoing colorectal procedures [2–5, 11, 12]. Risk factors for POI are multiple and are related both to the patient and to the procedure (Table 12.1). Consistently, male gender, pulmonary comorbidity, and creation of a new ostomy have been reported [2, 4]; the extent of surgery and the consequent surgical trauma also seem to have a direct influence on the incidence and duration of POI [2, 3, 11–13]. Surrogates for more extensive surgery such as the duration of surgery (>3 h), emergency procedure, and transfusion requirements have all been shown to increase the risk [2, 3]. On the other hand, minimally invasive techniques appear to be protective [12, 13]. Interestingly, the type of surgery (e.g., right-sided vs. left-sided etc.) seems to be less important than surgical approach (laparoscopy to be preferred) and anastomotique technique; a recent meta-analysis on ileostomy closure suggested faster return of bowel function of stapled vs. hand-sewn technique [2, 14].

Perioperative management has an important impact on POI, and can be either a major risk factor for POI or protect against it (Table 12.1). Perioperative fluid management shall serve as one example. Administration of excess perioperative intravenous fluid, especially saline, has a profound pathological effect on intestinal physiology [15]. Common pathophysiological features are intestinal edema, acidosis, and increased abdominal pressure resulting in wound healing problems, anastomotic complications, and POI (Fig. 12.1). Many different efforts have been undertaken over the recent years to shift the paradigm from POI being an inevitable part of abdominal surgery towards instead thinking of POI as a "preventable event" [16], as will be outlined in this chapter.

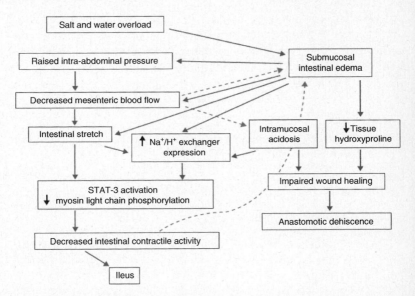

Fig. 12.1. Pathophysiology of postoperative ileus related to salt and water overload. The effects of the physiologic stress response to surgical trauma can be exacerbated by the approach to perioperative care. When excessive saline is administered, overloading the patient with salt and fluids, intestinal edema and an increase of the intraabdominal pressure result, contributing to the occurrence of postoperative ileus. With permission from Chowdhury AH, Lobo DN. Fluids and gastrointestinal function. Current Opinion in Clinical Nutrition and Metabolic Care 14:469–476 © 2011 Wolters Kluwer Health | Lippincott Williams & Wilkins 1363-1950

Prevention of Postoperative Ileus

1. Early oral feeding. Malnutrition affects up to 30–40 % of patients undergoing major surgery. It is perhaps *the* most important potentially modifiable risk factor for morbidity and for infectious complications in particular. Nutritional interventions have proven effective to correct this risk constellation and thus to improve surgical outcomes. However, artificial nutrition entails its own risks and is costly. It is therefore appealing to instead maintain and support normal nutritional intake pre- and postoperatively [17–19].

   Traditionally, patients were kept nil per os (NPO) the day before surgery and until full return of bowel function, which was often nearly a week thereafter [20]. The rationale behind this dogma was (1) to empty the stomach and decrease the risk of aspiration at induction of anesthesia (see Chap. 4); (2) to keep the bowel clean for surgery after a full anterograde bowel preparation; and (3) to avoid mechanical stress to a fresh anastomosis in the postoperative phase. Nasogastric tubes were widely used to decompress the digestive tract aiming to avoid distension of the anastomosis and to prevent pulmonary complications [20]. Meanwhile evidence has accumulated testing these assumptions. In fact, prophylactic nasogastric tube placement delays return of normal gastrointestinal function and increases pulmonary complications, without having a positive impact on anastomotic leak or wound complications [21, 22]. Early oral food intake has been shown to be safe and is well tolerated by 80–90 % of the patients [21, 23]. It also enhances patients' comfort, decreases complications, and facilitates early discharge [21, 24]. It should be emphasized that early feeding is just one of multiple preventive measures that needs to be embedded within a comprehensive perioperative care pathway.

2. Fluid management. Optimal perioperative fluid administration has been a matter of debate over the last decade (see Chap. 11), and multiple randomized trials have been conducted to compare liberal versus more restricted fluid regimens. Traditionally, surgeons and anesthetists both opted for rather liberal administration of intravenous fluids in order to prevent hypotension and hypoperfusion of organs and of the anastomosis in particular. These are potentially devastating complications, but excess administration of fluids and especially of saline also has profound pathological effects which have been summarized recently [15]. These include pulmonary edema, metabolic acidosis, and acute kidney dysfunction. Furthermore, splanchnic edema was shown by a German group to jeopardize anastomotic safety [25]. Maintaining gut perfusion both with adequate oxygen and nutrient delivery but also perfusion pressure is important to maintain gut function. Studies showing extreme fluid restriction demonstrate poor return of gut function [26], likely due to hypoperfusion, whereas "liberal" fluid regimes can lead to mucosal edema and gut dysfunction.

Lobo and coworkers clearly demonstrated in a randomized study from 2002 that fluid overload had significant effect on intestinal recovery [27]. Gastric emptying times were nearly doubled in the "liberal" group, delaying first flatus and stool by 1 and 2.5 days respectively. Compared with the restricted group, patients in the liberal group suffered from more complications and stayed 3 days longer in hospital after colonic resection. The same group summarized the available evidence in 2012 and pointed out confusion that has resulted from the terms "liberal" and "restricted." Both inadequate hydration and fluid overload have negative impact on complications and length of stay [28]. The aim of perioperative fluid management should be to maintain normovolemia (fluid balance) while avoiding salt and water excess. They suggest that fluid administration between 1.75 and 2.5 l/day for patients without on-going losses is optimal and found significantly worse outcomes in patients gaining more than 3 kg in the postoperative period [27, 28].

Proper fluid administration is likely important in the optimal perioperative care for the prevention of ileus. Intravenous administration can be limited within enhanced recovery pathways and should aim for "zero fluid balance" with minimal weight gain only. A balanced crystalloid solution should be preferred over normal saline and can be combined in the early postoperative period with low dose vasopressors or boluses of colloids if needed [15, 28–30]. Issues remain with how to treat low blood pressure postoperatively, which may be exacerbated by the neuraxial blockade. Recent studies have shown that intraoperative and early postoperative hypotension is transient and can be counteracted by administration of low dose vasoactive agents without increased risks for renal insufficiency [31, 32]. However, the use of these agents is generally limited to patients in monitored settings.

Current recommendations for how to achieve "zero fluid balance" are somewhat vague in terms of concrete numbers but result in no or only minimal weight gain (in the region of 2 % or 1.5 kg for a 70 kg man) in the postoperative period. The value of "Goal-directed therapy" using a hemodynamic monitoring tool and a management protocol to optimize cardiac performance has not been demonstrated in non-high-risk colorectal surgery patients [29, 30, 33]. Modern perioperative pathways include a whole array of measures to maintain homeostasis and to avoid electrolyte and fluid imbalance in the perioperative phase (Fig. 12.2, Table 12.1); these include allowing clear fluids up to 2 h of surgery, no bowel preparation, carbohydrate loading, early oral intake, and early discontinuation of IV fluids.

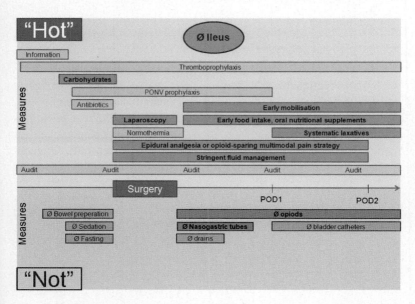

Fig. 12.2. Enhanced recovery pathway for prevention of postoperative ileus. Modern enhanced recovery strategies bundle a multitude of preventive measures ("Hot") in order to prevent postoperative ileus. Omission of counterproductive actions ("Not") complements the comprehensive perioperative pathway. Best results are obtained by complete application of the protocol. The most relevant measures for the prevention of ileus are highlighted (*bold*, *dark*) and refer directly to the pathophysiological risk factors displayed in Fig. 12.1.

3. Surgical considerations: The incidence and duration of POI appears to be commensurate with the degree of surgical trauma [2, 3, 11, 12]. It is therefore partially "in the surgeon's hands" to diminish the surgical aggression by gentle handling of tissues and minimizing manipulation of adjacent organs and reducing blood loss. Minimally invasive surgery assumes a particularly important role. In a retrospective analysis, postoperative nasogastric decompression was required in 17.8 % of patients after open colectomy while this was necessary in only 3.7 and 4.5 % of patients after straight laparoscopic and hand-assisted resections, respectively [12]. Small bowel obstruction/ileus appeared to be the most frequent cause for readmission after ileostomy closure [7]. A recent systematic review summarizes the available evidence of 4 RCTs and 645 patients of stapled versus hand-sewn anastomosis. One of the main

findings was a significantly reduced risk for small bowel obstruction in the stapled group attaining an OR of 0.54 (95 % CI 0.30–0.95).

4. Anesthetic considerations: The anesthetist also has a role in the prevention of POI. Perioperative anesthetic drugs, analgesic techniques, and the timing and quantity of intravenous fluid therapy can affect the incidence of ileus. The use of nitrous oxide has been shown to increase the risk of postoperative nausea and vomiting (PONV) and is best avoided [34]. Oxygen-enriched air combined with a short-acting anesthetic agent such as Desflurane or Sevoflurane is standard practice although the use of Total Intravenous Anesthesia (TIVA) using target-controlled propofol infusions may reduce the incidence of postoperative nausea and vomiting. Whilst PONV itself does not directly increase the incidence of ileus, it does prevent the patient taking oral opioid-sparing analgesics which results in the administration of higher doses of parenteral opiates (which are a risk factor for POI). Early enteral feeding also promotes gut function and enables the cessation of intravenous fluids which if continued are a risk factor for ileus. PONV is a significant problem after major surgery and prophylaxis using a 5HT3 antagonist such as Ondansetron should be routinely administered (see Chap. 8). The use of a single dose of dexamethasone as an antiemetic is also useful but there is still uncertainty in its routine use in cancer surgery.

5. Opioid-sparing analgesia: Thoracic epidural anesthesia (TEA) has traditionally been used in open surgery as the gold standard for postoperative analgesia as well as having other proven benefits of reducing the stress response (Level 1 evidence), reducing deep vein thrombosis (level 1 evidence), reducing pulmonary complications (level 1 evidence), reducing the incidence of ileus (level 1), and reducing negative nitrogen balance and fatigue (level 2 evidence). The sympathetic block achieved by TEA can improve gut motility by unopposed parasympathetic activity; however the arteriolar dilatation which also occurs can lead to hypotension and a reduction in gut perfusion so it is imperative to ensure the patient is normovolemic and maintains the blood pressure with vasopressor infusions rather than give lots of intravenous fluid which otherwise predisposes to ileus. This hypotensive side effect is minimized by using a thoracic epidural. The use of intravenous lidocaine as the main analgesic

component has been shown to be both efficacious and improve the return of gut function, and adding opioid slows down gastrointestinal recovery [35, 36].

Optimal postoperative pain management allows for early mobilization and food intake and provides comfort to the patients. Opioids can cause nausea and delay intestinal recovery and are therefore avoided as much as possible in enhanced recovery pathways [29, 30, 37]. Marret's large systematic review of 16 RCTs showed a 1.5 day (95 % CI 0.84–2.27) shortened duration of ileus by use of epidural analgesia. However, this analysis included only two small studies on laparoscopic resections which are nowadays the standard in most expert centers. Minimally invasive techniques alone have been successful in reducing POI [12, 13]. The value of epidural analgesia for laparoscopic resections was meanwhile addressed in several RCTs where epidural rather impeded recovery due to inherent side effects of the techniques, notably arterial hypotension [38, 39]. This is in line with a large-scale US review showing increased hospital stay and costs without obvious benefits for epidurals [40]. For laparoscopic colorectal resections, epidural analgesia should therefore not be routinely used but be reserved for specific indications only. Several promising alternatives have been proposed and tested in prospective trials [37, 39]. Large-scale studies have not been published though and individual pain strategies should be tailored for every patient from an array of diverse options to achieve multimodal, opioid-sparing analgesia (see Chap. 13).

6.   Other interventions. Routine use of laxative and prokinetic drugs are often included in enhanced recovery guidelines [29, 30]. In general terms, increased adherence to the recommended pathway interventions is associated with improved outcomes [41]. But the evidence supporting the benefits of laxatives such as magnesium oxide or bisacodyl is quite scarce. Some groups recommend the use of chewing gum and the morphine-antagonist alvimopan [1, 6]. Chewing gum stimulates the cephalic-vagal response and is a form of sham-feeding. A systematic review of 9 RCTs including 437 patients did not show a striking effect of chewing gum on bowel recovery [42]. However, some benefit was noted and the intervention is inexpensive, and well tolerated, without side effects.

Alvimopan is a peripheral mu opioid-receptor blocker. It is not currently available in Europe or Canada. The drug has been extensively tested in the USA mostly showing an acceleration of bowel recovery and prevention of postoperative ileus in the context of open colorectal surgery when opioid-based analgesia is used [1, 43]. The place of alvimopan within multimodal pathways remains yet to be determined, especially after laparoscopic resection.

Treating Postoperative Ileus

Treatment of POI is not standardized and varies widely according to institutional practice [9]. Nasogastric decompression and short-term bowel rest are basic measures to comfort the patient, avoid aspiration, and help to reduce abdominal pressure and intestinal edema. Timing for NG tube placement and algorithms for removal are not established. Imaging is not mandatory but in selected cases can be useful to exclude mechanical obstruction, or an abdominal or pelvic abscess that may be causing a secondary ileus. Administration of water-soluble contrast agent can be used as diagnostic tool and therapeutic attempt at the same time [44]. Several stimulants of the gastrointestinal tract have been tested but the clinical effects are rather disappointing [1, 43, 45–47]. No benefit has been shown for widely used prokinetics such as metoclopramide and erythromycin. Certainly *prevention is better than treatment* [16] and this can be best approached by application of multimodal enhanced recovery pathways (Fig. 12.2).

Take Home Messages

- Postoperative ileus is a transient cessation of normal bowel activity after surgery. It affects about 10–20 % of patients after colorectal resections.
- There is no uniformly accepted method of diagnosis. A pragmatic suggestion includes absence of stool and intolerance of solid food by postoperative day 4.
- Pathophysiology is multifactorial and includes intestinal edema, electrolyte imbalance, surgical manipulation, and medication use such as opioids.

- Several drugs have shown some effect and can be used as preventive therapy.
- Avoidance and treatment of risk factors can best be realized by application of multimodal pathways incorporating minimally invasive surgery, a stringent fluid regimen, modern opioid-sparing pain strategies, and early mobilization.

References

1. Barletta JF, Senagore AJ. Reducing the burden of postoperative ileus: evaluating and implementing an evidence-based strategy. World J Surg. 2014;38(8):1966–77.
2. Chapuis PH, Bokey L, Keshava A, Rickard MJ, Stewart P, Young CJ, et al. Risk factors for prolonged ileus after resection of colorectal cancer: an observational study of 2400 consecutive patients. Ann Surg. 2013;257(5):909–15.
3. Fesharakizadeh M, Taheri D, Dolatkhah S, Wexner SD. Postoperative ileus in colorectal surgery: is there any difference between laparoscopic and open surgery? Gastroenterol Rep. 2013;1(2):138–43.
4. Millan M, Biondo S, Fraccalvieri D, Frago R, Golda T, Kreisler E. Risk factors for prolonged postoperative ileus after colorectal cancer surgery. World J Surg. 2012;36(1):179–85.
5. Asgeirsson T, El-Badawi KI, Mahmood A, Barletta J, Luchtefeld M, Senagore AJ. Postoperative ileus: it costs more than you expect. J Am Coll Surg. 2010;210(2):228–31.
6. Keller D, Stein SL. Facilitating return of bowel function after colorectal surgery: alvimopan and gum chewing. Clin Colon Rectal Surg. 2013;26(3):186–90.
7. Keller DS, Swendseid B, Khan S, Delaney CP. Readmissions after ileostomy closure: cause to revisit a standardized enhanced recovery pathway? Am J Surg. 2014;208(4):650–5.
8. Huebner M, Hubner M, Cima RR, Larson DW. Timing of complications and length of stay after rectal cancer surgery. J Am Coll Surg. 2014;218(5):914–9.
9. Kehlet H, Williamson R, Buchler MW, Beart RW. A survey of perceptions and attitudes among European surgeons towards the clinical impact and management of postoperative ileus. Colorectal Dis. 2005;7(3):245–50.
10. Vather R, Trivedi S, Bissett I. Defining postoperative ileus: results of a systematic review and global survey. J Gastrointestinal Surg. 2013;17(5):962–72.
11. Baig MK, Wexner SD. Postoperative ileus: a review. Dis Colon Rectum. 2004;47(4):516–26.
12. Shussman N, Brown MR, Johnson MC, Da Silva G, Wexner SD, Weiss EG. Does nasogastric tube decompression get used less often with laparoscopic and hand-assisted compared with open colectomy? Surg Endosc. 2013;27(12):4564–8.
13. Abraham NS, Young JM, Solomon MJ. Meta-analysis of short-term outcomes after laparoscopic resection for colorectal cancer. Br J Surg. 2004;91(9):1111–24.

14. Sajid MS, Craciunas L, Baig MK, Sains P. Systematic review and meta-analysis of published, randomized, controlled trials comparing suture anastomosis to stapled anastomosis for ileostomy closure. Tech Coloproctol. 2013;17(6):631–9.

15. Lobo DN. Fluid, electrolytes and nutrition: physiological and clinical aspects. Proc Nutr Soc. 2004;63(3):453–66.

16. Holte K, Kehlet H. Postoperative ileus: a preventable event. Br J Surg. 2000; 87(11):1480–93.

17. Cerantola Y, Grass F, Cristaudi A, Demartines N, Schafer M, Hubner M. Perioperative nutrition in abdominal surgery: recommendations and reality. Gastroenterol Res Pract. 2011;2011:739347.

18. Cerantola Y, Hubner M, Grass F, Demartines N, Schafer M. Immunonutrition in gastrointestinal surgery. Br J Surg. 2011;98(1):37–48.

19. Weimann A, Braga M, Harsanyi L, Laviano A, Ljungqvist O, Soeters P, et al. ESPEN guidelines on enteral nutrition: surgery including organ transplantation. Clin Nutr. 2006;25(2):224–44.

20. Kehlet H, Buchler MW, Beart Jr RW, Billingham RP, Williamson R. Care after colonic operation—is it evidence-based? Results from a multinational survey in Europe and the United States. J Am Coll Surg. 2006;202(1):45–54.

21. Bauer VP. The evidence against prophylactic nasogastric intubation and oral restriction. Clin Colon Rectal Surg. 2013;26(3):182–5.

22. Wolff BG, Pembeton JH, van Heerden JA, Beart Jr RW, Nivatvongs S, Devine RM, et al. Elective colon and rectal surgery without nasogastric decompression. A prospective, randomized trial. Ann Surg. 1989;209(6):670–3. discussion 3–5.

23. Lassen K, Kjaeve J, Fetveit T, Trano G, Sigurdsson HK, Horn A, et al. Allowing normal food at will after major upper gastrointestinal surgery does not increase morbidity: a randomized multicenter trial. Ann Surg. 2008;247(5):721–9.

24. Greco M, Capretti G, Beretta L, Gemma M, Pecorelli N, Braga M. Enhanced recovery program in colorectal surgery: a meta-analysis of randomized controlled trials. World J Surg. 2014;38(6):1531–41.

25. Marjanovic G, Villain C, Juettner E, zur Hausen A, Hoeppner J, Hopt UT, et al. Impact of different crystalloid volume regimes on intestinal anastomotic stability. Ann surg. 2009;249(2):181–5.

26. MacKay G, Fearon K, McConnachie A, Serpell MG, Molloy RG, O'Dwyer PJ. Randomized clinical trial of the effect of postoperative intravenous fluid restriction on recovery after elective colorectal surgery. Br J Surg. 2006;93(12):1469–74.

27. Lobo DN, Bostock KA, Neal KR, Perkins AC, Rowlands BJ, Allison SP. Effect of salt and water balance on recovery of gastrointestinal function after elective colonic resection: a randomised controlled trial. Lancet. 2002;359(9320):1812–8.

28. Varadhan KK, Lobo DN. A meta-analysis of randomised controlled trials of intravenous fluid therapy in major elective open abdominal surgery: getting the balance right. Proc Nutr Soc. 2010;69(4):488–98.

29. Gustafsson UO, Scott MJ, Schwenk W, Demartines N, Roulin D, Francis N, et al. Guidelines for perioperative care in elective colonic surgery: Enhanced Recovery After Surgery (ERAS((R))) Society recommendations. World J Surg. 2013;37(2):259–84.

30. Nygren J, Thacker J, Carli F, Fearon KC, Norderval S, Lobo DN, et al. Guidelines for perioperative care in elective rectal/pelvic surgery: Enhanced Recovery After Surgery (ERAS(R)) Society recommendations. Clin Nutr. 2012;31(6):801–16.

31. Hubner M, Lovely JK, Huebner M, Slettedahl SW, Jacob AK, Larson DW. Intrathecal analgesia and restrictive perioperative fluid management within enhanced recovery pathway: hemodynamic implications. J Am Coll Surg. 2013;216(6):1124–34.

32. Hubner M, Schafer M, Demartines N, Muller S, Maurer K, Baulig W, et al. Impact of restrictive intravenous fluid replacement and combined epidural analgesia on perioperative volume balance and renal function within a fast track program. J Surg Res. 2012;173(1):68–74.

33. Pearse RM, Harrison DA, MacDonald N, Gillies MA, Blunt M, Ackland G, et al. Effect of a perioperative, cardiac output-guided hemodynamic therapy algorithm on outcomes following major gastrointestinal surgery: a randomized clinical trial and systematic review. JAMA. 2014;311(21):2181–90.

34. Fernandez-Guisasola J, Gomez-Arnau JI, Cabrera Y, del Valle SG. Association between nitrous oxide and the incidence of postoperative nausea and vomiting in adults: a systematic review and meta-analysis. Anaesthesia. 2010;65(4):379–87.

35. McCarthy GC, Megalla SA, Habib AS. Impact of intravenous lidocaine infusion on postoperative analgesia and recovery from surgery: a systematic review of randomized controlled trials. Drugs. 2010;70(9):1149–63.

36. Sun Y, Li T, Wang N, Yun Y, Gan TJ. Perioperative systemic lidocaine for postoperative analgesia and recovery after abdominal surgery: a meta-analysis of randomized controlled trials. Dis Colon Rectum. 2012;55(11):1183–94.

37. Joshi GP, Bonnet F, Kehlet H, Collaboration PROSPECT. Evidence-based postoperative pain management after laparoscopic colorectal surgery. Colorectal Dis. 2013; 15(2):146–55.

38. Hubner M, Blanc C, Roulin D, Winiker M, Gander S, Demartines N. Randomized clinical trial on epidural versus patient-controlled analgesia for laparoscopic colorectal surgery within an enhanced recovery pathway. Ann Surg. 2015;261(4):648–53.

39. Levy BF, Scott MJ, Fawcett W, Fry C, Rockall TA. Randomized clinical trial of epidural, spinal or patient-controlled analgesia for patients undergoing laparoscopic colorectal surgery. Br J Surg. 2011;98(8):1068–78.

40. Halabi WJ, Kang CY, Nguyen VQ, Carmichael JC, Mills S, Stamos MJ, et al. Epidural analgesia in laparoscopic colorectal surgery: a nationwide analysis of use and outcomes. JAMA Surg. 2014;149(2):130–6.

41. Gustafsson UO, Hausel J, Thorell A, Ljungqvist O, Soop M, Nygren J, et al. Adherence to the enhanced recovery after surgery protocol and outcomes after colorectal cancer surgery. Arch Surg. 2011;146(5):571–7.

42. Noble EJ, Harris R, Hosie KB, Thomas S, Lewis SJ. Gum chewing reduces postoperative ileus? a systematic review and meta-analysis. Int J Surg. 2009;7(2):100–5.

43. Story SK, Chamberlain RS. A comprehensive review of evidence-based strategies to prevent and treat postoperative ileus. Dig Surg. 2009;26(4):265–75.

44. Branco BC, Barmparas G, Schnuriger B, Inaba K, Chan LS, Demetriades D. Systematic review and meta-analysis of the diagnostic and therapeutic role of

146   M. Hübner et al.

water-soluble contrast agent in adhesive small bowel obstruction. Br J Surg. 2010;97(4):470–8.

45. Luckey A, Livingston E, Tache Y. Mechanisms and treatment of postoperative ileus. Arch Surg. 2003;138(2):206–14.

46. Stewart D, Waxman K. Management of postoperative ileus. Dis Mon. 2010; 56(4):204–14.

47. Traut U, Brugger L, Kunz R, Pauli-Magnus C, Haug K, Bucher HC, et al. Systemic prokinetic pharmacologic treatment for postoperative adynamic ileus following abdominal surgery in adults. Cochrane Database Syst Rev. 2008;1:CD004930.

13. Choosing Analgesia to Facilitate Recovery

Kyle G. Cologne and Gabriele Baldini

Perioperative Pain and Multimodal Analgesia

Pathophysiology of Surgical Pain

Surgical incision and manipulation of tissues lead to cell disruption and activation of humoral and cell-mediated inflammatory responses. A variety of intracellular chemical mediators including potassium, adenosine, prostanoids, bradykinin, nerve growth factors, cytokines, and chemokines are released from the injured tissues, then activate and sensitize peripheral nociceptors such as Aδ and c-fibers to mechanical stimuli (primary hyperalgesia). These pro-inflammatory substances together with the release of substance P and calcitonin gene-related peptide also sensitize silent Aδ nociceptors in the adjacent noninjured tissues (secondary hyperalgesia). Repeated and prolonged stimulation of peripheral nociceptors in the injured area and in the surrounding noninjured tissues leads to an increased firing of neurons at the level of the dorsal horn of the spinal cord, mediated by the activation of N-methyl-D-aspartate (NMDA) receptors (central sensitization). Clinically these pathophysiologic changes manifest with hyperalgesia, allodynia in the area of the surgical incision, with or without late persistent postsurgical pain. Descending sympathetic inhibitory pathways also take an important role at the level of the spinal cord by modulating transmission of noxious inputs. Acute surgical pain can therefore be somatic, visceral, or neuropathic depending on the type of surgery and on the surgical approach. Response to nociception contributes to activate and potentiate the stress response associated with surgery. These stress responses have consequences, such as activation of the hypothalamic-pituitary-adrenal

L.S. Feldman et al. (eds.), *The SAGES / ERAS®*
Society Manual of Enhanced Recovery Programs for
Gastrointestinal Surgery, DOI 10.1007/978-3-319-20364-5_13,
© Springer International Publishing Switzerland 2015

	CNS	CVS	Respiratory function	GI function	Genitourinary function	Musculo-skeletal function		Metabolism	Immune system
Mechanism	Activation of the HPA axis ↑ cortisol	↑ HR ↑SVR ↑MRO2	↓ movements of thoracic and abdominal respiratory muscles ↓ FRC, ↓VC ↓ MV Weak cough Retention of sputum and secretions	Spinal cord reflexes Sympathetic hyperactivity	Activation of the HPA axis ↑ cortisol ↑ ADH ↑ aldosterone ↑catecholamines ↑ angiotensine ↑ PG ↑ sympathetic stimulation	Splinting	↓ Fibrinolysis	Activation of the HPA axis ↑ cortisol ↑glucagone ↑catecholamines	Inflammation
Outcomes	Anxiety Insomnia Disorentation	Myocardial ischemia	Atelectasis Pneumonia Hypoxia	Paralytic ileus	↓ UO UR	VTE	VTE	IR	Wound infection Pneumonia Sepsis
Impaired ERAS elements	Mobilization Oral feeding	Mobilization	Mobilization	Mobilization Oral feeding	Mobilization Foley catheter	Mobilization	Mobilization	Mobilization Oral feeding	Mobilization Oral feeding

Delayed surgical recovery

Fig. 13.1. Impact of inadequate analgesia on organ functions and surgical recovery.

axis (HPA), sympathetic stimulation, and systemic release of pro-inflammatory cytokines, which are major determinants of post operative insulin resistance and other downstream effects, that if not attenuated potentially lead to multi-organ dysfunction (Fig. 13.1) [1].

These pathophysiologic mechanisms can be targeted as part of a multimodal approach to minimize the impact of these biologic processes. A key component of an enhanced recovery after surgery therefore includes analgesic strategies to prevent multi-organ dysfunction induced by unrelieved pain and ultimately facilitate enhanced recovery.

Preemptive Analgesia

Early studies suggested that analgesic treatments are more effective if administered before surgical incision (preemptive analgesia). However, the role of preemptive analgesic strategies such as preoperative administration of acetaminophen, Cox-2 inhibitors, NMDA antagonists, and/or gabapentinoids still remains unclear, especially in the context of an enhanced recovery program (ERP) for colorectal surgery [2].

Epidural analgesia appears the only preemptive analgesic technique that consistently reduces postoperative pain, analgesic consumption, and time to rescue analgesia [2].

Components of Multimodality Strategy

Several options exist for devising a multimodal pain management strategy as part of ERP. The main goal is to minimize or, when possible, avoid systemic opioids, which remain a cornerstone in the pharmacological treatment of acute postoperative pain. When considering the pathophysiology of pain origin, it seems intuitive that administering opioids alone is not sufficient to control the multiple aspects of postoperative pain. Systemic opioids block nociception by acting on central and peripheral G protein receptors (μ, δ, σ). They have undesirable side effects such as inducing ileus, by their action on μ receptors in the gastrointestinal tract, and nausea and vomiting, by their action on the chemoreceptor trigger zone (CTZ). These side effects significantly impair the recovery of patients undergoing gastrointestinal surgery, as they delay the return of gastrointestinal function and prevent early feeding. It is therefore paramount to use alternative forms of pain control to spare opioids.

There are a variety of non-opioid medications that are included in a multimodal approach to enhance analgesia, and each targets specific pathophysiologic mechanisms. Nonsteroidal anti-inflammatory drugs (NSAIDs), cyclooxygenases-2 inhibitors (COX-2), and systemic steroids attenuate the inflammatory component of surgical pain. Systemic local anesthetics, including lidocaine, have also shown to have analgesic properties by reducing the excessive release of inflammatory mediators (Il-6, Il-1β, and IL-1RA) and by attenuating the upregulation of inflammatory cells. Anti-NMDA agents such as ketamine, dextromethorphan, and magnesium attenuate central sensitization by reducing the neuron firing in the dorsal horn of the spinal cord. Gabapentinoids by binding the alpha-2-delta-1 subunit of the voltage-gated calcium channel in the central nervous system reduce the release of important excitatory neurotransmitters participating in nociception, especially in the development of neuropathic pain. Alpha-2 agonist such as clonidine and dexmedetomidine, by activating presynaptic and postsynaptic α2 receptors of the spinal cord, modulates the transmission of noxious stimuli. Local anesthetics block neural transmission by antagonizing sodium channels and therefore preventing the transmission of noxious stimuli from the periphery to the central nervous system [3]. Finally, peripheral μ-receptor antagonists such as alvimopan can be used in conjunction with narcotic medications to limit the gastrointestinal side effects. Each of these will be discussed in more detail below.

Thoracic Epidural Analgesia (TEA)

TEA (T6–T11) is one method to provide optimal analgesia and decrease narcotic requirements following gastrointestinal surgery, particularly if done with an open approach. Continuous epidural analgesia (CEA) or patient-controlled epidural analgesia (PCEA) for 48–72 h provides superior static and dynamic analgesia compared to systemic opioids [4]. Combining local anesthetic with lipophilic opioids [5, 6] and/or epidural epinephrine (2 μg/ml) [7, 8] improves the quality of analgesia. Epidural solution containing epidural morphine (0.02 mg/ml) increases segmental analgesia spread and could be recommended for long midline incisions [9]. Epidural catheters should be inserted in the mid-thoracic region (T6–T8) in patients undergoing upper gastrointestinal surgery and in the low-thoracic region (T9–T11) in patients undergoing lower gastrointestinal surgery. Supplement analgesia is required in patients undergoing abdominal perianal resection, in whom perianal pain (S1–S3 dermatomes) is not controlled by TEA.

Besides its analgesic properties TEA also plays a pivotal role in attenuating the stress response induced by surgery and facilitating early surgical recovery. Through the inhibition of hypothalamus-hypophysis-adrenal axis and thoracic sympathetic fibers, TEA decreases insulin resistance and protein breakdown [10, 11], and furthermore decreases the need for anesthetic agents, opioids, and muscle relaxants [10]. Finally, inhibition of thoracic sympathetic fibers and avoidance of systemic opioids facilitate the recovery of bowel function [12]. Despite these favorable effects, TEA is associated with higher risk of hypotension, pruritus, and lower limb motor weakness. PCEA provides similar analgesia but with less side effects than CEA [13]. Arterial hypotension caused by TEA can be particularly dangerous, especially when primary gastrointestinal anastomoses are created [14]. Interestingly, treating hypotension induced by TEA with intravenous fluids does not restore splanchnic blood flow. On the contrary, administration of small doses of vasopressors has been shown to be safe [15] and increase splanchnic circulation [16]. Orthostatic hypotension associated with TEA does not impair the ability to ambulate [17]. Although TEA impairs bladder functions, urinary catheters can be safely removed the day after the surgery, reducing the incidence of urinary tract infections and without increasing the risk of bladder recatheterization [18]. More rare but more serious complications such as post-dural puncture headache, epidural hematoma, and abscess can also occur. Main contraindications include patient refusal, coagulopathy, thrombocytopenia or platelets dysfunction, and systemic infections. In patients receiving antithrombotic or thrombolytic agents, insertion and removal of epidural catheters should be timed according to international guidelines (Table 13.1) [19, 20].

The benefits of TEA have not been observed after laparoscopic gastrointestinal surgery, where alternative techniques have provided satisfactory analgesia. In fact, two recent RCTs found that in colorectal patients undergoing laparoscopic surgery in a context of an enhanced recovery program, TEA delays hospital discharge [21] and prolongs medical recovery [22] compared with patients receiving intrathecal analgesia or systemic opioids. The use of TEA may remain valuable in patients at high risk of postoperative respiratory complications [23], in those with high probability of conversion to laparotomy, and in patients with an 8–10 cm Pfannenstiel-like incision after laparoscopic rectal surgery in whom pain is better controlled with TEA in the first 24 h [24].

When one considers that up to 1/3 of catheters can dislodge, block, leak [25], or not be correctly inserted [26], these modalities are best used as part of a team approach with highly specialized and experienced providers, including specialized nurses and acute pain service, where the success rates can be much higher, and epidurals not providing adequate analgesia quickly troubleshot. One must assess whether such a program exists at a particular institution before deciding on the use of routine thoracic epidurals. Given these largely equivocal results, and potential difficulties in postoperative management, the authors do not use TEA as a routine part of our practice following laparoscopic gastrointestinal surgery, unlike for open abdominal surgery.

Spinal Analgesia

Single-shot spinal analgesia with local anesthetic and intrathecal opioids is a valuable analgesic technique in patients undergoing laparoscopic procedures in whom wound pain relief requirements are more modest, as its analgesic effect is limited to the first postoperative 24 h. Although systemic opioid requirements are significantly decreased [27] compared with patients receiving systemic opioids, the risk of pruritus

Table 13.1. Perioperative use of antithrombotic agents and neuroaxial blockade.

	Time before puncture/ catheter manipulation or removal	Time after puncture/ catheter manipulation or removal	Comments
UFH (for prophylaxis) (sc)	4–6 h	1 h	Platelet count should be checked after 4 days of treatment (risk of HIT)
UFH (for treatment) (iv)	4–6 h	1 h	Platelet count should be checked after 4 days of treatment (risk of HIT)
LMWH (for prophylaxis)	12 h	2 h	Platelet count should be checked after 4 days of treatment (risk of HIT)
Low molecular weight heparin (for treatment)	24 h	2 h	Half-life of LMWH can be significantly prolonged in patients with impaired kidney function
Fondaparinux (for prophylaxis)	36–42 h	6–12 h	Platelet count should be checked after 4 days of treatment (risk of HIT)
Rivaroxaban	22–26 h	4–6 h	ASRA guidelines suggests avoidance of indwelling epidural catheters
Apixaban	26–30 h	4–6 h	
Dabigatran	Contraindicated according to the manufacture	6 h	
Warfarin	4 days (INR must be normal)	After catheter removal	If warfarin is used as thromboprophylaxis, catheter should be removed before INR > 1.5
Clopidogrel	7 days	After catheter removal	

(continued)

Table 13.1. (continued)

	Time before puncture/ catheter manipulation or removal	Time after puncture/ catheter manipulation or removal	Comments
Ticlopidine	10 days	After catheter removal	
Prasugrel	7–10 days	6 h after catheter removal	
Ticagrelor	5 days	6 h after catheter removal	
Glycoprotein IIb/IIIa inhibitors, Abciximab[a]	48 h[a]	–	Only to remove epidural catheter after Abciximab has been discontinued. Neuroaxial blockade is contraindicated in patients receiving Abciximab
ASA/ dipyridamole	None	None	
NSAIDs/COX-2 inhibitors	None	None	

Data from ASRA [19] and ESRA [20] recommendations

HIT heparin induced thrombocytopenia, *aPTT* activated partial thromboplastin time, *iv* intravenous, *UH* unfractionated heparin, *LMWH* low molecular weight heparin

[a]Only for Abciximab, as other glycoprotein IIb/IIIa inhibitors have different plasma half-life and different duration of action

(OR=3.85, 95 % CI 2.40–6.15) and respiratory depression (although rare) (OR=2.35, 95 % CI=1.00–5.51) is higher. Postoperative urinary retention is also more frequent after intrathecal morphine [28]. Similarly, arterial hypotension is higher and persists in the early postoperative period [29]. Contraindications are similar to those of TEA, but the risk of severe complications associated with this technique is significantly lower [30].

Behind providing excellent analgesia [27], spinal analgesia with intrathecal morphine or diamorphine seems an appealing technique to shorten hospital stay in patients undergoing laparoscopic colorectal surgery with an ERP protocol [21, 31].

Intravenous Lidocaine (IVL) Infusion

In view of its antinociceptive and anti-inflammatory properties, systemic administration of IVL as adjuvant to systemic opioids has been shown to improve postoperative analgesia, reduce opioid consumption, accelerate gastrointestinal function [32], and speed surgical recovery [33, 34]. Similar benefits have been observed after laparoscopic abdominal surgeries when compared to systemic opioids [35], but not when compared to TEA [24], and especially in absence of an ERP [24, 36]. A loading dose of 1.5 mg/kg (ideal body weight) should be initiated 30 min before or at the induction of anesthesia and continued until the end of surgery or in the recovery room (2 mg/kg/h-IBW). The exact duration of the infusion providing optimal analgesia and facilitating also recovery remains unknown. Systemic toxicity is rare, and continuous cardiovascular monitoring is required, limiting its use to the operating rooms or to high-dependency intensive care units [34].

Continuous Wound Infusion (CWI) of Local Anesthetic

CWI of local anesthetic after open abdominal surgery has been shown to improve postoperative analgesia and reduce opioid consumption [37, 38]; however the effect on the recovery of bowel function is unclear [37, 39]. Two recent RCTs have compared the analgesic efficacy of CWI of local anesthetic with TEA but the results are contrasting [40, 41]. Although preperitoneal multihole catheters have consistently provided satisfactory analgesia, and subfascial catheters have provided better results than suprafascial catheters [42], the anatomical location associated with optimal recovery remains undetermined [38, 42]. A recent feasibility study has compared the analgesic efficacy of CWI of local anesthetic with epidural analgesia after laparoscopic abdominal surgery. Pain intensity was similar among patients receiving epidural and CWI of local anesthetic [43]. Continuous infusion of ropivacaine 0.2 % (10 ml/h) for 48–72 h has been used in the majority of the studies. Other amide local anesthetics have also been used. Systemic opioids are still required to control visceral pain. Unfortunately, they do have a tendency to dislodge, so nursing and patient education are key to proper use.

Abdominal Trunk Blocks: Transversus-Abdominis Plane (TAP) Block and Rectus Sheath Block

Abdominal trunk blocks such as transversus-abdominis plane (TAP) block and rectus sheath block have been used to control surgical somatic pain originating from the abdominal wall. Significant reduction of pain intensity and opioid consumption after ultrasound-guided single-shot TAP blocks has been observed in the first 24 h after surgery [44–47]. TAP blocks can also be performed by surgeons from the peritoneal cavity before closing the abdominal wall [48, 49] or using laparoscopic guidance [50–52]. Few studies have reported a reduction of some of the opioid side effects such as nausea and vomiting [46] or sedation [48, 53], but these results have not been consistently reproduced [44]. Others have infused local anesthetic through multihole catheters inserted in the transversus-abdominis plane to improve and prolong opioid-based postoperative analgesia up to 48–72 h after abdominal surgery [54–56]. Niraj et al. found that epidural analgesia did not provide better visual analogue scores during coughing than intermittent local anesthetic boluses through bilateral subcostal TAP catheters in the first 72 h after upper abdominal surgery [57]. However the epidural failure rate was high (22 %) and almost half of the TAP catheters had to be replaced in the postoperative period.

Similar benefits have been reported in abdominal laparoscopic procedures [45, 47, 50–52] and in the context of ERPs [50–52, 58]. Despite facilitating hospital discharge [52], bilateral single-shot TAP blocks do not seem to reduce hospital stay after laparoscopic colorectal surgery [58]. A recent RCT has shown that the analgesic efficacy of four-quadrant TAP blocks in adjunct to bilateral posterior continuous TAP blocks was not inferior to TEA after laparoscopic colorectal surgery [59].

A minimal volume of 15 ml of long-acting local anesthetic injected under ultrasound guidance or at the level of the triangle of Petit is required to achieve satisfactory analgesia with single-shot TAP block [60]. A recent meta-analysis showed that preoperative TAP blocks provide greater analgesia than postoperative TAP blocks [50]. Ropivacaine 0.2 % (8–10 ml/h) can be infused for 48–72 h through a multihole catheter. A bilateral infusion (8–10 ml/h each side) is required with a midline incision. A second injection may be performed just beneath the rib cage (subcostal approach). It is unclear what, if any, effect TAP blocks have on length of stay [52]. Early evidence is encouraging regarding the use of these techniques. A meta-analysis of nine studies including 413 patients showed significant reduction in morphine requirements [46] and a potential for reduced length of stay [52].

Rectus sheath blocks have also been used but the evidence is limited in patients undergoing gastrointestinal surgery. Rectus sheath blocks (15–20 ml of long-acting local anesthetic, bilaterally) are particularly useful to control pain originating from midline incisions, as they provide sensory block for the whole midline of the abdomen. Like TAP blocks they can be inserted under ultrasound guidance or without, using a loss of resistance as verification of the correct plane, although surgeons can also insert them under direct vision. Very commonly a catheter is left in situ and local anesthetic can be administered either by bolus dosing or via continuous infusion, as the analgesic effect is shorter than TAP blocks.

Intraperitoneal Local Anesthetic (IPLA)

IPLA has been shown to improve postoperative analgesia but not reduce opioid consumption after laparoscopic abdominal procedures [61]. The type of procedure seems to influence this as beneficial effects are seen after upper GI procedures [62] but not after colorectal surgery [63]. This effect might be the result of intraperitoneal deafferentation as indicated by low cortisol and cytokine levels after IPLA instillation [64].

Nonsteroidal Anti-inflammatory Drugs (NSAIDs)

NSAIDs and COX-2 inhibitors have been shown to improve postoperative analgesia and reduce opioid consumption and some of their side effects by 30 % [65]. There have been recent concerns about the risk of anastomotic leakage and the use of NSAIDs or COX-2 inhibitors after colorectal surgeries based on experimental, retrospective, and case series studies [66]. Large RCTs are needed to confirm these results. Although not statistically significant, a trend towards higher risk of developing anastomotic leakage after bowel surgery was reported in a recent meta-analysis of six RCTs (480 patients) of patients receiving at least one dose of NSAIDs or COX-2 inhibitors within 48 h of surgery (Peto OR=2.16 [0.85–5.53]) [67]. Proper use of these and other oral medications for the multimodal treatment of postoperative pain requires routine (rather than PRN) use. This requires education of the entire treatment team to prevent noncompliance. NSAIDs should be stopped or avoided in the setting of renal dysfunction [68]. An additional concern with NSAIDs is the theoretical increased risk of bleeding. The largest published experience comes from the tonsillectomy literature, where large series suggest that the avoidance of these medications is equivocal at best for avoiding postoperative bleeding episodes [69–71].

Acetaminophen

Acetaminophen improves postoperative analgesia, and has an opioid sparing effect, but does not reduce opioids side effects [72–75]. An IV formulation (propacetamol) is also available and can be used in patients who are unable to tolerate oral medication. These have been shown to significantly decrease PCA-morphine consumption [76]. The maximum dose is 1 g four times per day. There is some evidence to support a 2 g loading dose, with better pain relief with no increase in toxicity. Use of acetaminophen in conjunction with an NSAID has been shown to be superior to either alone [77]. Acetaminophen dose should be reduced (<2 g/day) in patients with pre-existing liver disease [78, 79].

Gabapentanoids and Other Analgesics

Perioperative intravenous ketamine and gabapentinoids have also shown opioid sparing properties [80, 81], but they have been poorly studied in patients undergoing gastrointestinal surgery and in the context of an ERP. The risk of side effects such as dizziness and sedation potentially limiting early ambulation should be considered. An opioid-free multimodal analgesic strategy based mainly on analgesic adjuvants would be appealing but more studies are warranted to establish the feasibility, efficacy, and safety of such analgesic approaches [82]. The effect of gabapentanoids seems to be most beneficial when given pre-procedurally, and work through modulation of neuropathic pain [83–85]. There is some evidence that narcotic requirements are decreased [85, 86] and progression to chronic pain states seems to be diminished [87, 88].

Peripherally Acting Opioid Receptor Antagonist (Alvimopan)

The use of a peripherally acting μ-opioid receptor antagonist (e.g., alvimopan) can be used to counteract the intestinal (ileus) side effects of opioid medications. It does not cross the blood brain barrier so it does not alter the therapeutic effects of these medications [89]. Use of this receptor blocker has been shown to enhance the return of bowel function and hospital discharge by 11–26 h [90, 91]. The effect appears to be much more profound in open surgical patients than in laparoscopic procedures [92, 93]. One approach is to give a single dose of alvimopan preoperatively to block the effects of opioid administration intraoperatively for all patients, but only continue it postoperatively in open colectomy cases. Some hospitals have a restriction that a preoperative dose must be given, and this allows continued administration postoperatively in the event of conversion from a laparoscopic to an open procedure.

Common Comorbid Conditions and Alterations in Medication Regimen

Some potential problems occur which may require modification of ERP medication regimens. Intolerance of feeds and development of an ileus may require use of IV formulations, which are available with acetaminophen (propacetamol) and NSAIDS (ketorolac). Patients with renal failure (pre-existing or acute) and asthma should not receive NSAIDS. Patients with inflammatory bowel disease may have exacerbations in the severity of their disease with NSAIDS. Similarly, acetaminophen doses should be reduced in patients with liver failure [78].

Conclusions

A Multimodal analgesic approach including regional analgesia techniques when indicated, regular non-opioid analgesics, and breakthrough opioids is recommended to provide optimal analgesia, minimize opioids side effects, and facilitate surgical recovery.

Take Home Messages

- Enhanced recovery after surgery pathways includes a multimodal pain relief strategy. Common components include NSAIDS, acetaminophen, gabapentanoids, local and regional anesthesia blocks, and epidural anesthesia adjuncts [94–96].
- Opioid analgesics should be used with a μ receptor antagonist to minimize the effect on ileus, which has a more profound effect when an open approach is used [91, 92].
- Effective use of a multimodal pain relief strategy requires engagement of all team members, including surgery, anesthesia, nursing, pharmacy, and administrative components [25].

References

1. Kehlet H. Manipulation of the metabolic response in clinical practice. World J Surg. 2000;24(6):690–5.
2. Ong CK, Lirk P, Seymour RA, et al. The efficacy of preemptive analgesia for acute postoperative pain management: a meta-analysis. Anesth Analg. 2005;100(3):757–73. table of contents.
3. Buvanendran A, Kroin JS. Useful adjuvants for postoperative pain management. Best Pract Res Clin Anaesthesiol. 2007;21(1):31–49.
4. Werawatganon T, Charuluxanun S. Patient controlled intravenous opioid analgesia versus continuous epidural analgesia for pain after intra-abdominal surgery. Cochrane Database Syst Rev 2005;(1):CD004088.
5. Finucane BT, Ganapathy S, Carli F, et al. Prolonged epidural infusions of ropivacaine (2 mg/mL) after colonic surgery: the impact of adding fentanyl. Anesth Analg. 2001; 92(5):1276–85.
6. Block BM, Liu SS, Rowlingson AJ, et al. Efficacy of postoperative epidural analgesia: a meta-analysis. JAMA. 2003;290(18):2455–63.
7. Niemi G, Breivik H. The minimally effective concentration of adrenaline in a low-concentration thoracic epidural analgesic infusion of bupivacaine, fentanyl and adrenaline after major surgery. A randomized, double-blind, dose-finding study. Acta Anaesthesiol Scand. 2003;47(4):439–50.
8. Sakaguchi Y, Sakura S, Shinzawa M, et al. Does adrenaline improve epidural bupivacaine and fentanyl analgesia after abdominal surgery? Anaesth Intensive Care. 2000;28(5):522–6.
9. Rawal N, Allvin R. Epidural and intrathecal opioids for postoperative pain management in Europe—a 17-nation questionnaire study of selected hospitals. Euro Pain Study Group on Acute Pain. Acta Anaesthesiol Scand. 1996;40(9):1119–26.
10. Carli F, Kehlet H, Baldini G, et al. Evidence basis for regional anesthesia in multidisciplinary fast-track surgical care pathways. Reg Anesth Pain Med. 2011;36(1):63–72.

11. Uchida I, Asoh T, Shirasaka C, et al. Effect of epidural analgesia on postoperative insulin resistance as evaluated by insulin clamp technique. Br J Surg. 1988; 75(6):557–62.

12. Jorgensen H, Wetterslev J, Moiniche S, et al. Epidural local anaesthetics versus opioid-based analgesic regimens on postoperative gastrointestinal paralysis, PONV and pain after abdominal surgery. Cochrane Database Syst Rev 2000;(4):CD001893.

13. Wu CL, Cohen SR, Richman JM, et al. Efficacy of postoperative patient-controlled and continuous infusion epidural analgesia versus intravenous patient-controlled analgesia with opioids: a meta-analysis. Anesthesiology. 2005;103(5):1079–88. quiz 1109–10.

14. Rigg JR, Jamrozik K, Myles PS, et al. Epidural anaesthesia and analgesia and outcome of major surgery: a randomised trial. Lancet. 2002;359(9314):1276–82.

15. Hiltebrand LB, Koepfli E, Kimberger O, et al. Hypotension during fluid-restricted abdominal surgery: effects of norepinephrine treatment on regional and microcirculatory blood flow in the intestinal tract. Anesthesiology. 2011;114(3):557–64.

16. Gould TH, Grace K, Thorne G, et al. Effect of thoracic epidural anaesthesia on colonic blood flow. Br J Anaesth. 2002;89(3):446–51.

17. Gramigni E, Bracco D, Carli F. Epidural analgesia and postoperative orthostatic haemodynamic changes. Eur J Anaesthesiol. 2013;30(7):398–404.

18. Zaouter C, Kaneva P, Carli F. Less urinary tract infection by earlier removal of bladder catheter in surgical patients receiving thoracic epidural analgesia. Reg Anesth Pain Med. 2009;34(6):542–8.

19. Horlocker TT, Wedel DJ, Rowlingson JC, et al. Regional anesthesia in the patient receiving antithrombotic or thrombolytic therapy: American Society of Regional Anesthesia and Pain Medicine Evidence-Based Guidelines (Third Edition). Reg Anesth Pain Med. 2010;35(1):64–101.

20. Gogarten W, Vandermeulen E, Van Aken H, et al. Regional anaesthesia and antithrombotic agents: recommendations of the European Society of Anaesthesiology. Eur J Anaesthesiol. 2010;27(12):999–1015.

21. Levy BF, Scott MJ, Fawcett W, et al. Randomized clinical trial of epidural, spinal or patient-controlled analgesia for patients undergoing laparoscopic colorectal surgery. Br J Surg. 2011;98(8):1068–78.

22. Halabi WJ, Kang CY, Nguyen VQ, et al. Epidural analgesia in laparoscopic colorectal surgery: a nationwide analysis of use and outcomes. JAMA Surg. 2014;149(2): 130–6.

23. Popping DM, Elia N, Marret E, et al. Protective effects of epidural analgesia on pulmonary complications after abdominal and thoracic surgery: a meta-analysis. Arch Surg. 2008;143(10):990–9. discussion 1000.

24. Wongyingsinn M, Baldini G, Charlebois P, et al. Intravenous lidocaine versus thoracic epidural analgesia: a randomized controlled trial in patients undergoing laparoscopic colorectal surgery using an enhanced recovery program. Reg Anesth Pain Med. 2011;36(3):241–8.

25. Saclarides TJ. Current choices — good or bad — for the proactive management of postoperative ileus: a surgeon's view. J Perianesth Nurs. 2006;21(2A Suppl):S7–15.

26. Hermanides J, Hollmann MW, Stevens MF, et al. Failed epidural: causes and management. Br J Anaesth. 2012;109(2):144–54.

27. Wongyingsinn M, Baldini G, Stein B, et al. Spinal analgesia for laparoscopic colonic resection using an enhanced recovery after surgery programme: better analgesia, but no benefits on postoperative recovery: a randomized controlled trial. Br J Anaesth. 2012;108(5):850–6.

28. Meylan N, Elia N, Lysakowski C, et al. Benefit and risk of intrathecal morphine without local anaesthetic in patients undergoing major surgery: meta-analysis of randomized trials. Br J Anaesth. 2009;102(2):156–67.

29. Hubner M, Lovely JK, Huebner M, et al. Intrathecal analgesia and restrictive perioperative fluid management within enhanced recovery pathway: hemodynamic implications. J Am Coll Surg. 2013;216(6):1124–34.

30. 3rd National Audit Project of the Royal College of Anaesthetists (NAP3): major complications of central neuraxial block.

31. Levy BF, Scott MJ, Fawcett WJ, et al. 23-Hour-stay laparoscopic colectomy. Dis Colon Rectum. 2009;52(7):1239–43.

32. Sridhar P, Sistla SC, Ali SM, et al. Effect of intravenous lignocaine on perioperative stress response and post-surgical ileus in elective open abdominal surgeries: a double-blind randomized controlled trial. ANZ J Surg. 2014. doi:10.1111/ans.12783.

33. Marret E, Rolin M, Beaussier M, et al. Meta-analysis of intravenous lidocaine and postoperative recovery after abdominal surgery. Br J Surg. 2008;95(11):1331–8.

34. Vigneault L, Turgeon AF, Cote D, et al. Perioperative intravenous lidocaine infusion for postoperative pain control: a meta-analysis of randomized controlled trials. Can J Anaesth. 2011;58(1):22–37.

35. McCarthy GC, Megalla SA, Habib AS. Impact of intravenous lidocaine infusion on postoperative analgesia and recovery from surgery: a systematic review of randomized controlled trials. Drugs. 2010;70(9):1149–63.

36. Kaba A, Laurent SR, Detroz BJ, et al. Intravenous lidocaine infusion facilitates acute rehabilitation after laparoscopic colectomy. Anesthesiology. 2007;106(1):11–8. discussion 15–6.

37. Karthikesalingam A, Walsh SR, Markar SR, et al. Continuous wound infusion of local anaesthetic agents following colorectal surgery: systematic review and meta-analysis. World J Gastroenterol. 2008;14(34):5301–5.

38. Liu SS, Richman JM, Thirlby RC, et al. Efficacy of continuous wound catheters delivering local anesthetic for postoperative analgesia: a quantitative and qualitative systematic review of randomized controlled trials. J Am Coll Surg. 2006;203(6):914–32.

39. Beaussier M, El'Ayoubi H, Schiffer E, et al. Continuous preperitoneal infusion of ropivacaine provides effective analgesia and accelerates recovery after colorectal surgery: a randomized, double-blind, placebo-controlled study. Anesthesiology. 2007;107(3):461–8.

40. Bertoglio S, Fabiani F, Negri PD, et al. The postoperative analgesic efficacy of preperitoneal continuous wound infusion compared to epidural continuous infusion with local anesthetics after colorectal cancer surgery: a randomized controlled multicenter study. Anesth Analg. 2012;115(6):1442–50.

41. Jouve P, Bazin JE, Petit A, et al. Epidural versus continuous preperitoneal analgesia during fast-track open colorectal surgery: a randomized controlled trial. Anesthesiology. 2013;118(3):622–30.
42. Ventham NT, O'Neill S, Johns N, et al. Evaluation of novel local anesthetic wound infiltration techniques for postoperative pain following colorectal resection surgery: a meta-analysis. Dis Colon Rectum. 2014;57(2):237–50.
43. Boulind CE, Ewings P, Bulley SH, et al. Feasibility study of analgesia via epidural versus continuous wound infusion after laparoscopic colorectal resection. Br J Surg. 2013;100(3):395–402.
44. Charlton S, Cyna AM, Middleton P, et al. Perioperative transversus abdominis plane (TAP) blocks for analgesia after abdominal surgery. Cochrane Database Syst Rev 2010;(12):CD007705.
45. Siddiqui MR, Sajid MS, Uncles DR, et al. A meta-analysis on the clinical effectiveness of transversus abdominis plane block. J Clin Anesth. 2011;23(1):7–14.
46. Johns N, O'Neill S, Ventham NT, et al. Clinical effectiveness of transversus abdominis plane (TAP) block in abdominal surgery: a systematic review and meta-analysis. Colorectal Dis. 2012;14(10):e635–42.
47. De Oliveira Jr GS, Castro-Alves LJ, Nader A, et al. Transversus abdominis plane block to ameliorate postoperative pain outcomes after laparoscopic surgery: a meta-analysis of randomized controlled trials. Anesth Analg. 2014;118(2):454–63.
48. Bharti N, Kumar P, Bala I, et al. The efficacy of a novel approach to transversus abdominis plane block for postoperative analgesia after colorectal surgery. Anesth Analg. 2011;112(6):1504–8.
49. Owen DJ, Harrod I, Ford J, et al. The surgical transversus abdominis plane block—a novel approach for performing an established technique. BJOG. 2011;118(1):24–7.
50. Favuzza J, Delaney CP. Outcomes of discharge after elective laparoscopic colorectal surgery with transversus abdominis plane blocks and enhanced recovery pathway. J Am Coll Surg. 2013;217(3):503–6.
51. Keller DS, Stulberg JJ, Lawrence JK, et al. Process control to measure process improvement in colorectal surgery: modifications to an established enhanced recovery pathway. Dis Colon Rectum. 2014;57(2):194–200.
52. Favuzza J, Brady K, Delaney CP. Transversus abdominis plane blocks and enhanced recovery pathways: making the 23-h hospital stay a realistic goal after laparoscopic colorectal surgery. Surg Endosc. 2013;27(7):2481–6.
53. Brady RR, Ventham NT, Roberts DM, et al. Open transversus abdominis plane block and analgesic requirements in patients following right hemicolectomy. Ann R Coll Surg Engl. 2012;94(5):327–30.
54. Allcock E, Spencer E, Frazer R, et al. Continuous transversus abdominis plane (TAP) block catheters in a combat surgical environment. Pain Med. 2010;11(9):1426–9.
55. Kadam RV, Field JB. Ultrasound-guided continuous transverse abdominis plane block for abdominal surgery. J Anaesthesiol Clin Pharmacol. 2011;27(3):333–6.
56. Bjerregaard N, Nikolajsen L, Bendtsen TF, et al. Transversus abdominis plane catheter bolus analgesia after major abdominal surgery. Anesthesiol Res Pract. 2012;2012:596536.

57. Niraj G, Kelkar A, Jeyapalan I, et al. Comparison of analgesic efficacy of subcostal transversus abdominis plane blocks with epidural analgesia following upper abdominal surgery. Anaesthesia. 2011;66(6):465–71.

58. Walter CJ, Maxwell-Armstrong C, Pinkney TD, et al. A randomised controlled trial of the efficacy of ultrasound-guided transversus abdominis plane (TAP) block in laparoscopic colorectal surgery. Surg Endosc. 2013;27(7):2366–72.

59. Niraj G, Kelkar A, Hart E, et al. Comparison of analgesic efficacy of four-quadrant transversus abdominis plane (TAP) block and continuous posterior TAP analgesia with epidural analgesia in patients undergoing laparoscopic colorectal surgery: an open-label, randomised, non-inferiority trial. Anaesthesia. 2014;69(4):348–55.

60. Abdallah FW, Chan VW, Brull R. Transversus abdominis plane block: a systematic review. Reg Anesth Pain Med. 2012;37(2):193–209.

61. Kahokehr A, Sammour T, Soop M, et al. Intraperitoneal local anaesthetic in abdominal surgery—a systematic review. ANZ J Surg. 2011;81(4):237–45.

62. Kahokehr A, Sammour T, Srinivasa S, et al. Systematic review and meta-analysis of intraperitoneal local anaesthetic for pain reduction after laparoscopic gastric procedures. Br J Surg. 2011;98(1):29–36.

63. Moiniche S, Jorgensen H, Wetterslev J, et al. Local anesthetic infiltration for postoperative pain relief after laparoscopy: a qualitative and quantitative systematic review of intraperitoneal, port-site infiltration and mesosalpinx block. Anesth Analg. 2000;90(4):899–912.

64. Kahokehr A, Sammour T, Shoshtari KZ, et al. Intraperitoneal local anesthetic improves recovery after colon resection: a double-blinded randomized controlled trial. Ann Surg. 2011;254(1):28–38.

65. Marret E, Kurdi O, Zufferey P, et al. Effects of nonsteroidal antiinflammatory drugs on patient-controlled analgesia morphine side effects: meta-analysis of randomized controlled trials. Anesthesiology. 2005;102(6):1249–60.

66. Klein M. Postoperative non-steroidal anti-inflammatory drugs and colorectal anastomotic leakage. NSAIDs and anastomotic leakage. Dan Med J. 2012;59(3):B4420.

67. Burton TP, Mittal A, Soop M. Nonsteroidal anti-inflammatory drugs and anastomotic dehiscence in bowel surgery: systematic review and meta-analysis of randomized, controlled trials. Dis Colon Rectum. 2013;56(1):126–34.

68. Souter AJ, Fredman B, White PF. Controversies in the perioperative use of nonsteroidal antiinflammatory drugs. Anesth Analg. 1994;79(6):1178–90.

69. Gunter JB, Varughese AM, Harrington JF, et al. Recovery and complications after tonsillectomy in children: a comparison of ketorolac and morphine. Anesth Analg. 1995;81(6):1136–41.

70. Moiniche S, Romsing J, Dahl JB, et al. Nonsteroidal antiinflammatory drugs and the risk of operative site bleeding after tonsillectomy: a quantitative systematic review. Anesth Analg. 2003;96(1):68–77. table of contents.

71. Rusy LM, Houck CS, Sullivan LJ, et al. A double-blind evaluation of ketorolac tromethamine versus acetaminophen in pediatric tonsillectomy: analgesia and bleeding. Anesth Analg. 1995;80(2):226–9.

72. Remy C, Marret E, Bonnet F. Effects of acetaminophen on morphine side-effects and consumption after major surgery: meta-analysis of randomized controlled trials. Br J Anaesth. 2005;94(4):505–13.

73. Delaney CP, Fazio VW, Senagore AJ, et al. 'Fast track' postoperative management protocol for patients with high co-morbidity undergoing complex abdominal and pelvic colorectal surgery. Br J Surg. 2001;88(11):1533–8.

74. Maund E, McDaid C, Rice S, et al. Paracetamol and selective and non-selective non-steroidal anti-inflammatory drugs for the reduction in morphine-related side-effects after major surgery: a systematic review. Br J Anaesth. 2011;106(3):292–7.

75. McNicol ED, Tzortzopoulou A, Cepeda MS, et al. Single-dose intravenous paracetamol or propacetamol for prevention or treatment of postoperative pain: a systematic review and meta-analysis. Br J Anaesth. 2011;106(6):764–75.

76. Hernandez-Palazon J, Tortosa JA, Martinez-Lage JF, et al. Intravenous administration of propacetamol reduces morphine consumption after spinal fusion surgery. Anesth Analg. 2001;92(6):1473–6.

77. Issioui T, Klein KW, White PF, et al. The efficacy of premedication with celecoxib and acetaminophen in preventing pain after otolaryngologic surgery. Anesth Analg. 2002;94(5):1188–93. table of contents.

78. Chandok N, Watt KD. Pain management in the cirrhotic patient: the clinical challenge. Mayo Clin Proc. 2010;85(5):451–8.

79. Jones C, Kelliher L, Dickinson M, et al. Randomized clinical trial on enhanced recovery versus standard care following open liver resection. Br J Surg. 2013;100(8): 1015–24.

80. Bell RF, Dahl JB, Moore RA, et al. Perioperative ketamine for acute postoperative pain. Cochrane Database Syst Rev 2006;(1):CD004603.

81. Weinbroum AA. Non-opioid IV, adjuvants in the perioperative period: pharmacological and clinical aspects of ketamine and gabapentinoids. Pharmacol Res. 2012;65(4): 411–29.

82. White PF. The changing role of non-opioid analgesic techniques in the management of postoperative pain. Anesth Analg. 2005;101(5 Suppl):S5–22.

83. Dauri M, Faria S, Gatti A, et al. Gabapentin and pregabalin for the acute post-operative pain management. A systematic-narrative review of the recent clinical evidences. Curr Drug Targets. 2009;10(8):716–33.

84. Ho KY, Gan TJ, Habib AS. Gabapentin and postoperative pain—a systematic review of randomized controlled trials. Pain. 2006;126(1–3):91–101.

85. Zhang J, Ho KY, Wang Y. Efficacy of pregabalin in acute postoperative pain: a meta-analysis. Br J Anaesth. 2011;106(4):454–62.

86. Dahl JB, Mathiesen O, Kehlet H. An expert opinion on postoperative pain management, with special reference to new developments. Expert Opin Pharmacother. 2010; 11(15):2459–70.

87. Buvanendran A, Kroin JS, Della Valle CJ, et al. Perioperative oral pregabalin reduces chronic pain after total knee arthroplasty: a prospective, randomized, controlled trial. Anesth Analg. 2010;110(1):199–207.

88. Macrae WA. Chronic pain after surgery. Br J Anaesth. 2001;87(1):88–98.

89. Becker G, Blum HE. Novel opioid antagonists for opioid-induced bowel dysfunction and postoperative ileus. Lancet. 2009;373(9670):1198–206.

90. Kraft M, Maclaren R, Du W, et al. Alvimopan (entereg) for the management of postoperative ileus in patients undergoing bowel resection. P T. 2010;35(1):44–9.

91. Senagore AJ, Bauer JJ, Du W, et al. Alvimopan accelerates gastrointestinal recovery after bowel resection regardless of age, gender, race, or concomitant medication use. Surgery. 2007;142(4):478–86.

92. Obokhare ID, Champagne B, Stein SL, et al. The effect of alvimopan on recovery after laparoscopic segmental colectomy. Dis Colon Rectum. 2011;54(6):743–6.

93. Touchette DR, Yang Y, Tiryaki F, et al. Economic analysis of alvimopan for prevention and management of postoperative ileus. Pharmacotherapy. 2012;32(2):120–8.

94. Esteban F, Cerdan FJ, Garcia-Alonso M, et al. A multicentre comparison of a fast track or conventional postoperative protocol following laparoscopic or open elective surgery for colorectal cancer surgery. Colorectal Dis. 2014;16(2):134–40.

95. Zhuang CL, Ye XZ, Zhang XD, et al. Enhanced recovery after surgery programs versus traditional care for colorectal surgery: a meta-analysis of randomized controlled trials. Dis Colon Rectum. 2013;56(5):667–78.

96. Spanjersberg WR, Reurings J, Keus F et al. Fast track surgery versus conventional recovery strategies for colorectal surgery. Cochrane Database Syst Rev. 2011; (2):CD007635.

14. Early Nutrition and Early Mobilization: Why They Are Important and How to Make It Happen

Yuliya Y. Yurko, Kenneth C.H. Fearon, and Tonia M. Young-Fadok

This chapter will be subdivided into a first section regarding the theoretical basis behind early nutrition and early ambulation within the overall setting of an enhanced recovery program. Here it may be useful to consider some definitions: an enhanced recovery *protocol* involves sets of clinical instructions (orders, written, or electronic) that embody the components of evidence-based enhanced recovery research. An enhanced recovery *program* requires education of patients, nurses, and doctors, who need to be able to amend order sets to take into account how each individual upon whom we operate responds. These are not recipes. The latter half of the chapter will discuss practical, common sense measures that have worked in busy clinical practice settings to achieve these aims.

Enhanced Recovery Program in Theory

In the present digital era, patients turn to the Internet to find information about where and by whom to undergo surgical treatment. Increased patient expectations, cost of the treatment, and attention to safety outcomes by national regulatory bodies have generated significant interest in quantitative assessment of the quality of health care. One way of assessing the quality of surgical care is by using direct outcomes measures. These indicators include length of stay, readmission rate, complication rate, patient satisfaction, functional health status, etc.

L.S. Feldman et al. (eds.), *The SAGES / ERAS®*
Society Manual of Enhanced Recovery Programs for
Gastrointestinal Surgery, DOI 10.1007/978-3-319-20364-5_14,
© Springer International Publishing Switzerland 2015

168   Y.Y. Yurko et al.

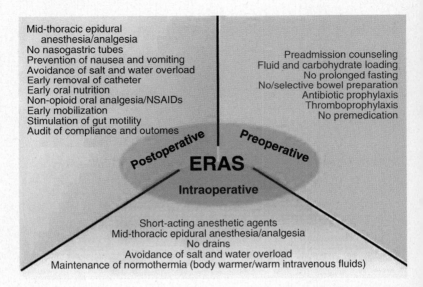

Fig. 14.1. ERAS multidisciplinary approach. (Courtesy of the ERAS Society [www.erassociety.org].).

The operation itself has long been perceived to be the single most important factor that influences surgical outcomes, but in reality pre-, intra- and postoperative care may be equally as important as the operation.

The concept of fast-track protocols was introduced by Kehlet in the 1990s to achieve early recovery after major surgical procedures [1]. Subsequently, the concept was modified by the Enhanced Recovery After Surgery (ERAS) Study Group, with a focus more on enhancing recovery than shortening length of stay [2]. Using a multidisciplinary team approach, enhanced recovery program (ERP) protocols focus on key elements including preoperative patient counseling, optimization of perioperative nutrition, standardized analgesic and anesthetic regimens, and early mobilization. A downstream effect is potential minimization of health care costs by reducing complications, use of tests, and hospital stay [2–6] (Fig. 14.1).

Early Nutrition

Preoperative fasting, previously one of the most important dogmas prior to surgery, has been dramatically changed by the ERP approach (see Chap. 4, preoperative fasting and carbohydrate treatment). In contrast to prior instruction regarding having nothing to eat or drink after midnight before an operation, patients are allowed to drink clear liquids up to 2 h before the surgical intervention. Carefully performed studies have shown that drinking clear liquids up to 2 h before the induction of anesthesia does not increase the volume of gastric contents or acidity, and does not increase the risk of aspiration [7–9]. In a study performed by Nygren et al., gastric emptying was not affected by carbohydrate-rich drinks consumed before elective surgery, and did not differ between experimental and control group [10]. According to a study performed by Gustaffson et al. on 25 patients with type 2 uncomplicated diabetes and 10 healthy volunteers, carbohydrate-rich drinks given 180 min before the induction of anesthesia did not increase the risk of aspiration, hyperglycemia, or delay gastric emptying in patients with diabetes compared with healthy volunteers [11]. Thus, the diagnosis of diabetes is not a contraindication for enrollment into an ERP protocol, in the absence of an additional diagnosis of gastroparesis.

Intake of complex carbohydrate-rich drinks up to 2 h before operation has been shown to reduce hunger, anxiety, and thirst in surgical patients in perioperative period [12–14]. A study performed by Wang et al. demonstrated that patients who received preoperative carbohydrate-rich beverages also had a reduced degree of insulin resistance, a marker of physiologic stress, in the postoperative period [15]. The clinical significance of postoperative insulin resistance was further illustrated in a prospective randomized study performed by a Belgian group in the setting of the surgical ICU [16]. Maintenance of euglycemia (the blood glucose concentration 80–110 mg/dl) in surgical patients in the intensive care unit resulted in a significant reduction in postoperative mortality, risk of infection, and use of antibiotics. Postoperative insulin resistance is most pronounced at postoperative day zero and lasts for about 3 weeks after uncomplicated elective major abdominal operations. It can be an important factor determining the length of postoperative hospital stay [17, 18]. Tamura et al. showed that fasting-induced insulin resistance in healthy participants could be reversed by preoperative oral administration of an 18 % carbohydrate solution [19]. It is essential to appreciate that the beneficial effect of carbohydrate loading is time dependent and that if the carbohydrate load is given longer than 2 h before surgery, the reduction of post-op insulin resistance secondary to the insulin peak induced by the CHO load is lost. This is a major practice point that is often forgotten.

Avoiding preoperative fasting also lowers the extent of the catabolic state as indicated by a reduction in blood ketone body levels [19], and reduced postoperative loss of urinary nitrogen [20]. The early initiation of postoperative nutrition can also ameliorate the metabolic response to surgery by reducing insulin resistance, loss of muscle strength, and negative nitrogen balance [21, 22]. With respect to postoperative care, Kehlet pioneered a dramatic change from nil per mouth to early implementation of diet in the immediate postoperative period [4, 5]. All patients are allowed clear liquid diet (water, juice, protein-enriched juices) as soon as they are awake and can advance to low residue diet on postoperative day 1 with supplementation of a protein drink with each meal. In some centers the emphasis is more on normal food than the use of oral supplements, but with the goal of achieving the same net intake. Normal food should be easily accessible to patients and should be of an attractive nature to further encourage spontaneous intake. Some programs rearrange the ward environment so that patients eat at a common dining table rather than being immobilized and isolated in their own beds. This encourages early mobilization and communication of common experiences between patients. It is important to appreciate that within an ERP protocol, although patients are encouraged to eat, this is not tolerated by all patients. Gastrointestinal dysfunction with nausea, vomiting, and paralytic ileus still occurs in a proportion of patients and it is important to modify the program according to patient progress. Equally it is vital that patients are closely supervised so that the rare case of acute gastric dilatation is promptly and correctly managed with placement of a nasogastric tube.

Clearly, maintenance of gut function in the post-op period is vital if early return of spontaneous dietary intake is to be achieved. To this end, the ERP protocols generally emphasize the use of nausea and vomiting prophylaxis especially in high-risk groups and avoidance/minimal use of systemic opiates.

Despite the fact that most of the patients have no limitations in their diet before an elective colonic resection, it is important to obtain information regarding nutritional status and make plans before surgery. In a randomized clinical trial involving patients undergoing moderate to major lower gastrointestinal abdominal surgery, Smedley et al. showed significantly lower weight loss and a reduced complication rate in the group receiving oral nutritional supplements in the form of protein drinks before and after the surgical intervention [23]. Following discharge from the hospital, patients taking oral nutritional supplements had better nutritional intake at 2 weeks, but by 4 weeks the total intake was similar to that in the control group. The latter trial was undertaken in the context of traditional rather than ERP perioperative care and it may be that if all patients are provided with optimal nutritional and metabolic care in the perioperative period (i.e., ERP), then the impact of malnutrition may be less than previously thought.

Early Mobilization

Prolonged bed rest is associated with pulmonary complications, insulin resistance, reduced work capacity, and loss of muscle mass and strength [24, 25]. In older patients, deconditioning can be seen after as little as 2 days of hospitalization [26]. Early mobilization is an important step in accelerating postoperative recovery and is a key component of ERPs. A multivariate linear regression analysis of data collected during the LAFA trial supported the hypothesis that mobilization on postoperative days 1–3 is significantly associated with successful outcome of ERP [27]. Patients in ERPs spend more time out of bed compared to traditional care [28] but even within established programs, overall adherence to mobilization may be low [29].

However, there are no standard definitions of mobilization, and programs may set very different goals for activity using different benchmarks such as time (hours out of bed, sitting or walking) or distance (e.g., number of "laps" in the hallway, meters, or steps to achieve). There are no randomized trials comparing one approach to another. It is unclear whether patient outcomes are improved if physiotherapists or other caregivers are involved in mobilization. It is important to involve nurses in all phases of the development of the protocol so that there is support for helping patients mobilize as early as possible. Patients who begin an exercise program preoperatively ("prehabilitation") remain more active postoperatively compared to controls [30]. Compliance may be improved by setting out daily goals in the preoperative patient education, and reinforcing these goals with posters on the ward, diaries, or pedometers. Pain, drains, and IVs reduce ambulation and demonstrate the interrelationship between several aspects of the pathway.

ERPs in Practice

The title of this chapter sounds easy: Early Mobilization and Early Feeding. Why do we not just give the patient a tray of food and get them out of bed! In reality this is considerably more complex. Achieving a successful protocol and program requires a champion or dedicated team who understand that all the components are intertwined as a complex intervention. Planning for a successful outcome starts in the preoperative period, continues through the intraoperative period, and postoperatively, and really only ends when the patient has returned to his or her expected functional status.

All patients receive detailed instructions regarding nutrition, ambulation goals, perioperative pain control, and anticipation of early discharge before the surgery (Table 14.1). They are aware that early eating and early mobilization are part of their recovery plan. Yet one of the most common reasons for deviation from an ERAS protocol in the early postoperative period is failure to mobilize the patient. Failure to mobilize the patient on postoperative day zero can be due to uncontrolled pain, pre-existing conditions, nausea/vomiting, lack of patient motivation, and lack of resources, such as nursing:patient ratios. Deviations from the program as early as the end of the first postoperative day are associated with delays in discharge [31].

The main roadblocks to early nutrition and mobilization have been addressed in other chapters of the book and include nausea/vomiting and/or poorly controlled pain, highlighting the interconnectedness of the multiple interventions included in the program. During the perioperative period, multimodal analgesic regimens should be used to decrease the use of opioids. Such regimens are dependent on local institutional expertise. The laparoscopic approach helps minimize handling of the bowel, reduces tissue trauma and the systemic inflammatory response, reduces the need for opiate analgesics, and facilitates early mobilization. In contrast with major open surgery, epidural analgesia is not required for laparoscopic colorectal surgery and may delay recovery [32]. Patients may receive pre-emptive analgesia in the preoperative setting including acetaminophen (paracetamol), celecoxib, and gabapentin. Currently there is debate about the influence of NSAIDs on increased rates of anastomotic leak and some centers now avoid NSAIDs. In the postoperative period, the protocol may include scheduled intravenous acetaminophen and ketorolac (except for elderly patients and those with impaired renal function) to decrease the use of narcotics. Some centers use an intravenous lidocaine infusion to reduce post-op nausea and vomiting by sparing the use of systemic opiates. Others emphasize a regional block involving bilateral infiltration of the transversus abdominis plane (TAP) with liposomal bupivacaine. This is used in open laparotomy and also in laparoscopic operations, being especially helpful in patients

Table 14.1. ERP booklet.

What is "Enhanced Recovery"?

- You might hear your surgical team talk about "enhanced recovery." This phrase refers to a special approach carefully designed by your colon and rectal surgical team to help improve your recovery. Your colon and rectal surgical team includes surgeons, anesthesiologists, nurses, pharmacists, and many others.

- Most people who have colon and rectal surgery with enhanced recovery approach stay in the hospital for 2–3 days. For example, if your surgery is on Tuesday, you will probably leave the hospital on Thursday or Friday. Keep this in mind as you make plans for care and for travel.

- You may be given a special drink that is rich in carbohydrates. This drink helps your body use insulin more effectively.

- You may need to have an enema to remove stool from your colon. You can give it to yourself or if you are in the hospital, a nurse can provide assistance.

- Your surgeon may give you instructions on how to do a bowel prep.

While in the Hospital After Surgery

Nutrition

- Your surgical team will let you know when you can begin eating and drinking after surgery. Typically it is within 4 h.

- You may have been given some pain medicine before surgery in an effort to manage pain ahead of time. Your surgical team will try to make you as comfortable as possible so that you can participate in your recovery.

- Several methods are used for giving pain medicine. Initially you may receive pain medicine intravenously (through a vein or by "IV"). As soon as you are able to eat, you will be given pain medicine in tablet form. Your surgical team will decide what is best for you.

Preventing Complications

To help reduce the risk of blood clots forming:

- During surgery:
  - You will have devices on your legs that gently squeeze your legs.
  - You may be given injections of a blood-thinning medicine.

- Regular activity helps shorten your recovery time by:
  - Keeping muscles active.
  - Improving the return of bowel function.
  - Preventing complications such as the formation of blood clots and pneumonia.

After You Leave the Hospital

Follow the guidelines carefully that you were given in your discharge instructions.

Nutrition

- When you leave the hospital, you will have diet instructions. You may continue drinking the supplement beverages you received in the hospital if you wish. The supplements are available over the counter from most grocery stores and pharmacies.

(continued)

Table 14.1. (continued)

The Goals of the Enhanced Recovery Approach are to:
- Keep you well hydrated and well nourished.
- Help you prepare mentally and emotionally for surgery and recovery.
- Reduce your risk of surgical site infection.
- Reduce the risk of medicine-related problems.
- Help you manage your other health conditions.
- Help you manage pain.
- Help you plan for the time after surgery while your activity is restricted.

Before Surgery
- Your surgeon will talk with you about the kind of surgery you are going to have and will review the side effects and risks of surgery.

- Your surgical team will recommend that you drink supplemental carbohydrate beverage while you are still in the hospital.
- Begin by eating only small amounts of food. You may find that eating small amounts more often helps you tolerate food easier the first few days after surgery.
- It is common to have some nausea while you are in the hospital. Be sure to tell a member of your surgical team if you are nauseated. They may give you medicine to help you feel better.

Pain Management
- Most people have some pain or discomfort after surgery which will be managed by pain medication. You will be asked to rate your pain according to a number scale.

After surgery:
- The leg-squeezing devices may be used for short periods of time when you are in bed.
- You may be given more injections of blood-thinning medicine.
- You will be asked to get up and walk early and frequently. You will be helped out of bed on the day of surgery, as early mobility is important to your recovery.

Activity
Activity is important for these reasons:
- Every day that you lie in bed leads to a loss of muscle mass, so you will be expected to get out of bed the same day as your surgery. You will also be expected to be out of bed in a chair for all meals.

Pain Management
- Follow the instructions you have been given about managing pain. Managing pain is important in your recovery. Do not feel like you have to "tough it out." If you are in pain, you will not be able to do the activities you need to for getting well.

Activity
- Follow the activity guidelines you have been given and the goals you have made.

If you have any questions about this Information, please call your doctor.

with preoperative use of narcotics or marijuana. Due to elimination of postoperative fasting, the transition to oral pain management is more efficient with ERAS protocols.

Postoperative nausea and vomiting (PONV) can affect 25–35 % of surgical patients and delay nutrition, ambulation, and discharge from the hospital. Minimal preoperative fasting, carbohydrate loading, and reduced postoperative opiate use all have a positive effect on postoperative nausea and vomiting (PONV). A multimodal approach should be adopted to prevent PONV, starting in the preoperative area.

Most patients have decreased appetite after the surgery, or are nervous about oral intake. Their nutrition intake has been driven by the information given before the operation on the importance of nutrition balance in the perioperative period. Some centers use oral nutritional supplements (200 ml carton of protein-rich drink containing 9 g of protein) three times a day starting on the day of surgery for at least the first two postoperative days (or longer if they are still in the hospital) to achieve target intakes of calories and protein during the very early postoperative phase. All patients are encouraged to start mobilization on postoperative day zero and continue ambulation at least three times a day.

In our program, patients receive a clear liquid diet as soon as they are awake and if well tolerated, the diet is advanced to low residue with the next meal. Intake of nutritional supplements and time of ambulation are recorded each day by the patient on a paper form provided in their bedside "welcome package" which encourages them to eat, drink, and get out of bed.

Take Home Messages

- Early nutrition and ambulation are key drivers of recovery
- Successful implementation of an Enhanced Recovery program requires full investment by a multidisciplinary team and understanding of the evidence led by surgical, anesthesia, and nursing champions
- Patient engagement with early ambulation and nutrition is key and begins in the preoperative period
- An enhanced recovery protocol is not a "cookbook" and not all patients tolerate early feeding. The patient is *not* "noncompliant" if their physiology means that the protocol is delayed.

References

1. Kehlet H. Multimodal approach to control postoperative pathophysiology and rehabilitation. Br J Anaesth. 1997;78:606–17.
2. Fearon KC, Ljungqvist O, Von Meyenfeldt M, Revhaug A, Dejong CH, Lassen K, Nygren J, Hausel J, Soop M, Andersen J, Kehlet H. Enhanced recovery after surgery: a consensus review of clinical care for patients undergoing colonic resection. Clin Nutr. 2005;24:466–77.
3. Wilmore DW, Kehlet H. Management of patients in fast track surgery. BMJ. 2001;322:473–6.
4. Kehlet H, Wilmore DW. Multimodal strategies to improve surgical outcome. Am J Surg. 2002;183:630–41.
5. Kehlet H, Dahl JB. Anaesthesia, surgery, and challenges in postoperative recovery. Lancet. 2003;362:1921–8.
6. Arumainayagam N, McGrath J, Jefferson KP, et al. Introduction of an enhanced recovery protocol for radical cystectomy. BJU Int. 2008;101:698–701.
7. Kehlet H, Mogensen T. Hospital stay of 2 days after open sigmoidectomy with a multimodal rehabilitation programme. Br J Surg. 1999;86:227–30.
8. Scabini S, Rimini E, Romairone E, Scordamaglia R, Damiani G, Pertile D, Ferrando V. Colon and rectal surgery for cancer without mechanical bowel preparation: one-center randomized prospective trial. World J Surg Oncol. 2010;8:35.
9. Ljungqvist O, Søreide E. Preoperative fasting. Br J Surg. 2003;90:400–6.
10. Nygren J, Thorell A, Jacobsson H, et al. Preoperative gastric emptying. Effects of anxiety and oral carbohydrate administration. Ann Surg. 1995;222:728–34.
11. Gustafsson UO, Nygren J, Thorell A, et al. Preoperative carbohydrate loading may be used in type 2 diabetes patients. Acta Anaesthesiol Scand. 2008;52:946–51.
12. Ljungqvist O, Nygren J, Thorell A. Modulation of post-operative insulin resistance by pre-operative carbohydrate loading. Proc Nutr Soc. 2002;61:329–36.
13. Hausel J, Nygren J, Lagerkranser M, Hellstrom PM, Hammarqvist F, Almstrom C, et al. A carbohydrate-rich drink reduces preoperative discomfort in elective surgery patients. Anesth Analg. 2001;93:1344–50.
14. Helminen H, Viitanen H, Sajanti J. Effect of preoperative intravenous carbohydrate loading on preoperative discomfort in elective surgery patients. Eur J Anaesthesiol. 2009;26:123–7.
15. Wang ZG, Wang Q, Wang WJ, Qin HL. Randomized clinical trial to compare the effects of preoperative oral carbohydrate versus placebo on insulin resistance after colorectal surgery. Br J Surg. 2010;97(3):317–23.
16. Van den Berghe G. Insulin therapy for the critically ill patient. Clin Cornerstone. 2003;5(2):56–63.
17. Thorell A, Nygren J, Ljungqvist O. Insulin resistance: a marker of surgical stress. Curr Opin Clin Nutr Metab Care. 1999;2:69–78.
18. Ljungqvist O, Nygren J, Soop M, Thorell A. Metabolic perioperative management: novel concepts. Curr Opin Crit Care. 2005;11:295–9.

19. Tamura T, Yatabe T, et al. Oral carbohydrate loading with 18% carbohydrate beverages alleviates insulin resistance. Asia Pac J Clin Nutr. 2013;22(1):48–53.

20. Svanfeldt M, Thorell A, Hausel J, Soop M, Rooyackers O, Nygren J, et al. Randomized clinical trial of the effect of preoperative oral carbohydrate treatment on postoperative whole-body protein and glucose kinetics. Br J Surg. 2007;94(11):1342e50.

21. Lewis SJ, Egger M, Sylvester PA, Thomas S. Early enteral feeding versus "nil by mouth" after gastrointestinal surgery: systematic review and meta-analysis of controlled trials. BMJ. 2001;323:773–6.

22. Correia MI, da Silva RG. The impact of early nutrition on metabolic response and postoperative ileus. Curr Opin Clin Nutr Metab Care. 2004;7:577–83.

23. Smedley F, Bowling T, James M, Stokes E, Goodger C, O'Connor O, et al. Randomized clinical trial of the effects of preoperative and postoperative oral nutritional supplements on clinical course and cost of care. Br J Surg. 2004;91(8): 983–90.

24. Houborg KB, Jensen MB, Hessov I, Laurberg S. Little effect of physical training on body composition and nutritional intake following colorectal surgery—a randomised placebo-controlled trial. Eur J Clin Nutr. 2005;59(8):969–77.

25. Jensen MB, Houborg KB, Norager CB, Henriksen MG, Laurberg S. Postoperative changes in fatigue, physical function and body composition: an analysis of the amalgamated data from five randomized trials on patients undergoing colorectal surgery. Colorectal Dis. 2011;13(5):588–93.

26. Hirsch CH, Sommers L, Olsen A, Mullen L, Winograd CH. The natural history of functional morbidity in hospitalized older patients. J Am Geriatr Soc. 1990;38: 1296–303.

27. Vlug MS, Wind J, Hollmann MW, Ubbink DT, Cense HA, Engel AF, et al. Laparoscopy in combination with fast track multimodal management is the best perioperative strategy in patients undergoing colonic surgery: a randomized clinical trial (LAFA-study). Ann Surg. 2011;254(6):868–75.

28. Basse L, Hjort Jakobsen D, Billesbolle P, Werner M, Kehlet H. A clinical pathway to accelerate recovery after colonic resection. Ann Surg. 2000;232:51–7.

29. Gustafsson UO, Hausel J, Thorell A, Ljungqvist O, Soop M, Nygren J. Adherence to the enhanced recovery after surgery protocol and outcomes after colorectal cancer surgery. Arch Surg. 2011;146:571–7.

30. Gillis C, Li C, Lee L, Rashami A, Berson A, Liberman AS, Stein B, Charlebois P, Feldman LS, Carli F. Prehabilitation vs. rehabilitation: a randomized control trial in patients undergoing colorectal resection for cancer. Anesthesiology. 2014;121(5): 937–47.

31. Smart NJ, White P, Allison AS, Ockrim JB, Kennedy RH, Francis NK. Deviation and failure of enhanced recovery after surgery (ERAS) following laparoscopic colorectal surgery: early prediction model. Colorectal Dis. 2012;14(10):e727–34.

32. Hübner M, Blanc C, Roulin D, Winiker M, Gander S, Demartines N. Randomized clinical trial on epidural versus patient-controlled analgesia for laparoscopic colorectal surgery within an enhanced recovery pathway. Ann Surg. 2015;261(4):648–53.

15. Management of Tubes, Drains, and Catheters

William S. Richardson

Rounding on patients the day after surgery we frequently know that the patient has not moved since they left the recovery room except from the stretcher to the bed. In addition, the nurse has told them not to get up until they have time to help them. In part this is due to the effects of sedation and making sure that they are safe to ambulate but the patients and their family members how to take care of the drains and tubes properly. The drains also cause pain to the patient immobilizing him further. In this regard we have tied the patient to the bed which we know is bad for recovery. In addition, each tube has risks as well as benefits and although they should be removed as soon as medically unnecessary this timing is difficult to determine. In this chapter we discuss the use of tube drains and catheters in various surgical situations. Table 15.1 summarizes suggested uses of drains and tubes within enhanced recovery programs.

Nasogastric Tubes

Benefits

Prophylactic gastric decompression using nasogastric tubes aims to decrease aspiration risk from reflux of gastrointestinal fluid, decrease risk of stretching of an anastomosis on the stomach, and remove gastric fluid to prevent symptoms of ileus. The theoretical benefits of prophylactic gastric decompression are not born out in many circumstances. Routine use of nasogastric tubes should be replaced with selective use.

L.S. Feldman et al. (eds.), *The SAGES / ERAS®*
Society Manual of Enhanced Recovery Programs for
Gastrointestinal Surgery, DOI 10.1007/978-3-319-20364-5_15,
© Springer International Publishing Switzerland 2015

Table 15.1. Recommended use of drain, tube, and catheters for routine surgery.

	Drain	NG	Foley
Bariatrics	−	−	−
Colon and rectal	−	−	−
Gallbladder	−	−	−
Appendix	−	−	−
Liver	−	−	−
Stomach	−	−	−
Perforated ulcer	+/−	+/−	−
Pancreas	+	−	−
Hernia	+/−	−	−

From Zaouter C, Kaneva P, Carli F. Less urinary tract infection by earlier removal of bladder catheter in surgical patients receiving thoracic epidural analgesia. Reg Anesth Pain Med 2009 Nov–Dec;34(6):542–8, with permission

Risks

These are likely the most irritating tubes that we use and cause nausea, sore throat, and pain at the patient's nose. They must be periodically assessed to make sure that they are working properly. Other risks include misplacement which can rarely lead to pneumothorax or brain injury. Side effects include sinusitis which can be a cause of fever of unknown origin, loss of nasal septum, and ulcers from gastric irritation. The percent risk of these complications is low but not well elucidated.

Alternatives

When the need for prolonged gastric decompression is predicted, consider a gastrostomy tube (placed endoscopically or at the time of surgery).

Specific Clinical Situations

Colon and Rectal Surgery

Current literature suggests that the routine use of nasogastric tubes for uncomplicated surgery does not decrease anastomotic leak, wound complications, pulmonary complications, or length of hospital stay and should be abandoned. Avoiding a nasogastric tube encourages early feeding which has been shown to decrease recovery time without worsening ileus or vomiting. Without routine use only 10 % of patients will need postoperative placement of nasogastric tubes—essentially the same number that need to be reinserted if they are used routinely and removed several days after surgery. Risk factors predicting the need for postoperative NG tubes include age greater than 60, preoperative use of narcotics, previous abdominal surgery (requiring lysis of adhesion), low albumin, low hemoglobin, low potassium, low calcium, and deep vein thrombosis.

Liver Resection

Routine placement of nasogastric tubes has no value in liver surgery and may increase the risk of pulmonary complications. Risk factors for need of postoperative placement in one randomized trial are female patients, current smokers, and left hepatectomy with 30 % risk with all three factors present.

Gastric Resection

One randomized controlled trial has shown that avoiding a nasogastric at the time of surgery decreased time to flatus, time to oral intake, and length of hospital stay. In this trial 12 % of patients required placement of a nasogastric tube postoperatively. A meta-analysis of studies of the need for routine nasogastric or nasojejunal decompression after gastrectomy for gastric cancer found no difference in leaks, respiratory complications, length of stay, or complications with their use while time to oral diet was significantly longer when routine decompression was used. The role for nasogastric decompression after esophagectomy requires more study, with contradictory findings related to pulmonary complications.

Bariatrics

Good evidence suggests that routine use of a nasogastric tube is not necessary.

NG Take-Home Messages

Nasogastric tubes should not be used routinely. However, we should consider it routine to assess our patients for their need postoperatively. Postoperative placement of a nasogastric tube should not be considered a failure, just like conversion from laparoscopic to open should not be considered a complication. If 10–15 % of patients will have a nasogastric tube inserted postoperatively, 85–90 % of patients will have avoided it. Remember that nasogastric tubes are some of the most painful treatments we inflict on our patients. Consider placement of a nasogastric tube, gastrostomy tube, or feeding jejunostomy tube at the time of surgery in patients who have had difficult, long, or redo cases where there may be a higher risk of ileus or aspiration or who have multiple risk factors identified in this section.

Intra-abdominal Drains

Benefits

Drains are used in the hope of detecting bowel or organ leak or bleeding at a surgical site and may help in early detection or prevent abscess formation. They may detect high rates of leak or bleeding which can assist in operative decision making. They can easily be placed through a trocar site at the time of laparoscopic surgery. Many papers have shown that there is no need to "cover" a drain with antibiotics. Yet generally when patients develop a significant complication, they manifest clinical symptoms (elevated respiration rate, elevated heart rate, fever, or abdominal tenderness) for which we would typically obtain a CT, giving us better information than our drainage tubes alone.

Risks

Drains cause inflammation with elevated cytokines detected in drainage fluid at 7 days and 80 % are colonized with bacteria at the same time, so they may themselves cause inflammation and infection, which could possibly lead to leak and abscess formation. They can get trapped in facial closure and require operative removal, may cause bleeding at the incision site for placement, and may migrate from the site of placement, thereby not giving you the information you want from the site of original placement. In general, they stop draining about a week postoperatively as they get covered with fibrinous material, clot, or omentum.

Specific Clinical Situations

Cholecystectomy

Many prospective trials and randomized trials have shown that routine use of drains in cholecystectomy is unnecessary.

Appendectomy

Good evidence suggests that no drains are necessary after surgery for any stage of appendicitis. There is increased risk with their use.

Bariatric Surgery

For uncomplicated cases, early detection of complication is on the basis of changes in vital signs (for example, respiration rate greater than 20, heart rate greater than 120, and fever or persistent elevation in vital signs over baseline) and need for operation should be based on vital signs and not on suction drainage. Intraluminal bleeding will not be detected by drains but by melena. Typically, any change in management will be based on symptoms and signs and not with changes in drainage.

Pancreatic Surgery

Here the literature presents a mixed picture. On the one hand a very good randomized trial has shown that total nonuse of drains increases the risk of complication with pancreatic leak compared to routine usage. Outcome for Whipple procedure was improved with drains in one randomized trial but other trials reported increased risk of pancreatic fistula and abscess within the drain group. Another randomized trial demonstrated that outcomes were improved with external pancreatic duct stenting in soft pancreases or with nondilated pancreatic ducts. Certainly some pancreas resections should be drained but we are still working out which ones and as an alternative or for extra protection stenting can be used in high-risk pancreas cases (soft pancreas, small duct). Also, consider early removal of drains at 3 days postop to decrease the risk of complication from the drain.

Gastric Resection

A randomized controlled trial demonstrated that length of hospital stay was lower when drains were used, and a large meta-analysis showed that both length of hospital stay and complications were higher in the drained groups (in this paper there was no significant difference in anastomotic leak rates of fistulas). There may be subgroups of complicated cases where drainage should be used.

Colon and Rectal Surgery

Many papers have shown no benefit of drains on mortality, anastomotic dehiscence, wound infection, reoperation rates, or length of hospital stay.

Liver Resection

Several randomized trials have shown that routine use of drains for liver surgery is unnecessary. However for larger resections, where bile leak is more likely, they may be beneficial.

Hernia Repair

Here the data are inconclusive and there is no significant difference in length of hospital stay or postoperative pain with drain use. Because of the risk of causing infection routine use should be discouraged and early removal encouraged.

Perforated Peptic Ulcer

Data are inconclusive. Certainly drainage may be useful where a relatively high risk of leak is suspected.

Appendectomy

A meta-analysis of four randomized trials showed higher rates of fecal fistula and wound infection in the drained group whereas the rate of intra-abdominal abscess was the same.

Drains Take-Home Message

Drains may be helpful in complicated or redo cases where the risk of bleeding or leakage is higher and in particular where the risk is 20–30 % such as in pancreatectomy. Otherwise, routine abdominal drainage is not recommended.

Urinary Catheter

Benefits

Urinary output has been used to assess intravascular volume and the need and amount of resuscitation fluid. However urine output, particularly during laparoscopic surgery, is not a good monitor of intravascular volume. Several noninvasive hemodynamic measurement tools including the esophageal Doppler probe and the arterial pulse contour devices are available to more reliably guide goal-directed fluid therapy (see Chap. 11). Urinary catheters also help prevent bladder overdistention or rupture in long cases or in patients who are immobile.

Risks

The risk of urinary tract infection increases with the duration of catheterization. The catheters make it more difficult for the patient to safely ambulate and make it unnecessary to ambulate in order to urinate. A randomized trial in patients with thoracic epidural demonstrated that removal of the urinary catheter on postoperative day 1 in patients at low risk for urinary retention was associated with lower rates of urinary tract infection than a group in whom the urinary catheter was only removed after the epidural was removed. Using a bladder-scan protocol to guide management of urinary retention after catheter removal, 8 % of patients in the early removal group required in-and-out catheterization, but only 3 % required reinsertion of a urinary catheter.

Urinary Catheters Take-Home Message

Urinary catheters should not be left in place routinely and should not be used as a sole means to determine intraoperative intravascular volume. They may be safely removed on postoperative day 1 in patients at

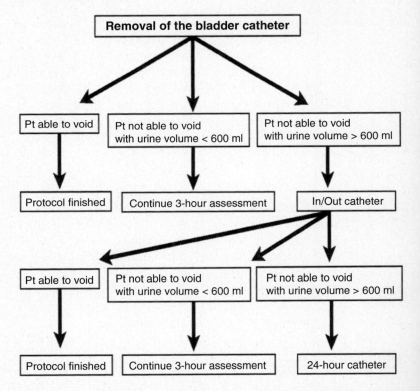

Fig. 15.1. Flowchart of urinary bladder volume assessment by ultrasound every 3 h from the removal of the bladder catheter (from Zaouter C, Kaneva P, Carli F. Less urinary tract infection by earlier removal of bladder catheter in surgical patients receiving thoracic epidural analgesia. Reg Anesth Pain Med 2009;34:542–548, with permission).

low risk for urinary retention even in the presence of a thoracic epidural. A bladder scan is helpful to guide management of urinary retention and avoid prolonged urinary catheterization (Fig. 15.1).

Conclusions

It has been traditional to liberally place drains, tubes, and catheters in surgical patients. Recent evidence has shown that in many cases they are not only irrelevant but can cause harm and lengthen hospital stay.

This is a changing field but in general surgeons should make sure that they are placing drains, tubes, and catheters for good reasons or the risks will outweigh the benefits.

Suggested Readings

1. Gurusamy KS, Allen VB. Wound drains after incisional hernia repair (review). Cochrane Collaboration. 2013;12:1–19.
2. Petrowsky H, Demartines N, Rousson V, Clavien PA. Evidence-based value of prophylactic drainage in gastrointestinal surgery a systematic review and meta-analysis. Ann Surg. 2004;240:1074–85.
3. Van Buren G, et al. A randomized prospective multicenter trial of pancreaticoduodenectomy with and without routine intraperitoneal drainage. Ann Surg. 2014;259:605–12.
4. De Jesus EC, Karliczek A, Matos D, Castro AA, Atallah AN. Prophylactic anastomotic drainage for colorectal surgery (review). Cochrane Collaboration. 2008;4:1–31.
5. Kronberg U, Kiran RP, Soliman MSM, Hammel JP, Galway U, Coffey JC, Fazio VW. A characterization of factors determining postoperative ileus after laparoscopic colectomy enables the generation of a novel predictive score. Ann Surg. 2011;253:78–81.

16. Hospital Recovery and Full Recovery

Colin F. Royse and Julio F. Fiore Jr.

The systematic evaluation and documentation of patient and healthcare outcomes is useful to determine the effectiveness of enhanced recovery after surgery programs (ERPs). Monitoring postoperative outcomes provides a feedback loop to evaluate the program results and facilitate a continual improvement process.

The aim of this chapter is to discuss outcomes relevant to patient recovery so as to measure the effectiveness of ERPs. Special focus is given to the Postoperative Quality of Recovery Scale (PostopQRS) [1], a tool specifically developed to assess multiple domains of recovery over time, appraising recovery both in-hospital and after discharge. The PostopQRS has been recently adopted by the ERAS Society as an outcome measurement tool.

Measuring Postoperative Recovery

As the primary objective of ERPs is to improve recovery after surgery, outcomes used within ERPs should reflect the process of postoperative recovery. This process has a specific trajectory involving a rapid decline in health status after the operation, followed by a gradual return towards or beyond preoperative levels of health (Fig. 16.1) [2]. Put simply, "recovery" is a return to baseline (pre-surgery) state or better. ERPs impact this recovery trajectory by attenuating health status decline and introducing interventions which may promote earlier recovery. Measuring recovery outcomes within ERPs, however, is not a simple or straightforward task. Recovery is a complex construct (i.e., theoretical concept) involving multiple dimensions of health including symptom

L.S. Feldman et al. (eds.), *The SAGES / ERAS®*
Society Manual of Enhanced Recovery Programs for
Gastrointestinal Surgery, DOI 10.1007/978-3-319-20364-5_16,
© Springer International Publishing Switzerland 2015

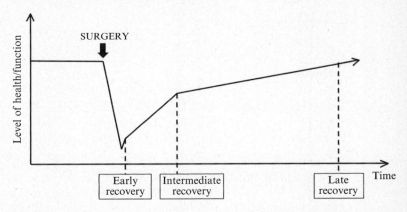

Fig. 16.1. Trajectory of postoperative recovery (adapted from Lee L, Tran T, Mayo NE, Carli F, Feldman LS. What does it really mean to "recover" from an operation? Surgery. 2014; 155(2):211–6, with permission).

experiences (e.g., pain, fatigue, nausea), functional status (e.g., walking capacity, bowel function) and postoperative well-being (e.g., physical, mental, social) [2]. This multidimensionality should be taken into account when recovery is measured.

The time frame of postoperative recovery can be divided into three distinct phases, named early recovery (period immediately after surgery until discharge from the post-anesthesia care unit (PACU)), intermediate recovery (the time from PACU discharge until hospital discharge), and late recovery (time from hospital discharge until return to normal or baseline health) (Fig. 16.1) [2]. Most of the evidence regarding the effectiveness of ERPs concerns outcomes evaluated during the hospitalization period (intermediate recovery phase), with studies using duration of hospital stay and postoperative complications as outcome measures [3]. However, it is recognized that the process of recovery extends after postoperative hospitalization, often lasting months [4].

Outcomes after surgery can be broadly classified into two groups:

1. Hospital/doctor outcomes:

    (a) Length of stay/readiness for discharge
    (b) Incidence of complications/readmission rates/requirement for long-term care
    (c) Safety indicators, such as morbidity or mortality events
    (d) Cost/resource utilization

2. Patient-focused outcomes:

    (a) Nociception (pain and nausea)
    (b) Emotive (anxiety and depression)
    (c) Functional recovery (ability to self-care)
    (d) Cognitive recovery
    (e) Physiological recovery
    (f) Satisfaction with the surgery and recovery

Both hospital/doctor and patient-focused outcomes are important in assessing the success of ERPs, as well as providing an audit loop for continual improvement. All of these outcomes are relevant to all phases of recovery, though each time period has a particular focus. It is important to appreciate that recovery indicators may not equate to quality. The term "quality of recovery" is a subjective assessment of recovery outcomes. For example, patient satisfaction is often used as a measure of quality, when it has very poor correlation with actual recovery indicators [5]. Satisfaction also has a ceiling effect whereby the majority of patients are satisfied whatever the outcome, and therefore lacks discriminant validity to determine differences in quality [5, 6].

In-Hospital Recovery

Early Recovery

The phase of early recovery is of particular interest to anesthesiologists and nurses involved in post-anesthesia care. This phase can be broadly defined as the time required for patients to sufficiently recover from anesthesia enabling discharge from PACU to the surgical ward [2]. The time can be further subdivided to immediate and early. The immediate phase is typically the first 15 min after cessation of anesthesia when emergence occurs and the predominant focus is on safety. The physiological recovery domain predominates including airway, consciousness, hemodynamic stability, temperature, and treatment of pain and nausea. After this, the early phase generally focuses on criteria to define readiness for PACU discharge. However, there is little agreement on which are the optimal criteria [7]. The American Society of Anesthesiologists, for example, recommend that minimal requirements for discharge are defined for each PACU, but do not endorse a specific set of criteria [8].

Making discharge decisions based on post-anesthesia recovery scores is a common practice in PACUs and, of the different scoring systems described in the literature, the Aldrete score is arguably the most popular [9]. This scoring system involves the assessment of five parameters (respiration, oxygen saturation, blood pressure, level of consciousness, and activity) scored at three levels [10]. Patients are considered ready to be discharged to the ward when a score of 9 is achieved (of 10 maximal possible). The time to achieve readiness for PACU discharge based on Aldrete scores is often used as a measure of recovery in studies comparing different anesthetic regimens [11–13]. A common criticism to the Aldrete scoring system is that its measurement properties (e.g., validity, reliability) were not broadly studied [9].

Intermediate Recovery

Most of the research evaluating the effectiveness of ERPs focuses on the phase of intermediate recovery, which comprises the period spent in the surgical ward from PACU discharge until readiness for hospital discharge [2]. The focus in this phase is physiological stability, return of organ function and patient mobility, resolution of pain and nausea, and cognitive recovery. Hospital length of stay (LOS) is the outcome most frequently reported in ERP studies [3], essentially presuming that patients leave the hospital as soon as they achieve discharge criteria and are able to manage independently at home. The validity of LOS as a measure of recovery, however, is debatable as length of hospitalization can be influenced by fixed protocols or social circumstances (health care system, hospital culture, surgeon's preferences, patient's expectations, and availability of post-discharge support). Research shows that patients often leave the hospital 1–3 days after achieving minimal requirements for discharge [14–16]. For this reason, several authors advocate that, although still relevant as an audit measure for organizational purposes, LOS should not be taken as an index of recovery [2, 3, 15].

Considering the limitations involved in the assessment of LOS, an alternative measure of intermediate recovery may be obtained by assessing the time to achieve standardized hospital discharge criteria ("time to readiness for discharge") [15]. The main advantage of this measure is that multiple factors related to in-hospital recovery are taken into account (e.g., pain, mobility, gastrointestinal function), without the influence of non-clinical factors that affect LOS. In colorectal surgery, minimal criteria for hospital discharge were suggested by consensus (Table 16.1) [17] and a subsequent study supported the validity and reliability of these criteria when measuring intermediate recovery [15].

Table 16.1. Criteria to determine readiness for hospital discharge after colorectal surgery.

Criteria	Endpoints to determine when criteria should be considered to have been achieved
Tolerance of oral intake	Patient should be able to tolerate at least one solid meal without nausea, vomiting, bloating, or worsening abdominal pain. Patient should drink liquids actively (ideally >800–1000 ml/day) and not require intravenous fluid infusion to maintain hydration
Recovery of lower gastrointestinal function	Patient should have passed flatus
Adequate pain control with oral analgesia	Patient should be able to rest and mobilise (sit up and walk, unless unable preoperatively) without significant pain (i.e., patient reports pain is controlled or pain score ≤ 4 on a scale from 0 to 10) while taking oral analgesics
Ability to mobilise and self-care	Patient should be able to sit up, walk, and perform activities of daily living (e.g., go to the toilet, dress, shower, and climb stairs if needed at home) unless unable preoperatively

Although these discharge criteria may be applicable to other gastrointestinal surgeries, further research is warranted to define procedure specific requirements for hospital discharge. A potential problem with this approach is that some criteria may be subjective rather than objective, leading to performance bias if the treating medical and nursing team has a strong early discharge philosophy.

Recovery After Discharge (Late Recovery)

The focus in the late recovery period changes from acute impact of surgery to the return to normality (i.e., return to preoperative health state or improvement). Although clinicians may consider that patients are "sufficiently" recovered when they are ready for hospital discharge, for patients, recovery is only achieved when they are able to "perform activities as they performed before surgery" [18]. Recovery to preoperative health extends way beyond hospital stay. Elderly patients undergoing major abdominal surgery, for example, may take up to 3 months to recover their ability to self-care and up to 6 months to return to preoperative levels of strength and conditioning [4]. In spite of the relevance of monitoring recovery after hospital discharge, late recovery outcomes are rarely reported in ERP research [3].

As late recovery implies return to normal health, this phase should be measured in relation the patient's preoperative (baseline) levels of symptoms, functional status and well-being. In the literature, measures of late recovery often take the form of patient-reported outcomes (PROs; reports coming directly from the patient, generally in the form of questionnaires) [3]. The main advantage of using PROs to measure recovery is that they allow a broad assessment of health status across various domains of health (e.g., pain, fatigue, organ function, physical function). PROs are also relatively inexpensive and easy to administer. A potential disadvantage is that changes in PRO scores may be confounded by postoperative cognitive decline [1], recall bias (i.e., inaccurate recollection of events), and response shift (i.e., change in patients' standards and values in relation to their health status over time) [19]. Multidimensional questionnaires of generic health status (e.g., Short-Form 36 [20]) and recovery-related health status (e.g., Quality of Recovery Score [21] and Postoperative Quality of Life [22]) had their validity supported in the context of late recovery. The validity of questionnaires specifically focused on postoperative fatigue (Identity–Consequence Fatigue Questionnaire) [23] and physical activity (CHAMPS) [24] has also been supported in the literature.

Performance-based outcomes are also often used to measure late recovery. These outcomes involve the objective assessment a patient's performance in a given task. The 6-min walk test (a test of functional walking capacity which measures the distance a patient is able to walk over 6 min in a straight corridor) showed favorable evidence of validity when measuring recovery after colorectal surgery [25]. Other performance-based outcomes previously used in the context of recovery include hand-grip strength (a test of muscle strength using a hand-dynamometer), timed up and go (a test of functional mobility which measures the time required to rise from a chair, walk 3 m, and return to the chair), and functional reach (a test of postural control which measures the maximal distance a patient can reach forward maintaining the feet planted) [4]. Theoretical advantages of performance-based measures include better reproducibility, greater sensitivity to change, and less vulnerability to external influences such as cognition. A potential disadvantage is that they are often too specific to the task being performed, not taking into account the multidimensionality of the postoperative recovery process. Performance-based measures can also be resource intensive, as they often require additional patient visits, trained examiners, and special equipment.

Other Measures Relevant to Recovery

Complication Rates

Although the safety of gastrointestinal surgery has improved considerably in recent years, postoperative complications still occur in a relatively large proportion of patients [26]. There is sound evidence showing that complications have an important negative impact on recovery [4, 27]. In ERP research, complications within 30 days of surgery are commonly reported as an outcome measure [3] and results from a meta-analysis suggest that implementation of ERP is associated with a reduction in complications [28]. Therefore, measuring complication rates is important for appraising the effectiveness of ERPs.

A major challenge when measuring complication rates is the lack of universal consensus on how complications should be defined. This often hampers comparison of data within and between institutions. In the absence of a stable and agreed definition, researchers and clinicians often adopt definitions previously reported in the literature. In the ERP Audit System for example, postoperative complications are defined according to criteria proposed by Buzby et al. [29]. Complications can also be reported in regards to their grade of severity using classification systems such as the Clavien-Dindo [30]. In this system, complications are defined as any deviation from the normal postoperative course and graded from I to V, according to the therapy needed for treatment. The Clavien-Dindo classification has been extensively used in the literature and was validated across various fields of surgery [31]. A more recent configuration incorporates the number and severity of multiple complications occurring in a single patient into a single score from 0 to 100 [32].

Readmission Rates

Readmission rate is also often reported as an outcome in studies evaluating the effectiveness of ERP. This possibly reflects concerns that shortening hospital length of stay may lead to premature discharge and thus increase the risk of hospital readmission. However, evidence suggests that readmission rates are comparable when treating patients with ERPs versus traditional care [28].

Hospital readmission is an unwanted outcome of surgery as it interferes with normal recovery, conflicts with patient expectations, and increases the cost of care. Therefore, monitoring readmission rates is relevant to ensure that patients are discharged when they are sufficiently recovered to manage independently at home. In the ERP literature, readmission rates between 5 and 10 % have been reported [33, 34]. Readmissions above these expected rates indicate the need to review discharge policies and/or post-discharge follow-up schedules. Furthermore, the need for long-term care (e.g., rehabilitation or nursing home placement) is also relevant for institutions implementing ERPs, but often determined by providers other than the hospital or treating surgeons. Long-term care has consequences to the patient, family, and community and capture of this data may not be recorded in hospital records.

Measuring Quality of Recovery

Quality is a subjective assessment and varies with who is asked to rate quality. Operations with a high complication rate may be rated as poor quality by the surgeons, postoperative infarction may be rated as poor quality by the anesthesiologist or intensivist, poor mobility may be rated as poor recovery by nursing staff, severe pain or nausea may be rated as poor quality by the patient, cognitive decline and requirement for nursing home care as poor quality by the patient's family, and high cost of treatment may be rated as poor quality by the hospital administrators. The reader is invited to read a recent comparative review on quality of recovery measurement tools [35].

Interestingly, satisfaction is a poor metric of quality as most patients are satisfied with care despite failure of recovery in multiple domains [5, 6]. Healthcare providers and insurers use satisfaction because it is easy to perform rather than because it is a well-validated metric of quality. The desire to have a simple measurement that will ensure high use with patients (e.g., satisfaction) must be counterbalanced with the poor data output and lack of discriminant validity. Poor data collection will inevitably lead to poor data output.

Patient-reported outcomes are convenient because the survey is completed by the patient and can be done online or via mail. However, the data that is recorded is usually based on patient recall of events and is therefore subjective. For example "please rate your worst pain on the last day" is a different question from the objective question "please rate your pain now." Subjective data is less reliable than objective data, and therefore of less validity than objective data. Recovery is not a single event, but rather a process over time. Many surveys are not designed for repeated measurements over multiple time periods, nor adapted to the changing focus of recovery as time progresses.

The PostopQRS [1] was designed to measure patient-focused outcomes over multiple time periods from surgery to the long term. It was designed to measure recovery in multiple domains (physiological, nociceptive, emotive, cognitive, function (ADLs)) and to report the patient's subjective perspective as well. It is objective rather than subjective (not reliant on recall), and cognitive tests include parallel forms to reduce the impact of learning. It has been validated for face-to-face as well as telephone follow-up [36] and shows good discriminant validity in a number of different patient cohorts [37–39].

Fundamental to detecting poor recovery is the ability to drill down to identify which domains were affected (such as nociception versus cognition). The PostopQRS is designed to report recovery in individual domains enabling diagnosis of which aspect of recovery is poor. This is contrary to many other scales, including the Aldrete scores and traditional health status questionnaires (e.g., Short-Form 36) where a composite numerical outcome is used to represent recovery. Whilst this is statistically convenient, a composite score transforms a data-rich input to a data-poor output. For example, compare a group of patients where cognition is predominantly affected but other recovery domains are normal. The diagnosis of cognitive problems is clinically meaningful compared to "the recovery score was lower in group A."

Quality relates to recovery, which is broadly defined as "a return to baseline values or better." Recovery can be reported for groups or individuals. Individual patient recovery may be useful in real time, as automated scoring systems of recovery (as exists in the online database; see www.pqrsonline.org) allow the clinicians to identify patients with poor recovery, and facilitate interventions to improve their recovery. The concept of identifying early failure of recovery and changing management to improve recovery is a very exciting prospect for patient care, but requires further research to validate that a change in management does produce improvement in recovery.

Summary

Recovery is a complex interplay of outcomes that relate to conventional healthcare metric as well as the more recent recognition of the importance of assessing recovery from the patients' perspective.

Both outcome approaches are important and are complementary to the ERP goal of continually improving protocols based on the best evidence available. Increasingly, recovery after hospital discharge (late recovery) is being recognized as an important aspect of the postoperative recovery process.

Take-Home Messages

- Postoperative recovery is a complex multidimensional construct that is difficult to measure.
- Research has traditionally focused on the impact of ERAS on hospital length of stay, but this outcome is influenced by several confounders and may not reflect recovery.
- Recovery after hospital discharge (late recovery) is rarely reported in ERAS research.
- Outcomes of late recovery reported in the literature include patient-reported and performance-based measures. These types of measure have both strengths and limitations.
- The PostopQRS is a promising tool to appraise recovery both in-hospital and after discharge.

References

1. Royse CF, Newman S, Chung F, et al. Development and feasibility of a scale to assess postoperative recovery the post-operative quality recovery scale. Anesthesiology. 2010;113:892–905.
2. Lee L, Tran T, Mayo NE, et al. What does it really mean to "recover" from an operation? Surgery. 2014;155:211–6.
3. Neville A, Lee L, Antonescu I, et al. Systematic review of outcomes used to evaluate enhanced recovery after surgery. Br J Surg. 2014;101:159–71.
4. Lawrence VA, Hazuda HP, Cornell JE, et al. Functional independence after major abdominal surgery in the elderly. J Am Coll Surg. 2004;199:762–72.
5. Royse CF, Chung F, Newman S, et al. Predictors of patient satisfaction with anaesthesia and surgery care: a cohort study using the postoperative quality of recovery scale. Eur J Anaesthesiol. 2013;30:106–10.
6. Myles PS, Weitkamp B, Jones K, et al. Validity and reliability of a postoperative quality of recovery score: the QoR-40. Br J Anaesth. 2000;84:11–5.
7. Phillips NM, Street M, Kent B, et al. Determining criteria to assess patient readiness for discharge from postanaesthetic care: an international Delphi study. J Clin Nurs. 2014;23(23–24):3345–55.

8. Apfelbaum JL, Silverstein JH, Chung FF, et al. Practice guidelines for postanesthetic care: an updated report by the American Society of Anesthesiologists Task Force on Postanesthetic Care. Anesthesiology. 2013;118:291–307.

9. Phillips NM, Street M, Kent B, et al. Post-anaesthetic discharge scoring criteria: key findings from a systematic review. Int J Evid Based Healthc. 2013;11:275–84.

10. Aldrete JA. The post-anesthesia recovery score revisited. J Clin Anesth. 1995; 7:89–91.

11. Kochs E, Cote D, Deruyck L, et al. Postoperative pain management and recovery after remifentanil-based anaesthesia with isoflurane or propofol for major abdominal surgery. Br J Anaesth. 2000;84:169–73.

12. Strum EM, Szenohradszki J, Kaufman WA, et al. Emergence and recovery characteristics of desflurane versus sevoflurane in morbidly obese adult surgical patients: a prospective, randomized study. Anesth Analg. 2004;99:1848–53.

13. De Baerdemaeker LEC, Jacobs S, Pattyn P, et al. Influence of intraoperative opioid on postoperative pain and pulmonary function after laparoscopic gastric banding: remifentanil TCI vs. sufentanil TO in morbid obesity. Br J Anaesth. 2007;99: 404–11.

14. Maessen JM, Dejong CH, Kessels AG, et al. Length of stay: an inappropriate readout of the success of enhanced recovery programs. World J Surg. 2008;32:971–5.

15. Fiore Jr J, Faragher I, Bialocerkowski A, et al. Time to readiness for discharge' is a valid and reliable measure of short-term recovery after colorectal surgery. World J Surg. 2013;37:2927–34.

16. Gillissen F, Hoff C, Maessen JC, et al. Structured synchronous implementation of an enhanced recovery program in elective colonic surgery in 33 hospitals in the Netherlands. World J Surg. 2013;37:1082–93.

17. Fiore JFJ, Bialocerkowski A, Browning L, et al. Criteria to determine readiness for hospital discharge following colorectal surgery: an international consensus using the Delphi technique. Dis Colon Rectum. 2012;55:416–23.

18. Kleinbeck SV, Hoffart N. Outpatient recovery after laparoscopic cholecystectomy. AORN J. 1994;60:394. 397–8, 401–2.

19. McPhail S, Haines T. Response shift, recall bias and their effect on measuring change in health-related quality of life amongst older hospital patients. Health Qual Life Outcomes. 2010;8:65.

20. Antonescu I, Carli F, Mayo N, et al. Validation of the SF-36 as a measure of postoperative recovery after colorectal surgery. Surg Endosc. 2014;28:3168–78.

21. Paddison JS, Sammour T, Kahokehr A, et al. Development and validation of the surgical recovery scale (SRS). J Surg Res. 2011;167:e85–91.

22. Keller DS, McGee MF, Goyal S, et al. Construct validation and comparison of a novel postoperative quality-of-life metric and the Short Form-36 in colorectal surgery patients. Surgery. 2013;154:690–6.

23. Paddison JS, Booth RJ, Hill AG, et al. Comprehensive assessment of peri-operative fatigue: development of the Identity-Consequence Fatigue Scale. J Psychosom Res. 2006;60:615–22.

24. Feldman LS, Kaneva P, Demyttenaere S, et al. Validation of a physical activity questionnaire (CHAMPS) as an indicator of postoperative recovery after laparoscopic cholecystectomy. Surgery. 2009;146:31–9.

25. Moriello C, Mayo NE, Feldman L, et al. Validating the six-minute walk test as a measure of recovery after elective colon resection surgery. Arch Phys Med Rehabil. 2008;89:1083–9.

26. Schilling PL, Dimick JB, Birkmeyer JD. Prioritizing quality improvement in general surgery. J Am Coll Surg. 2008;207:698–704.

27. Brown SR, Mathew R, Keding A, et al. The impact of postoperative complications on long-term quality of life after curative colorectal cancer surgery. Ann Surg. 2014; 259:916–23.

28. Nicholson A, Lowe MC, Parker J, et al. Systematic review and meta-analysis of enhanced recovery programmes in surgical patients. Br J Surg. 2014;101:172–88.

29. Buzby GP, Knox LS, Crosby LO, et al. Study protocol: a randomized clinical trial of total parenteral nutrition in malnourished surgical patients. Am J Clin Nutr. 1988; 47:366–81.

30. Dindo D, Demartines N, Clavien PA. Classification of surgical complications—a new proposal with evaluation in a cohort of 6336 patients and results of a survey. Ann Surg. 2004;240:205–13.

31. Clavien PA, Barkun J, de Oliveira ML, et al. The Clavien-Dindo classification of surgical complications: five-year experience. Ann Surg. 2009;250:187–96.

32. Slankamenac K, Graf R, Barkun J, et al. The comprehensive complication index: a novel continuous scale to measure surgical morbidity. Ann Surg. 2013; 258(1):1–7.

33. Lawrence JK, Keller DS, Samia H, et al. Discharge within 24 to 72 hours of colorectal surgery is associated with low readmission rates when using Enhanced Recovery Pathways. J Am Coll Surg. 2013;216:390–4.

34. Gustafsson UO, Hausel J, Thorell A, et al. Adherence to the enhanced recovery after surgery protocol and outcomes after colorectal cancer surgery. Arch Surg. 2011; 146:571–7.

35. Bowyer A, Jakobsson J, Ljungqvist O, et al. A review of the scope and measurement of postoperative quality of recovery. Anaesthesia. 2014;69(11):1266–78.

36. Royse CF, Newman S, Williams Z, et al. A human volunteer study to identify variability in performance in the cognitive domain of the postoperative quality of recovery scale. Anesthesiology. 2013;119:576–81.

37. Newman S, Wilkinson DJ, Royse CF. Assessment of early cognitive recovery after surgery using the Post-operative Quality of Recovery Scale. Acta Anaesthesiol Scand. 2014;58:185–91.

38. Royse CF, Williams Z, Ye G, et al. Knee surgery recovery: Post-operative Quality of Recovery Scale comparison of age and complexity of surgery. Acta Anaesthesiol Scand. 2014;58:660–7.

39. Royse CF, Williams Z, Purser S, et al. Recovery after nasal surgery vs. tonsillectomy: discriminant validation of the Postoperative Quality of Recovery Scale. Acta Anaesthesiol Scand. 2014;58:345–51.

Key References

Lee L, Tran T, Mayo NE, Carli F, Feldman LS. What does it really mean to "recover" from an operation? Surgery. 2014;155(2):211–6.

Neville A, Lee L, Antonescu I, Mayo NE, Vassiliou MC, Fried GM, et al. Systematic review of outcomes used to evaluate enhanced recovery after surgery. Br J Surg. 2014;101(3):159–71.

Fiore Jr J, Faragher I, Bialocerkowski A, et al. Time to readiness for discharge' is a valid and reliable measure of short-term recovery after colorectal surgery. World J Surg. 2013;37:2927–34.

Royse CF, Newman S, Chung F, et al. Development and feasibility of a scale to assess postoperative recovery: the post-operative quality recovery scale. Anesthesiology. 2010;113:892–905.

Part II
Creation and Implementation
of an Enhanced Recovery Program

17. Overcoming Barriers to the Implementation of an Enhanced Recovery After Surgery Program

Emily Pearsall and Allan Okrainec

Despite the well-established benefits of enhanced recovery after surgery programs (ERPs) such as hastened recovery, reduced hospital costs, and increased patient satisfaction, the reported uptake of these programs can be slow and haphazard [1–4]. This chapter presents common barriers and enablers to implementation of an ERP as well as implementation strategies that may be used to effectively implement an ERP.

Evidence suggests that when uptake of a quality improvement program like ERP is slow, it may be important to identify and address local barriers and enablers [5–7]. The process of understanding barriers and enablers is thought to be important because they may be effective predictors of healthcare professionals' intentions to change behavior [8]. As well, assessing barriers and enablers can assist with developing tailored strategies that address these issues and support successful implementation. The assessment of barriers and enablers to knowledge use is an important component of the Knowledge to Action (KTA) framework described by Graham et al. as seen in Fig. 17.1 [5]. Of note is that different disciplines may identify specific barriers and enablers to their roles in the implementation of new evidence. Therefore, it is essential to identify the potential barriers and facilitators for different groups of stakeholders.

L.S. Feldman et al. (eds.), *The SAGES / ERAS®*
Society Manual of Enhanced Recovery Programs for
Gastrointestinal Surgery, DOI 10.1007/978-3-319-20364-5_17,
© Springer International Publishing Switzerland 2015

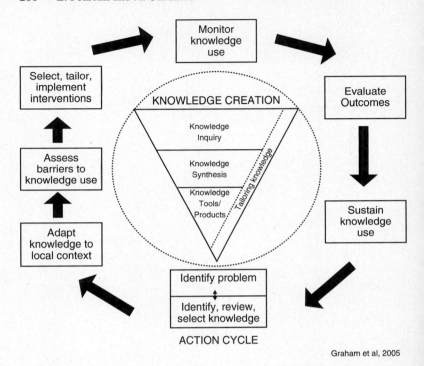

Fig. 17.1. Knowledge to Action Cycle (adapted from Graham ID, Logan J, Harrison MB, et al. Lost in knowledge translation: time for a map? J Contin Educ Health Prof 2006;26(1):13–24, with permission).

Common Barriers to Implementation of Enhanced Recovery Programs

Grol and Grimshaw suggest that three common issues affect whether new evidence is introduced into clinical practice: the attributes of the evidence itself, barriers and facilitators to changing practice, and the effectiveness of the implementation strategies [9]. The strength of the evidence supporting the individual elements included in ERPs is discussed throughout this manual and will not be further discussed here. The literature on barriers to adoption of new evidence suggests that it is important to be aware of all potential barriers prior to implementation. Different barriers to change can be identified at the level of the individual professional, the patient, the healthcare team, the organization, or the greater community [9]. As well, studies suggest that different healthcare professionals may perceive different factors as barriers. For physicians, commonly stated barriers include organizational constraints, prevailing practices and social opinions (i.e., current standard of practice, key opinion leaders disagreeing with the proposed change), and personal barriers such as not being aware of or believing the evidence, or not wanting to change practice [9, 10]. For nurses, barriers involve perceptions that they do not have the time, resources, and access to persons who can locate the evidence and translate it for use in practice. Other constraints include lack of support from administration and other healthcare professionals. Unfortunately, there is limited information available about barriers to implementing evidence as a multidisciplinary team.

To address this gap in knowledge, the implementation of enhanced recovery after surgery (iERAS) program at the University of Toronto conducted a qualitative study to better understand the multidisciplinary perioperative teams' current beliefs regarding enablers and barriers to successful adoption of a local, university-wide ERP. Semi-structured face-to-face audio-recorded interviews were conducted with general surgeons, anesthesiologists, and ward nurses at each of the seven University of Toronto affiliated adult teaching hospitals. The results suggested that overall, interviewees were supportive of the implementation of a standardized ERP.

The most commonly cited barriers to adoption of an ERP related to time and personnel restrictions required to develop the guideline, limited hospital resources (financial, staffing, space restrictions, and education), perceived resistance from other members of the perioperative team, necessity of engagement of the whole perioperative multidisciplinary team, lack of knowledge about the benefits of specific interventions in the program, perceptions about patients' social and cultural values, and institutional barriers. Institutional barriers such as lack of nursing staff and lack of financial resources from the hospital were seen as barriers by many interviewees. At an individual level, resistance to change by various members of the perioperative team was seen as the primary barrier. As well, many participants felt that poor communication and lack of collaboration among the team members were barriers.

When the data were analyzed at the discipline level, there were a few notable differences and similarities. Surgeons, anesthesiologists, and nurses all felt that their discipline and the others would be resistant to changing their practice and this would be the biggest barrier to adoption of an ERP. Interestingly, each discipline acknowledged their peers as being resistant to change and also suggested that other disciplines were also resistant to change, suggesting that resistance is a systemic issue and not discipline specific.

With respect to enablers, most participants suggested that in order for the program to succeed, they required a standardized guideline based on best evidence, standardized pre- and postoperative order sets, education for the entire perioperative multidisciplinary team, patients and families, and a hospital ERP champion. Surgeons and anesthesiologists placed a high level of importance on having the interventions based on high-quality evidence while the nurses were more concerned with patient education and patient satisfaction. All disciplines suggested that increased communication between disciplines would be required.

Overall, the findings from these interviews suggested that there are many barriers to implementation of an ERP; however the most common barriers related to the multidisciplinary nature of the program. Based on the many known barriers to adoption of new evidence, numerous strategies may be required in order to effectively implement an ERP.

Overcoming the Barriers: Selection of Strategies

There are many known strategies to increase the use of clinical practice guidelines in healthcare. Systematic reviews have evaluated the effectiveness of different strategies with each resulting in small-to-moderate changes in practice. Table 17.1 illustrates the overall effect of each major implementation strategy based on Cochrane reviews of effectiveness [11–16].

Table 17.1. Summary of Cochrane reviews on the effectiveness of interventions.

Intervention	Author, year	Included studies	Effect
Audit and feedback	Ivers et al. (2012) [11]	140 RCTs	4.3 % (0.5–16 %)
Reminders	Arditi et al. (2012) [12]	32 RCTs	7.0 % (4–16 %)
Continuing educational meetings and workshops	Forsetlund et al. (2009) [13]	81 RCTs	6.0 % (2–15 %)
Educational outreach visits	O'Brien et al. (2007) [14]	65 RCTs	6.0 % (4–16 %)
Opinion leaders	Flodgren et al. (2011) [15]	18 RCTs	12.0 % (6–15 %)
Printed educational meetings	Giguere et al. (2012) [16]	14 RCTs and 31 non-RCTs	2.0 % (0–11 %)

Due to the varied evidence to support implementation strategies and to be consistent with the Knowledge to Action Cycle, the enablers and barriers identified in our study were used to select implementation strategies [5]. As there were multiple barriers and enablers, the iERAS program developed a multipronged implementation strategy that involved all disciplines and that was applicable to all academic hospitals. The implementation strategy included assigning champions, development of standardized materials, development of educational tools, audit and feedback, support from hospital administration, and communication strategies.

Identification of Local Champions at Each Hospital

One of the most important strategies when implementing an ERP is the identification of local champions. It is important that a champion from each discipline be identified including a nurse champion, anesthesia champion and surgeon champion. Identifying a champion in hospital administration can also be a useful strategy to get institutional buy-in and help secure resources for the program. The main role of the champions is to lead implementation. The champions should meet regularly with members of the perioperative team and facilitate education and communication by presenting multidisciplinary educational rounds, in-services, and teaching sessions to increase awareness and acceptance of the guideline recommendations. Having discipline-specific champions is important to address a number of barriers. First, discipline-specific champions are the foundation and leaders of the local ERP team. Having a point person from each discipline allows for open communication between these leaders representing the key stakeholders. Second, discipline-specific champions are key to addressing discipline specific issues, and concerns. For example, nurses may be concerned about the amount of time it will take them to mobilize the patient starting on the day of surgery. The nurse champion would work with the team to discuss these issues specifically and come up with a plan that was agreeable to the rest of the unit. The champion also acts as a liaison between other disciplines. For example, ward nurses may be best able to identify issues with adherence to the guidelines specific to an individual surgeons. The nurse champion would communicate this to the surgeon champion who would then be responsible for following up with these surgeons to understand and address their concerns.

Engagement of Surgical Residents

In many institutions surgical residents are important members of the surgical team and play a central role in managing patients postoperatively. They rotate on and off services frequently. Thus, resident education, given as seminars as well as printed material, is an important aspect of an ERP. Providing material such as pathways, standardized orders, and guidelines in digital format, such as a smartphone app, may also be useful for residents since this is the usual tool used by residents to find information.

Development of Standardized Materials

Having standardized materials, such as pre-printed orders, is an essential strategy to increase compliance. These order sets act as a constant reminder to staff regarding prescription of antibiotics, thromboprophylaxis, early feeding, and early removal of drains and catheters. As each center will have its own order entry system, it is important for the organization to be willing to modify these orders to reflect the recommendations. In addition to order sets, clinical pathways are also an important element that may be of assistance to all healthcare professionals. Clinical pathways detail all guideline recommendations over the patient's entire surgical journey, whereas standardized orders only include recommendations that may be added to orders (e.g., choice of antibiotics or use of lidocaine). For example, a clinical pathway would outline recommendations such as preoperative patient education, fluid management, and postoperative mobilization. Clinical pathways outline daily goals and explicitly state each stakeholder's roles and responsibilities. These pathways allow members of the perioperative team to understand all steps in the patient's journey and provide the same information to all patients and families.

Development of Educational Tools

Providing education to the perioperative team as well as to patients and their families is a very important element in successful implementation of an ERP. Educational tools such as posters, reminder cards, and slide decks help champions provide a consistent educational message. Clinical pathways and care maps that provide a visual depiction of the pathway help decrease variability between practitioners and guide the care of common postoperative complications. An expamle of a clinical pathway in ERP is the management of urinary retention. Including anesthesia checklists to guide intraoperative fluid management, and creating daily flowcharts for nurses also support implementation.

An integrated patient education resource is also an essential element of this program. This should highlight information that the patient and their family need to know about the entire surgical journey. Examples of patient education resources included printed materials such as educational booklets or digital information such as videos or websites. More specifically, these resources should provide information on what is expected of them as active participants in their recovery and the proposed milestones. As part of the iERAS program, patients are asked to complete a daily "Patient Activity Log" that is included in their patient education booklet where information on their activity, oral intake, chewing gum, pain control, and elimination is recorded. This has been strongly embraced by patients and nurses as it provides information to healthcare workers while also reinforcing expectations of patients. As well, patients have felt that it empowers them in their recovery.

Audit and Feedback

Audit and feedback is an essential part of the implementation strategy as feeding back information assists with maintaining or increasing engagement of the perioperative team, as well as increasing compliance with ERP recommendations. A Cochrane review suggested that audit and feedback on average is associated with a 12 % increase in compliance with guideline recommendations. Many databases exist to assist centres to collect and feedback information [15]. Despite the audit mechanism, it is important to feedback these results to all members of the perioperative team on a regular basis. The reports should provide data on a variety of process and outcome measures, so individual hospitals can benchmark their performance against pre-implementation data. The data from the reports are also meant to be used to assess compliance and develop specific strategies to improve performance at their own hospital.

Support from Hospital Administration

Many barriers originate at the organizational level of the hospital. It is suggested to speak with the CEO and leaders of all related departments including surgery, nursing, and quality to ensure that members of administration are supportive and engaged. Having hospital administration buy-in to the program and communicating this support to the front-line staff proved to be a very useful strategy in the iERAS program to increase buy-in from healthcare professionals.

Conclusion

While there is support for implementation of ERP, many barriers exist. The most commonly cited barriers of ERP are time and personnel restrictions, limited hospital resources, resistance from members of the perioperative team, necessity of engagement of the whole perioperative multidisciplinary team, lack of education, patients' social and cultural values, and institutional barriers. The most common enablers are a standardized guideline based on best evidence, standardized pre- and postoperative order sets, education for the entire perioperative multidisciplinary team, patients and families, and a hospital ERP champion. The literature suggests that various implementation strategies must be used in order to increase uptake. Common strategies include identification of local champions (nursing, anesthesia, and surgery), engagement of surgical residents, development of standardized materials (order sets, care pathways, guidelines, etc), development of educational tools (posters, reminders, slide decks), educational booklet and video, audit and feedback, and eliciting support from hospital administration.

Take-Home Messages

- It is essential to understand and address local barriers and enablers prior to implementation.
- Multiple implementation strategies are required to successfully engage all members of the perioperative team.

References

1. Donohoe CL, Nguyen M, Cook J, et al. Fast-track protocols in colorectal surgery. Surgeon. 2011;9(2):95–103.
2. Maessen J, Dejong CH, Hausel J, et al. A protocol is not enough to implement an enhanced recovery programme for colorectal resection. Br J Surg. 2007;94:224–31.

3. Gustafsson UO, Hausel J, Thorell A, et al. Adherence to the enhanced recovery after surgery protocol and outcomes after colorectal cancer surgery. Arch Surg. 2011;146: 571–7.
4. Kahokehr A, Sammour T, Zargar-Shoshtari K, et al. Implementation of ERAS and how to overcome the barriers. Int J Surg. 2009;7:16–9.
5. Graham ID, Logan J, Harrison MB, et al. Lost in knowledge translation: time for a map? J Contin Educ Health Prof. 2006;26(1):13–24.
6. Straus S, Tetroe J, Graham I, editors. Knowledge translation in health care: moving from evidence to practice. 2nd ed. London: BMJ Books; 2013.
7. Pearsall EA, Meghji Z, Pitzul KB et al. A qualitative study to understand the barriers and enablers in implementing an Enhanced Recovery After Surgery program. Ann Surg. 2014; [Epub ahead of print].
8. Legare F, Zhang P. Barriers and facilitators – strategies for identification and measurement. In: Straus S, Tetroe J, Graham I, editors. Knowledge translation in health care: moving from evidence to practice. 2nd ed. London: BMJ Books; 2013.
9. Grol R, Grimshaw J. From best evidence to best practice: effective implementation of change in patients' care. Lancet. 2003;362(9391):1225–30.
10. Cabana MD, Rand CS, Powe NR, Wu AW, Wilson MH, Abboud PA, Rubin HR. Why don't physicians follow clinical practice guidelines? A framework for improvement. JAMA. 1999;282(15):1458–65.
11. Ivers N, Jamtvedt G, Flottorp S, et al. Audit and feedback: effects on professional practice and healthcare outcomes. Cochrane Database Syst Rev. 2012;6:CD000259.
12. Arditi C, Rege-Walther M, Wyatt JC, et al. Computer-generated reminders delivered on paper to healthcare professionals; effects on professional practice and health care outcomes. Cochrane Database Syst Rev. 2012;12:CD001175.
13. Forsetlund L, Bjorndal A, Rashidian A, et al. Continuing education meetings and workshops: effects on professional practice and health care outcomes. Cochrane Database Syst Rev. 2009;2:CD003030.
14. O'Brien MA, Rogers S, Jamtvedt G, et al. Educational outreach visits: effects on professional practice and health care outcomes. Cochrane Database Syst Rev. 2007; 4:CD000409.
15. Flodgren G, Parmelli E, Doumit G, et al. Local opinion leaders: effects on professional practice and health care outcomes. Cochrane Database Syst Rev. 2011;8: CD000125.
16. Giguere A, Legare F, Grimshaw J, et al. Printed educational materials: effects on professional practice and healthcare outcomes. Cochrane Database Syst Rev. 2012; 10:CD004398.

Key References

McLeod RS, Aarts MA, Chueng F, Eskicioglu C, Forbes SS, Gotlib Conn L et al. Development of an Enhanced Recovery After Surgery guideline and implementation strategy based on the knowledge-to-action cycle. Ann Surg. In Press.

Pearsall EA, Meghji Z, Pitzul KB, Aarts MA, McKenzie M, McLeod RS, Okrainec A. A qualitative study to understand the barriers and enablers in implementing an Enhanced Recovery After Surgery program. Ann Surg. Accessed 18 Mar 2014 [Epub ahead of print] PubMed.

Nadler A, Pearsall EA, Victor JC, Aarts MA, Okrainec A, McLeod RS. Understanding surgical residents' postoperative practices and barriers and enablers to the implementation of an Enhanced Recovery After Surgery (ERAS) guideline. J Surg Educ. 2014;71(4):632–8. doi: 10.1016/j.jsurg.2014.01.014. Epub 5 May 2014. PubMed.

18. Introducing Enhanced Recovery Programs into Practice: Lessons Learned from the ERAS® Society Implementation Program

Olle Ljungqvist and Martin Hübner

Apart from developing new knowledge, educational material, and creating network globally for these missions, a key focus of the ERAS® Society is to help units to implement best practice and make use of the guidelines. This chapter will discuss The ERAS® Society implementation program specifically, but the principles are applicable to any quality improvement or knowledge translation project, where planning, audit, and revision are fundamental to success.

Why ERAS Implementation Is Needed

From surveys [1] and national data on length of stay following defined procedures, it is obvious that best practice in perioperative care as summarized in ERAS® Society guidelines is not in wide use. For instance in the UK (Enhanced Recovery Partnership, NHS report 2013) and in Sweden (Swedish colonic cancer registry 2013), the average length of stay after colonic resections is still 8 days and if ERAS was in use, these figures would be 4–6 days or even shorter. That prompted the ERAS Group (see Chap. 28, "ERAS Society") to develop a program to help other units implement ERAS. This work was pioneered by the Dutch group led by Cornelius deJong and Jose Maessen in collaboration with the Dutch Institute for Healthcare Improvement Kwaliteitsinstituut (CBO).

L.S. Feldman et al. (eds.), *The SAGES / ERAS®*
Society Manual of Enhanced Recovery Programs for
Gastrointestinal Surgery, DOI 10.1007/978-3-319-20364-5_18,
© Springer International Publishing Switzerland 2015

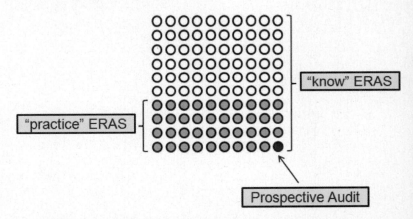

Fig. 18.1. ERAS implementation: wish and reality. Results of an informal survey among colorectal specialists in January 2012 and repeated with 200 US surgeons in February 2014: Every single surgeon was aware of the *enhanced recovery after surgery* (ERAS) concept. About 40 % of the respondents declared to have an ERAS program running in their unit. However, only 1 % of the departments performed a prospective audit in order to monitor clinical outcomes and the actual application of the intended protocol (compliance).

While many units employ parts of the ERAS protocols, and believe they are actually performing ERAS in their practice, it is impossible to know the details of ERAS protocol usage without an ongoing, in-depth continuous audit that includes process measures (Fig. 18.1). The patient goes through several departments and units in the care pathway and hundreds of employees may be involved in their care. This includes personnel in preoperative and outpatient facilities, operating units and theaters, postoperative care and postoperative recovery room (PACU), intensive care units, and surgical wards. In each unit the staff focus is on the care they provide during the period of time the patient is under their supervision. The specific focus varies greatly between units. For instance anesthesia has to secure vital functions such as circulation, breathing, pain management, and muscle relaxation during surgery, while the ward has the objective to facilitate the return of functions such as mobilization, gut function, and eating while also managing pain control and other specialized matters such as stomas. Rarely if ever do these two groups of professionals meet and exchange ideas around their respective objectives or how they achieve it. To an even lesser degree do they discuss, let alone make choices, to facilitate the objectives of each other's missions. The anesthesia personnel may not be aware to what extent their choices influence the return of gut function for instance, since they are rarely involved with this part of the recovery. Nor do the ward nurses know that there are choices made earlier in the pathway that have a major impact on their chances of helping patients eat normally. This is just one example of how important the overview and collaboration between the departments and professionals is to put optimal ERAS care in place in practice. There are many more if you start to scrutinize the care pathway for major surgical patients.

This is the fundamental starting point for improvement of care— understanding the complexity of the pathway and securing the involvement of everyone on staff along that pathway. This is also the starting point for the ERAS® Society's implementation program.

The ERAS Team

To participate in the ERAS® Implementation Program (EIP), each participating unit is asked to form a multiprofessional and multidisciplinary team. They are also required to have an administrator sign an agreement to confirm that the team will have sufficient time away from their other duties to perform the tasks involved in the ERAS® Implementation Program (see below).

Forming a team consisting of all the professionals involved in the entire patient journey is the key to successful implementation. That means that a surgeon, an anesthesiologist, PACU personnel and, importantly, nurses from each of the units involved in perioperative care form the basis for the local ERAS team. In addition, many units have very good dietitians and/or physiotherapists and they can also play an important part in an ERAS team.

The team will select a team leader, generally a physician, who will assume the overall medical responsibility for the group and the implementation process. They also select an ERAS coordinator, usually a nurse, who will be available about half time or longer, depending on the number of patients involved. The ERAS coordinator is reasonable for adapting provided material to produce local order sets, care paths, memos, slides, posters, and other information to support implementation. During the EIP, teams receive templates of these documents that conform with the ERAS® Society guidelines and the Interactive Audit System (see below). The ERAS coordinator also prepares presentations to educate and provide information to the different units involved. Finally, but very importantly, the ERAS coordinator will be tasked with collecting data for the Interactive Audit that is used as part of the implementation process (see below). The team leader and the ERAS coordinator will also be the main contact persons with the EIP trainers and coaches.

The ERAS team should make time available for weekly or biweekly meetings during the process of implementation. They will also require time to ensure that everyone involved in the care of the patient is fully informed about the changes that will be made with the introduction of the ERAS protocol. Listening to the various professionals during this information process is important to understanding local barriers (see Chap. 18, "Overcoming Barriers to the implementation of an ERAS program"). They will also establish a system to provide continuous feedback to all units involved in the care process. For this to happen, it is essential that the leadership of the surgical and anesthesia/intensive care departments agree to make this program a priority. In order to resource the team appropriately, leadership should be informed of the evidence suggesting the significant clinical and economic benefits achieved with proper implementation of ERAS.

As reviewed in the first section of this manual, each of the interventions included in the ERAS protocols is supported by evidence. They are treatments in use worldwide and there is ample data supporting the safety and benefits of the approach. The "magic" of ERAS is to have best practices being used in as many patients as possible. That said, compliance with each element in an ERAS protocol does not need be 100 % to achieve results. There will be exceptions to the use of some of the elements for certain patients. But then again, many units reporting the use of ERAS actually comply with only around 50 % of the interventions when they start out, and an increase in overall adherence even to the 70 % range is associated with improved outcomes (faster recovery and fewer complications) [2] (Fig. 18.2).

The ERAS® Implementation Program

The ERAS® Implementation Program (EIP) brings together several units from different hospitals to a series of four workshops over a period of 8–10 months (Fig. 18.3). During these workshops a very standardized process of implementation is used, developed and tailored for ERAS from the Breakthrough methodology described by the Institute of Health Improvement [3]. A medical expert in ERAS and a Change management coach trained in ERAS Implementation run the program. They are both

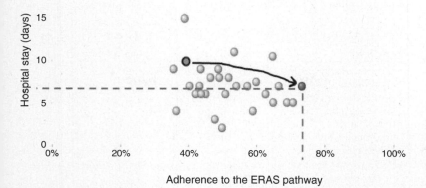

Adherence to the ERAS pathway

Fig. 18.2. Outcomes of systematic ERAS implementation. This example describes a typical evolution of performance by implementation of the *enhanced recovery after surgery* (ERAS) pathway. Adherence to all the elements of the ERAS pathway is plotted against hospital length of stay and every center is depicted by a *grey dot*. At the university hospital Lausanne, ERAS principles were already applied before systematic implementation but the actual adherence was only 40 % (*red dot*). After systematic implementation, compliance could be nearly doubled and hospital stay after colorectal resections was subsequently reduced from 10 to 6 days.

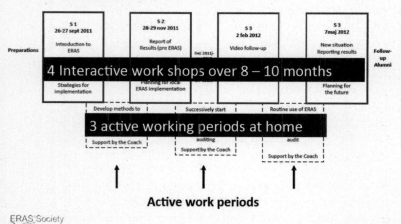

Fig. 18.3. Outline of the ERAS® Implementation Program. Over 8–10 months period, four workshops are run. In between workshops each group is active in their own hospital while being coached by the ERAS trainers. (Courtesy of the ERAS Society [www.erassociety.org]).

selected by the ERAS® Society and have their own personal experience in ERAS implementation and ERAS care. The hospitals get the basic information on what ERAS care is about, the outline of the implementation program, how they are to work, and how to use Interactive Audit to have the team continuously review their practice and their outcomes.

Between workshops the teams have tailored coaching from the Trainers helping them resolve their specific issues. When coming back to work shops each team reports about their progress, problems and how they are tackling them, and the results; they also make their plans for the next work period.

From the clinical perspective, the evidence-based ERAS guidelines need to be translated into clinical routine of the respective hospitals; the considerable change from traditional practice is best achieved using institutional protocols and integrated clinical care pathways (Fig. 18.4).

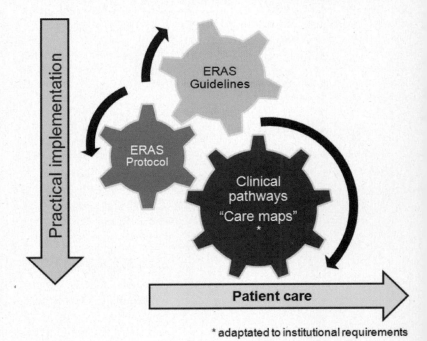

Fig. 18.4. Mechanism of ERAS implementation. For successful implementation of a comprehensive *enhanced recovery after surgery* (ERAS) pathway, several steps need to be performed. First, an institutional ERAS protocol is established which should adhere closely to the evidence-based ERAS recommendations. The protocol is then translated into daily routine by use of integrated clinical care pathways.

The teams are advised to spend ample time preparing for the changes by reviewing their actual care as captured by the Interactive Audit System. The work period between the first and second workshop is about 2 months during which time the teams gather the baseline data on their practice. The data collected during the first work period will be reviewed during Session 2. From then on the entire team will know where their practice needs to change based on real data.

During the second work period the team starts off with one patient that they aim to take through the care completely according to the ERAS protocol. They then review that first patient together and make changes, and identify problem and issues before continuing to have another couple of patients go through the process. After each week, they review their process and their outcomes together, and on a regular basis involve and report back to all units involved. Over time they gradually bring in more complex patients to have them all being treated according to the protocol of ERAS while continuously reviewing their outcomes and processes using the interactive audit.

During the work periods the teams stay in touch with the ERAS coaches and teachers on a regular basis, and the teams then come together and report in the last two workshops. The last one is usually held about 9 months after the start and by this time the teams usually have made substantial changes in practice and improved their outcomes. In the initial experience, the Dutch group implemented the ERAS protocol in over 35 hospitals in the Netherlands and managed to have the hospitals reduce length of stay from 9 to 6 days following colonic resections during a 1-year program [4]. Similar experiences have been reported by other centers (Fig. 18.2). Longer term follow-up suggests that these improvements in general are sustainable but variable between different units [5]. Most of the experience of the ERAS Implementation Program is from colorectal surgery [3], but improvements in recovery have also been shown after major gynecology [6] and preliminary data indicated success for ERAS implementation in cystectomy [7].

The cost for participation in the ERAS Implementation program varies between countries (so far the program has been run with hospitals form Sweden, Norway, Switzerland, France, UK, and Canada). The average cost for the entire team to participate in the training and use of the ERAS Interactive Audit System (see below) for 1 year is around 25,000 USD (for details : info@erassociety.org). It has been estimated that the total expenses for the course including personnel time etc. are covered by the first 20 ERAS patients and the average savings for the first 50 patients are around 2000 USD per patient [3].

Challenges of Implementing ERAS

As outlined above there are many people and professionals involved in the perioperative care of patients undergoing major surgery. All of them have had their training and all have their own habits and feel more or less comfortable doing things they are used to. Changing to a new way of managing a patient creates some anxiety in most health professionals, especially since their work involves the care of fellow men and women. While you know what to expect from a certain way of dealing with a problem, being asked to use another method makes you less certain and it will take time before you have reached the same comfort with the new method.

Given that in most units that have been through ERAS training the compliance with the ERAS protocol is around 50 %, this means many treatments need to be changed and a lot of people will need to be involved and asked to change their ways. This is the real challenge of the implementation. And this is why making the change needs very thorough preparation. That means there has to be proper information given to everyone well ahead of the start of the actual protocol being used. There needs to be time for discussions and for people to actually study the data behind some of the changes, as one can expect opposition both openly and also more silently. It is very important that this is dealt with the appropriate respect and understanding that people need time to make change and most people actually do not like change at all. And using actual data is very powerful as well by showing everyone what is actually happening and not allowing unfounded beliefs to rule.

So expect the change to take some time. It is important that the team running the ERAS project is fully on board and united and that they themselves feel comfortable with running the protocol. The ERAS team has to gain firsthand experience themselves to be able to help other colleagues to follow the pathways when they are to be more universally employed.

Essentials of a successful ERAS implementation are given in Fig. 18.5. A multidisciplinary team approach is pivotal and necessary to establish the institutional ERAS protocol and monitor its application and clinical outcomes. Critical analysis of the performance helps to overcome resistance and convince the skeptics. The crucial role of prospective audit is outlined below and in Chap. 20.

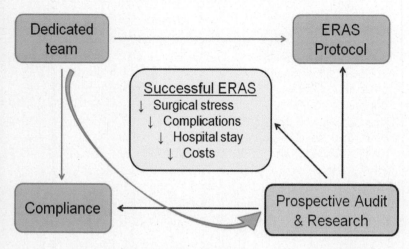

Fig. 18.5. Requirements for a successful ERAS program. A successful *enhanced recovery after surgery* (ERAS) program has been shown to improve surgical stress response and hence to reduce postoperative complications. Beneficial side effects are reduced hospital length of stay and costs. Considerable efforts are needed to implement and to maintain a successful ERAS program: First, a multidisciplinary team needs to be formed. Important members of the team are surgeons, anesthetists, nurses, nutritionists, and hospital administration; the team leader is typically a senior surgeon. The ERAS team establishes an institutional ERAS protocol based on published recommendations. The pathway should be applied with a high compliance to the various care processes. Application of the intended protocol and clinical outcomes are prospectively monitored in order to identify eventual problems and thus to improve the performance. Regular team meetings (every 2–4 weeks) help to sustain good clinical results after initial implementation. Finally, clinical research helps to develop ERAS care further.

ERAS® Interactive Audit System (EIAS)

Given the complexity of the perioperative care pathways for major surgery, a key to successful implementation is having the staff understand that what they do influences the next in line. The published ERAS Guidelines, as well as the first section of this manual, outline elements known to have impact on outcomes and each and every component has a role in the pathway. Understanding the impact of adherence to the guidelines and outcomes at the local level facilities the change process

Table 18.1. ERAS® Interactive Audit System has the system developed for a number of surgeries and more is under development.

Current	Under development	In planning
Colonic resection	Liver resection	ENT surgery
Rectal resection	Hip replacement	Breast reconstruction
Pancreatic resection	Knee replacement	Non cardiac thoracic surgery
Cystectomy	Obesity surgery	Esophageal resections
Gastric resection	Nephrectomy	
	Major gynecology	

to make the right choices. To support the teams in this process, the ERAS Society, working with its IT partner, Encare AB, created the ERAS® Interactive Audit System, an online software tool that is used during and after the ERAS implementation Program. The system is developed to help units implement ERAS but also to continuously update their practice and to have ongoing audit available in real time. The system is updated as the ERAS Society guidelines are modified and the number of available procedures is growing (Table 18.1).

In the Interactive audit system teams collect and input patient information, adherence to ERAS guidelines care processes, perioperative data (surgery and anesthesia), and recovery milestones. The follow-up is for 30 days postoperatively. Modules for longer follow-up are under construction.

The system manages the data so that the team can review all patients that have been discharged in real time. The system allows immediate access to all data and has a series of built-in features that let the users drill down into the data set to check their outcomes with regard to recovery of the patient, the length of stay, and complications and symptoms that may delay discharge (Fig. 18.6).

The ERAS® Interactive Audit System is a tool to help the team analyze underlying problems and find solutions. During the training period, the ERAS® Interactive Audit System allows the teams to see what is actually happening to their patients throughout the entire perioperative care period. This is usually the first time ever that the team can see what care process they actually collectively deliver. This is also the first time they can connect outcomes results with the processes of care and focus efforts on changes for treatment items that are not yet in place. As they make the changes, they can follow the changes in real time and report back to the units involved, including any impact with regard to patient outcomes. The system also allows comparison of the data with other units on the system.

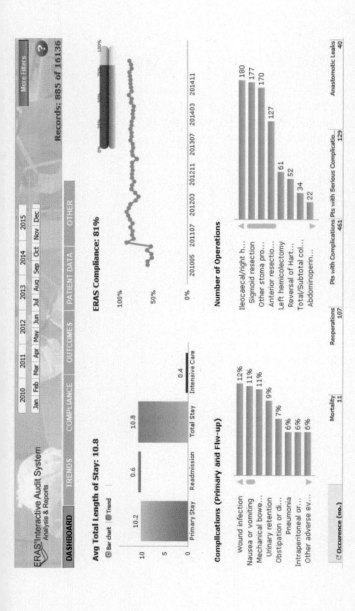

Fig. 18.6. ERAS® Interactive Audit System. The figure shows the Dashboard that gives the overview of the data with average length of stay, surgical approaches, complications, and main outcomes alongside the compliance with the ERAS Society guidelines over time. From the dashboard in-depth information is available momentarily for the ERAS team to review. (Courtesy of the ERAS Society [www.erassociety.org]).

The ERAS Society Implementation Network

The ERAS Society is building a network of ERAS trainers via the Societies Centers of Excellence. These Centers are selected on the basis of their experience and their capacity to help the Society train other units in their region or country. They may have undergone the Implementation program themselves. The process of becoming a Trainer in ERAS required use of ERAS principles at a high level and completing a "Train the Trainers" course run by the ERAS Society. ERAS Implementation programs are running in several countries all over the world including Norway, Sweden, Switzerland, UK, France, and Canada. In addition Centers of Excellence have been formed in a number of other countries including the USA, Poland, Spain, France, The Philippines, South Africa, Argentina, and with many more lining up to join the mission.

The vision is to have a large system available for many users to facilitate research and also have a system that can help units adopt new evidence as it emerges at a much faster rate than today.

References

1. Lassen K, et al. Patterns in current perioperative practice: survey of colorectal surgeons in five northern European countries. BMJ. 2005;330(7505):1420–1.
2. Gustafsson UO, et al. Adherence to the enhanced recovery after surgery protocol and outcomes after colorectal cancer surgery. Arch Surg. 2011;146(5):571–7.
3. Roulin D, et al. Cost-effectiveness of the implementation of an enhanced recovery protocol for colorectal surgery. Br J Surg. 2013;100(8):1108–14.
4. Gillissen F, et al. Structured synchronous implementation of an enhanced recovery program in elective colonic surgery in 33 hospitals in The Netherlands. World J Surg. 2013;37(5):1082–93.
5. Gillissen F, et al. Sustainability of an Enhanced Recovery After Surgery Program (ERAS) in colonic surgery. World J Surg. 2015;39(2):526–33.
6. Wijk L, et al. Implementing a structured Enhanced Recovery After Surgery (ERAS) protocol reduces length of stay after abdominal hysterectomy. Acta Obstet Gynecol Scand. 2014;93(8):749–56.
7. Persson B, Carringer M, Andrén O, Andersson SO, Carlsson J, Ljungqvist O. Initial experiences with the enhanced recovery after surgery (ERAS®) protocol in open radical cystectomy. Scand J Urol. 2015;7:1–6.

19. Enhanced Recovery Programs: Making the Business Case

Anthony J. Senagore

The various components and patient benefits of enhanced recovery after surgery protocols are more extensively discussed elsewhere in this publication. The focus of this discussion is on the institutional benefits related to adoption of a strong Enhanced Recovery Programs (ERP). The two major sources of institutional benefit are related to reductions in resource consumption and potentially avoidable complications. The net result of these benefits is improved quality of care and lower cost of care. There is often concern regarding the complexity and cost of adoption but in reality the principal components of care should be readily available and actually less expensive compared to standard care. The slow adoption of ERP strategies confirms the difficulties in transforming traditional approaches in health care systems, even in the face of simple, evidence based processes of care which benefit both patients and providers. This chapter focuses on colorectal surgery as an example, but the principles are applicable to other procedures.

ERP Impact on Length of Stay

Most Western healthcare systems are facing significant pressures to control the growth of health care expenses, especially in the surgical population. Because most colorectal pathology has a predictable incidence and prevalence of disease burden within a population, the only option to control costs at the provider level is to redesign the process, reduce variability of care, and decrease the rate of truly preventable complications. ERPs have been adopted broadly since the 2000s and the consistent benefit across all health care systems has been a reduction in

L.S. Feldman et al. (eds.), *The SAGES / ERAS®*
Society Manual of Enhanced Recovery Programs for
Gastrointestinal Surgery, DOI 10.1007/978-3-319-20364-5_19,
© Springer International Publishing Switzerland 2015

the duration of hospital stay which is the principal driver of institutional productivity gains and cost savings [1–5]. At a basic level, reducing the length of stay allows a greater number of patients to be managed within the constraints of fixed resources such as number of hospital beds and nursing care at the inpatient unit level. This benefit has been consistently demonstrated across all studies and accrues to both open and laparoscopic approaches [6]. Therefore, the data consistently demonstrate and confirm a reduction in length of stay by 2–5 days depending on the original process of care and the adoption of laparoscopic techniques.

Adoption of Laparoscopic Colectomy

The widespread adoption of laparoscopic colon resection was delayed because of concerns regarding the adequacy of oncologic resection; however, robust prospective randomized studies confirmed equipoise with the open technique [7, 8]. These studies also confirmed a reduced length of stay compared to open colectomy in the absence of a structured enhanced recovery program. However, it should be recognized that increasing the case mix in favor of laparoscopic resection is an important component of providing system benefits even within an ERP [6, 9–13]. The data is clear that laparoscopic surgery is a key enabler to safely and consistently reduce the length of stay and other outcomes within a healthcare system [9, 13]. At the system level, Archibald et al. showed that a 10 % shift towards laparoscopic colectomy, in addition to adoption of an ERP protocol, was an important component of reducing length of stay. Similarly, Bosio et al. showed in a case matched study that this combination of laparoscopy and ERP resulted in a 5 days reduction in length of stay [13]. Yet there remains large geographic variability in uptake of laparoscopic colectomy for colon cancer in the USA, from 0 to 67 % [14]. Given the breadth of data and the increased training opportunities for advanced laparoscopic techniques, the data support a broader adoption of laparoscopic colectomy whenever possible.

Specific Components

It is difficult to tease out the relative benefits of laparoscopic colectomy versus ERP components; however, the evidence does suggest a reduction in specific complications related to simple components of care. Cakir et al. assessed multiple ERP components and determined that laparoscopic surgery, removal of nasogastric tube before extubation, mobilization within 24 h after surgery, starting nonsteroidal anti-inflammatory drugs at day 1 and removal of thoracic epidural analgesia at day 2 were independent predictors of LOS [15].

Avoidance of postoperative ileus is a very important component of reducing a cause for unnecessary delay in discharge and a significant source of increased cost of care [16]. The two major approaches to reducing the rate of ileus are prophylaxis with alvimopan and narcotic sparing multimodality analgesia. Although alvimopan is not routinely mentioned as part of ERP protocols, there is a preponderance of data to suggest that use of this agent is associated with a reduction in both ileus rates and length of stay [17–19]. However, it should be understood that each team should assess the care plan used because the relative benefit of extended use (other than preoperative prophylaxis for intraoperative narcotic exposure) of alvimopan is dependent on the amount of narcotic used subsequently as ileus risk appears to be dose dependent [20–22].

The next major component of ERP is effective multimodal analgesia because it not only reduces ileus risk, but allows for early ambulation which conveys its own particular advantages. The various components vary by institution; however, commonly invoked strategies included epidural analgesia, transversus abdominis plane (TAP) blocks, nonsteroidal anti-inflammatory agents, gabepentin, and acetaminophen [23–27]. In laparoscopic colectomy it is not clear that epidural analgesia is an important adjunct and avoidance of the approach avoids one more additional procedure and its associated cost [28, 29]. Therefore, the literature suggest that inexpensive, oral analgesia combined with surgeon delivered TAP blocks provides for a very efficient means of perioperative analgesia. For open colectomy, there is more data to support the role of epidural analgesia within a structured ERP [30–33].

Surgical site infection (SSI) is another common complication associated with colectomy and results in patient morbidity, mortality, increased cost of care and prolonged length of stay. Once again laparoscopic colectomy appears to be associated with a relative reduction in SSI compared to open colectomy [34–36]. A major issue in the ERAS Society guidelines is the recommendation that mechanical bowel preparation be avoided, at least for open colon surgery [37]. This recommendation is based on systematic reviews finding no decrease in SSI rate with the use of mechanical bowel preparation versus no preparation, but a major limitation is that the bowel preparation groups did not include the use of oral antibiotics [37]. This gap has been exposed by studies which document higher SSI rates after abandoning the oral antibiotic/mechanical preparation strategy and lower rates after its reintroduction [38–41]. While the need for oral antibiotics is clear, whether oral antibiotics need a mechanical preparation in order to be effective has not been studied [42]. The issue of appropriate intravenous prophylactic antibiotics has been well studied and the appropriate options are evidence based [43]. These data support the role of inexpensive strategies to effectively reduce the risk of SSI following colectomy and surgeons should give strong consideration to adding these measures to their ERAS protocol.

Cost Benefits of ERP

The data associated with ERP clearly demonstrate many potential sources of cost containment with adoption of these inexpensive strategies. In fact, other than the often cumbersome process of adoption of ERP protocols, the individual components are relatively inexpensive and readily available even in cost constrained environments [44–48]. Sammour et al. identified an adoption cost of NZ$ 102,000 for an ERP protocol which produced and excellent rate of return of NZ$ 6900 per patient [49]. Delaney et al. demonstrated similar benefits and highlighted a variety of sources of cost reduction related to shortened length of stay, lower complication rates, and lower utilization of laboratory, imaging and pharmaceutical resources [11]. These cost benefits can be considered within the construct of a warranty process which allows providers to assess the financial risks associated with internal processes of care and the population managed [49, 50].

Summary

The data associated with ERP protocols, particularly when combined with laparoscopic techniques, has consistently demonstrated efficient cost reduction while producing superior clinical outcomes. The time has arrived for senior surgeon leadership and hospital administrative leadership to demand implementation of a "bundle" of inexpensive highly effective processes of care. Each team should then regularly assess and evaluate further opportunities guided by actual experience to resolve the remaining clinical issues which can be modified. These assessments should include both clinical and financial analyses, as well as the potential cost of risk mitigation. This practical approach to operational management will allow maximal innovation which should produce higher quality and lower cost of care for colorectal surgical patients.

Take Home Messages

Key take home messages based upon this review include:

- Introduction of an ERP will almost assuredly safely reduce the length of hospital stay by avoiding components of the care plan which negatively impact recovery.
- The addition of a significant volume of minimally invasive colorectal resection will be necessary for a system to see significant improvement even with the introduction on an ERP.
- Prophylaxis for postoperative ileus is an important adjunct because this factor disproportionately accounts for many unnecessary days of care within a colectomy population.
- A multimodal, narcotic minimized analgesic program is highly effective in managing postoperative pain while avoiding opioid related adverse events.
- The standardization of care and adoption of effective, inexpensive care components will yield a significant cost of care for the provider within ERP.

References

1. Kehlet H, Wilmore DW. Evidence-based surgical care and the evolution of fast-track surgery. Ann Surg. 2008;248:189–98.
2. Basse L, Thorbøl JE, Løssl K, Kehlet H. Colonic surgery with accelerated rehabilitation or conventional care. Dis Colon Rectum. 2004;47:217–71. discussion 277–8.
3. Abraham NS, Byrne CM, Young JM, Solomon MJ. Metaanalysis of non-randomized comparative studies of the short-term outcomes of laparoscopic resection for colorectal cancer. ANZ J Surg. 2007;77(7):508–16.
4. Wind J, Polle SW, Fung Kon Jin PH, Dejong CH, von Meyenfeldt MF, Ubbink DT, Gouma DJ, Bemelman WA. Systematic review of enhanced recovery programmes in colonic surgery. Br J Surg. 2006;93:800–9.
5. Gouvas N, Tan E, Windsor A, Xynos E, Tekkis PP. Fast-track vs standard care in colorectal surgery: a meta-analysis update. Int J Colorectal Dis. 2009;24:1119–31.
6. Vlug MS, Wind J, Hollmann MW, Ubbink DT, Cense HA, Engel AF, Gerhards MF, van Wagensveld BA, van der Zaag ES, van Geloven AA, Sprangers MA, Cuesta MA, Bemelman WA. Laparoscopy in combination with fast track multimodal management is the best perioperative strategy in patients undergoing colonic surgery: a randomized clinical trial (LAFA-study). Ann Surg. 2011;254:868–75.
7. Franks PJ, Bosanquet N, Thorpe H, Brown JM, Copeland J, Smith AM, Quirke P, Guillou PJ. CLASICC trial participants. Short-term costs of conventional vs

232   A.J. Senagore

laparoscopic assisted surgery in patients with colorectal cancer (MRC CLASICC trial). Br J Cancer. 2006;95(1):6–12.

8. Clinical Outcomes of Surgical Therapy Study Group. A comparison of laparoscopically assisted and open colectomy for colon cancer. N Engl J Med. 2004;350(20):2050–9.

9. Archibald LH, Ott MJ, Gale CM, Zhang J, Peters MS, Stroud GK. Enhanced recovery after colon surgery in a community hospital system. Dis Colon Rectum. 2011; 54(7):840–5.

10. Senagore AJ, Duepree HJ, Delaney CP, Dissanaike S, Brady KM, Fazio VW. Cost structure of laparoscopic and open sigmoid colectomy for diverticular disease: similarities and differences. Dis Colon Rectum. 2002;45(4):485–90.

11. Delaney CP, Kiran RP, Senagore AJ, Brady K, Fazio VW. Case-matched comparison of clinical and financial outcome after laparoscopic or open colorectal surgery. Ann Surg. 2003;238(1):67–72.

12. Senagore AJ, Duepree HJ, Delaney CP, Brady KM, Fazio VW. Results of a standardized technique and postoperative care plan for laparoscopic sigmoid colectomy: a 30-month experience. Dis Colon Rectum. 2003;46(4):503–9.

13. Bosio RM, Smith BM, Aybar PS, Senagore AJ. Implementation of laparoscopic colectomy with fast-track care in an academic medical center: benefits of a fully ascended learning curve and specialty expertise. Am J Surg. 2007;193(3):413–5. discussion 415–6.

14. Reames BN, Sheetz KH, Waits SA, Dimick JB, Regenbogen SE. Geographic variation in use of laparoscopic colectomy for colon cancer. J Clin Oncol. 2014;32:3667–72.

15. Cakir H, van Stijn MF, Lopes Cardozo AM, Langenhorst BL, Schreurs WH, van der Ploeg TJ, Bemelman WA, Houdijk AP. Adherence to Enhanced Recovery After Surgery and length of stay after colonic resection. Colorectal Dis. 2013;15(8): 1019–25.

16. Asgeirsson T, El-Badawi KI, Mahmood A, Barletta J, Luchtefeld M, Senagore AJ. Postoperative ileus: it costs more than you expect. J Am Coll Surg. 2010;210(2): 228–31.

17. Harbaugh CM, Al-Holou SN, Bander TS, Drews JD, Shah MM, Terjimanian MN, Cai S, Campbell Jr DA, Englesbe MJ. A statewide, community-based assessment of alvimopan's effect on surgical outcomes. Ann Surg. 2013;257(3):427–32.

18. Itawi EA, Savoie LM, Hanna AJ, Apostolides GY. Alvimopan addition to a standard perioperative recovery pathway. JSLS. 2011;15(4):492–8.

19. Delaney CP, Craver C, Gibbons MM, Rachfal AW, VandePol CJ, Cook SF, Poston SA, Calloway M, Techner L. Evaluation of clinical outcomes with alvimopan in clinical practice: a national matched-cohort study in patients undergoing bowel resection. Ann Surg. 2012;255(4):731–8.

20. Barletta JF, Asgeirsson T, El-Badawi KI, Senagore AJ. Introduction of alvimopan into an enhanced recovery protocol for colectomy offers benefit in open but not laparoscopic colectomy. J Laparoendosc Adv Surg Tech A. 2011;21(10):887–91.

21. Madbouly KM, Senagore AJ, Delaney CP. Endogenous morphine levels after laparoscopic versus open colectomy. Br J Surg. 2010;97(5):759–64. Erratum in: Br J Surg. 2010;97(8):1314.

22. Barletta JF, Asgeirsson T, Senagore AJ. Influence of intravenous opioid dose on postoperative ileus. Ann Pharmacother. 2011;45(7–8):916–23.

23. Gatt M, Anderson AD, Reddy BS, Hayward-Sampson P, Tring IC, MacFie J. Randomized clinical trial of multimodal optimization of surgical care in patients undergoing major colonic resection. Br J Surg. 2005;92(11):1354–62.

24. Zutshi M, Delaney CP, Senagore AJ, Mekhail N, Lewis B, Connor JT, Fazio VW. Randomized controlled trial comparing the controlled rehabilitation with early ambulation and diet pathway versus the controlled rehabilitation with early ambulation and diet with preemptive epidural anesthesia/analgesia after laparotomy and intestinal resection. Am J Surg. 2005;189(3):268–72.

25. Basse L, Thorbøl JE, Løssl K, Kehlet H. Colonic surgery with accelerated rehabilitation or conventional care. Dis Colon Rectum. 2004;47(3):271–7. discussion 277–8. Erratum in: Dis Colon Rectum. 2005;48(8):1673.

26. Keller DS, Ermlich BO, Schiltz N, Champagne BJ, Reynolds Jr HL, Stein SL, Delaney CP. The effect of transversus abdominis plane blocks on postoperative pain in laparoscopic colorectal surgery: a prospective, randomized, double-blind trial. Dis Colon Rectum. 2014;57(11):1290–7.

27. Keller DS, Stulberg JJ, Lawrence JK, Delaney CP. Process control to measure process improvement in colorectal surgery: modifications to an established enhanced recovery pathway. Dis Colon Rectum. 2014;57(2):194–200.

28. Senagore AJ, Delaney CP, Mekhail N, Dugan A, Fazio VW. Randomized clinical trial comparing epidural anaesthesia and patient-controlled analgesia after laparoscopic segmental colectomy. Br J Surg. 2003;90(10):1195–9.

29. Levy BF, Tilney HS, Dowson HM, Rockall TA. A systematic review of postoperative analgesia following laparoscopic colorectal surgery. Colorectal Dis. 2010;12(1):5–15.

30. Halabi WJ, Kang CY, Nguyen VQ, Carmichael JC, Mills S, Stamos MJ, Pigazzi A. Epidural analgesia in laparoscopic colorectal surgery: a nationwide analysis of use and outcomes. JAMA Surg. 2014;149(2):130–6.

31. Swenson BR, Gottschalk A, Wells LT, Rowlingson JC, Thompson PW, Barclay M, Sawyer RG, Friel CM, Foley E, Durieux ME. Intravenous lidocaine is as effective as epidural bupivacaine in reducing ileus duration, hospital stay, and pain after open colon resection: a randomized clinical trial. Reg Anesth Pain Med. 2010;35(4):370–6. 8151.

32. Feo CV, Lanzara S, Sortini D, Ragazzi R, De Pinto M, Pansini GC, Liboni A. Fast track postoperative management after elective colorectal surgery: a controlled trial. Am Surg. 2009;75(12):1247–51.

33. Braumann C, Guenther N, Wendling P, Engemann R, Germer CT, Probst W, Mayer HP, Rehnisch B, Schmid M, Nagel K, Schwenk W, Fast-Track Colon II Quality Assurance Group. Multimodal perioperative rehabilitation in elective conventional resection of colonic cancer: results from the German Multicenter Quality Assurance Program "Fast-Track Colon II". Dig Surg. 2009;26(2):123–9.

34. Kiran RP, El-Gazzaz GH, Vogel JD, Remzi FH. Laparoscopic approach significantly reduces surgical site infections after colorectal surgery: data from national surgical quality improvement program. J Am Coll Surg. 2010;211(2):232–8.

234   A.J. Senagore

35. Aimaq R, Akopian G, Kaufman HS. Surgical site infection rates in laparoscopic versus open colorectal surgery. Am Surg. 2011;77(10):1290–4.
36. Lawson EH, Hall BL, Ko CY. Risk factors for superficial vs deep/organ-space surgical site infections: implications for quality improvement initiatives. JAMA Surg. 2013;148(9):849–58.
37. Gustafsson UO, Scott MJ, Schwenk W, Demartines N, Roulin D, Francis N, McNaught CE, MacFie J, Liberman AS, Soop M, Hill A, Kennedy RH, Lobo DN, Fearon K, Ljungqvist O. Guidelines for perioperative care in elective colonic surgery: Enhanced Recovery After Surgery (ERAS®) Society recommendations. World J Surg. 2013;37:259–84.
38. Englesbe MJ, Brooks L, Kubus J, Luchtefeld M, Lynch J, Senagore A, Eggenberger JC, Velanovich V, Campbell Jr DA. A statewide assessment of surgical site infection following colectomy: the role of oral antibiotics. Ann Surg. 2010;252(3):514–9. discussion 519–20.
39. Wick EC, Hobson DB, Bennett JL, Demski R, Maragakis L, Gearhart SL, Efron J, Berenholtz SM, Makary MA. Implementation of a surgical comprehensive unit-based safety program to reduce surgical site infections. J Am Coll Surg. 2012;215(2):193–200.
40. Cannon JA, Altom LK, Deierhoi RJ, Morris M, Richman JS, Vick CC, Itani KM, Hawn MT. Preoperative oral antibiotics reduce surgical site infection following elective colorectal resections. Dis Colon Rectum. 2012;55(11):1160–6.
41. Crolla RM, van der Laan L, Veen EJ, Hendriks Y, van Schendel C, Kluytmans J. Reduction of surgical site infections after implementation of a bundle of care. PLoS One. 2012;7(9), e44599.
42. Hendren S, Fritze D, Banerjee M, Kubus J, Cleary RK, Englesbe MJ, Campbell Jr DA. Antibiotic choice is independently associated with risk of surgical site infection after colectomy: a population-based cohort study. Ann Surg. 2013;257(3):469–75.
43. Zelhart M, Hauch AT, Slakey DP, Nichols RL. Preoperative antibiotic colon preparation: have we had the answer all along? JACS. 2014;219(5):1070–7.
44. Nygren J, Soop M, Thorell A, Hausel J, Ljungqvist O, ERAS Group. An enhanced-recovery protocol improves outcome after colorectal resection already during the first year: a single-center experience in 168 consecutive patients. Dis Colon Rectum. 2009;52(5):978–85.
45. Maessen J, Dejong CH, Hausel J, Nygren J, Lassen K, Andersen J, Kessels AG, Revhaug A, Kehlet H, Ljungqvist O, Fearon KC, von Meyenfeldt MF. A protocol is not enough to implement an enhanced recovery programme for colorectal resection. Br J Surg. 2007;94(2):224–31.
46. Fearon KC, Ljungqvist O, Von Meyenfeldt M, Revhaug A, Dejong CH, Lassen K, Nygren J, Hausel J, Soop M, Andersen J, Kehlet H. Enhanced recovery after surgery: a consensus review of clinical care for patients undergoing colonic resection. Clin Nutr. 2005;24(3):466–77.
47. Hendry PO, Hausel J, Nygren J, Lassen K, Dejong CH, Ljungqvist O, Fearon KC, Enhanced Recovery After Surgery Study Group. Determinants of outcome after colorectal resection within an enhanced recovery programme. Br J Surg. 2009;96(2):197–205.

48. Rona K, Choi J, Sigle G, Kidd S, Ault G, Senagore AJ. Enhanced recovery protocol: implementation at a county institution with limited resources. Am Surg. 2012; 78(10):1041–4.

49. Sammour T, Zargar-Shoshtari K, Bhat A, Kahokehr A, Hill AG. A programme of Enhanced Recovery After Surgery (ERAS) is a cost-effective intervention in elective colonic surgery. N Z Med J. 2010;123(1319):61–70.

50. Asgeirsson T, Jrebi N, Feo L, Kerwel T, Luchtefeld M, Senagore AJ. Incremental cost of complications in colectomy: a warranty guided approach to surgical quality improvement. Am J Surg. 2014;207(3):422–6. discussion 425–6.

20. Audit: Why and How

Andrew Currie and Robin Kennedy

Clinical audit is a vital component of effective clinical governance. A surgical department that undertakes regular and comprehensive audit should be able to provide data to patients about the quality of care that it delivers, as well as reassurance to those who pay for and regulate health care. Well-constructed and conducted audit should also enable surgeons to continually improve the quality of care that they deliver.

Surgeons have been at the forefront of clinical audit historically. Ernest Codman, a surgeon at Massachusetts General Hospital was a prolific quality pioneer, developing the first intraoperative anesthetic record, the first tumor registry and the first record of individual surgeon's 1-year outcomes. Codman was quoted in his time as saying, "every hospital should follow every patient it treats long enough to determine whether or not the treatment has been successful and then to inquire, if not, why not?" Codman's zeal for measuring surgical outcomes, however, became his greatest professional liability as the surgical community expelled him from Boston—a pioneer simply ahead of his time. Modern surgery is embracing the clinical audit experience from cardiac and gastrointestinal surgery, which shows national audit practice has led to significant improvements in care. The Donabedian model conceptualizes health care quality into three interrelated components of structure, process, and outcome. "Structure" refers to the context in which care is provided, such as practitioner and institution experience, nursing ratios, and availability of an electronic medical record. Examples of structural measures specific to colon and rectal surgery include hospital and surgeon volume and specialist practice certification. "Process" refers to the activities of care provision. Process measures assess whether a specific intervention was performed for a defined patient population, such as preadmission patient education or preoperative antibiotics. "Outcomes" are the results of providing care. Examples include

L.S. Feldman et al. (eds.), *The SAGES / ERAS®*
Society Manual of Enhanced Recovery Programs for
Gastrointestinal Surgery, DOI 10.1007/978-3-319-20364-5_20,
© Springer International Publishing Switzerland 2015

mortality and morbidity, surgical site infections (SSIs), quality of life, and patient satisfaction. The underlying idea is that the structure of the system impacts the process of providing care, which then affects patient outcomes. Any one of these components can be evaluated in audit and then modified to improve overall quality of care.

This chapter will explore the different methods of surgical audit, illustrated with examples from clinical practice, define the relevance of audit to enhanced recovery care and describe the possible options for audit of enhanced recovery program (ERP) care. The basis for this chapter has been a narrative search of the Medline and EMBASE databases using the keywords and synonyms for "clinical audit" and "surgery" and/or enhanced recovery.

Why Conduct Audit

There are a number of reasons why surgeons might want to incorporate audit into their work. Local practice issues are a common driver as a result of special interest or concerns regarding particular patient outcomes or procedures. National initiatives, either driven by clinician groups or health-care regulators, are another common rationale for undertaking audit and the results can be used to drive local quality improvement projects. In a recent Cochrane review of 140 studies, clinical audit was shown to provide small but definite improvements in professional practice, especially when feedback was available in a structured and repetitive format. Quality improvement initiatives driven by clinicians have been shown to derive greater impact than those implemented by managerial process. The Surviving Sepsis initiative is a prime example of this. Through the implementation of a clinical management pathway for severly septic patients at 165 hospitals, there was an improvement in compliance (the measure of adherence to a set of practice measures) by 18 % in the initial period, rising to 36 % in the 2 years following set-up [1]. This translated into a substantial reduction in mortality from severe sepsis (36–30.8 %).

Audit and Quality Improvement in Gastrointestinal Surgery

Previous quality improvement initiatives in gastrointestinal cancer surgery have focused on selective referral, process compliance, and participation in an outcomes registry with data feedback. For example, from

1993 to 1997, Norway enacted a selective referral and national audit program for rectal cancer care that was based on compliance with the process of total mesorectal excision (TME). A single nominated surgeon at each hospital was responsible for submitting clinical and operative data. The national surgical society determined that only specialist gastrointestinal surgeons should undertake rectal cancer surgery. These surgeons underwent masterclass training under the auspices of Professor Bill Heald (who pioneered the technique) and the pathologists all received training on reporting of TME specimens by Professor Phil Quirke, University of Leeds. Follow-up and tracing of individuals was facilitated by a unique 11-digit personal identification number allocated to all Norwegian citizens at birth, which ensured comprehensive analysis and linkage to tumor registries. The intervention significantly reduced local recurrence rates from 12 to 6 % and improved 4 years survival rates from 60 to 73 %.

The American College of Surgeons (ACS) national surgical quality improvement project (NSQIP) is the most well studied quality improvement initiative in gastrointestinal surgery. Use of NSQIP from 1991 to 2001 was credited with significantly reducing 30 days surgical morbidity from 17.5 to 9.5 % and 30 days mortality from 3.1 to 2.3 % [2]. Currently, more than 400 hospitals in the USA and Canada participate in the ACS NSQIP. Each hospital is required to pay a participation fee to the program, and provide a surgeon champion and funding for a trained surgical clinical reviewer involved in data collection. All data are reported to NSQIP via a web-based data entry program. The validity of the 30-day outcomes is increased by direct communication with surgical patients by phone or letter, and by public record death searches to complete the 30-day follow-up. The program collects more than 130 preoperative, intraoperative, and postoperative data variables, and reports on more than 20 risk-adjusted outcomes, including 30-day mortality, thromboembolic disease, SSI (superficial, deep, and organ space), and unplanned reoperation, among other morbidities.

NSQIP provides participating institutions with reports to compare risk-adjusted outcomes to other participating hospitals. Participants also have access to best practice guidelines, risk calculators to help inform patients about operative risk, and a participant use data file for research. A number of more locally driven projects, such as The Better Colectomy project in Massachusetts, use NSQIP data to define collaborating surgeons' key evidence-based practices in colectomy and then evaluated practice within their network [3]. Nonadherence to these key practices predicted complication occurrence and each missed practice increased the odds of a complication by 60 %. The Enhanced Recovery in NSQIP (ERIN) is a new collaborative to help teams implement colorectal pathways. ERIN includes new process and outcomes measures embedded within the colorectal-specific NSQIP tool specific to enhanced recovery pathways such as multimodal analgesia, goal-directed fluid management, and early nutrition and ambulation.

Audit and Quality Improvement in Enhanced Recovery

Clinical pathways demonstrate efficacy in improving the quality of perioperative care. This is especially true for high volume, high morbidity procedures such as gastrointestinal surgery. The Enhanced Recovery After Surgery program is a multimodal synthesis of evidence-based care practices developed to reduce surgical stress and improve patient recovery. It can be highly complex incorporating up to 30 individual interventions, which means ensuring that all are delivered is challenging, and thus audit may help. Audits of enhanced recovery programs should include the recording of compliance with the individual care processes measures. The safety of Enhanced Recovery After Surgery protocols has been demonstrated in numerous randomized trials and a number of studies and meta-analyses have shown the efficacy of ERP [4]. Reduction in morbidity, faster return of bowel function, earlier mobilization, lower pain scores and reduced length of stay, have all been demonstrated. What is less well understood is how the ERP performs in clinical practice outside the trial setting.

A study undertaken in Scarborough, UK explored the outcomes of patients receiving ERP care within an RCT compared to outside an RCT, within the same surgical unit using the same protocol [5]. Whilst trial patients had marginally higher compliance, little difference was seen regarding the development of complications or length of postoperative hospital stay. However, in a larger single center study, Gustaffson and colleagues showed a positive relationship between compliance and outcome [6]. As the ERP protocol became more embedded at the hospital over time, compliance improved. This increased compliance was associated with a concomitant reduction in both postoperative complications and symptoms delaying recovery. More recently, the ERAS Compliance Group published outcomes on over 2300 patients undergoing elective colorectal cancer surgery [7]. As ERP perioperative factor

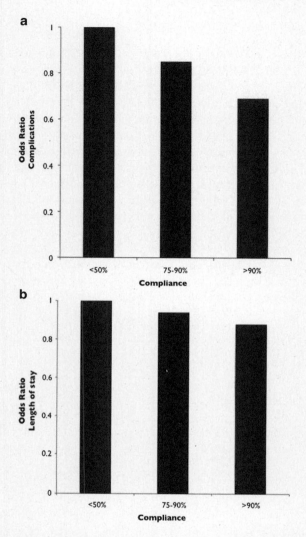

Fig. 20.1. (**a, b**) Impact of ERP compliance on the development of complications and length of stay. (Adapted from ERAS Compliance Group. The Impact of Enhanced Recovery Protocol Compliance on Elective Colorectal Cancer Resection: Results From an International Registry. *Annals of Surgery* 2015 Jan 23, with permission).

compliance increased, both complications and length of stay decreased in multivariate analysis (Fig. 20.1). The combined dataset of the ERAS Society allowed this analysis to be undertaken and is a prime example of how quality improvement can be defined and delivered within enhanced recovery care.

However, compliance can go up as well as down and just as important as implementation is sustainability. Innovations, such as ERP, require continual work, and it is often challenging to maintain early positive results. Around 40 % of public health interventions are not maintained after the implementation phase, and after funding has ended. ERP is a complex, multimodal, multidisciplinary intervention and presents a particular challenge for sustainability. A single center study in Holland demonstrated that during the implementation phase of ERP, significant improvements in hospital stay and reduction in complications were seen following colectomy for cancer [8]. However, in the 2 years after implementation, the compliance with a number of fields fell and there was a concomitant increase in overall length of stay. This unit would have had excellent ERP protocols and surgical ERP pioneers, and one of the Dutch authors concluded, "a protocol is not enough." Audit together with continual monitoring and analysis of data is essential to deliver and maintain the improvements in perioperative care that are offered by ERP.

Practical Tips on How to Conduct an Audit

What Makes a Good Audit?

- Prior consideration of an aspect of surgical care that is measurable and in which a change/improvement in practice will be beneficial.
- Formulating a question that is as simple as possible to aid clarification for others.
- Delivery of the outcome within available resources (staff, time, IT).
- By gaining local support, an alignment with the organization's overall audit priorities and early involvement of the local hospital clinical audit department can greatly improve quality.
- Contributing to national, regional or international audit has the significant benefits of per-to-peer comparisons so that local activity can concentrate on high quality data submission and actions arising from the findings.

Finding and Setting the Standards

- In establishing standards, a number of national reference sources/guidelines are available, e.g., "Guidelines for perioperative care in elective colonic surgery" and "Consensus guidelines for enhanced recovery after gastrectomy," both published by the ERAS Society.
- Having agreed a standard, define a baseline or criterion with the minimum expected level of performance.

Collecting the Data

- Minimize the collection of new data by using existing sources of collected data, possibly networking systems to allow access to data.
- Be clear about methodology before designing data collection proformas.
- Define who is collecting data—enhanced recovery facilitators are likely to be both motivated and accurate, but if other members of the team are involved the shared responsibility can be an advantage. NSQIP uses specially trained nurse data collectors.
- Collect the minimum amount of data to answer the audit question, opt for prospective collection whenever possible and avoid "mission creep" for "interesting" questions.
- Discuss with colleagues to avoid pitfalls and repetition, and to maximize benefit.
- Ensure that the audit collection and storage are compatible with local information governance procedures with regards to patient confidentially and data protection.

A highly developed database is commercially available from the ERAS Society that has many useful functions to help units to set up enhanced recovery care and track outcomes (www.erassociety.org/index.php/eras-care-system/eras-interactive-audit-system). Should teams not wish to use this then we suggest a minimum dataset of the enhanced recovery elements be measured as listed in Table 20.1. Compliance with these "interventions" can then be measured and benchmarked with established standards. Outcomes should include postoperative hospital stay, readmission, and reoperation as a minimum. If possible, an assessment of complications within 28 days of surgery should be included in order to allow a more sophisticated analysis of the effect of the program on outcomes, and thus quality.

Table 20.1. A suggested minimum dataset to audit for compliance to enhanced recovery care pathway.

Preoperative	Intraoperative	Postoperative
Preadmission patient education	Pre-incision antibiotics	Early feeding, drinking and mobilization
Selective bowel preparation in colonic surgery	Maintain normothermia	Early urinary catheter removal
	Appropriate use of epidurals	
Thromboembolic prophylaxis use	Restrictive fluid/sodium administration	Discontinuation of intravenous fluid
Carbohydrate loading	Routine nausea/vomiting prophylaxis	Multimodal analgesia (minimized opiate use)
	Avoid nasogastric/intra-abdominal drains	Routine laxative use
		Early outpatient review after early discharge

Analysis and Interpretation

- Seek statistical help if needed prior to starting data collection.
- Understand the range of variation—has the standard been reached? Has the target for improvement been met; if not, what are the contributory factors?
- Present data in a range of visual formats to improve understanding and analyze the data early in order to ensure the system is suitable.

Actions from Findings

- Having identified changes that are necessary in the program, share your findings with other team members and discuss the issues. Invite team members to contribute to the proposed solution, if appropriate, as it will strengthen the change management process. Agree an action plan, identify the time frame for change, clarify whether there are barriers to overcome, or resource implications.
- After implementation of change, revisit the standard and agree the next cycle of audit.

Initiating and maintaining an enhanced recovery program is a complex process due to the multimodal and multidisciplinary nature of the care pathway. It is also likely to be a constantly changing intervention, as it needs to be modified when new developments in clinical care appear. The benefits to patient care are considerable and a method of assessing the efficacy of this intervention is desirable, as without it optimal care is unlikely to be initiated or sustained.

Take Home Messages

- Audit is key tenet of ERP care and good surgical practice.
- Choose an audit topic that will produce change and benefit patient care.
- Keep the question(s) simple.
- Seek help early in the process from local clinical audit departments and register the audit with them.
- High quality data collection is key, either through a bespoke tool or by undertaking a pilot to ensure comprehensive, robust data capture.
- Present the findings in clear visual formats to engage others and influence successful change/improvement.

References

1. Levy MM, Dellinger RP, Townsend SR, Linde-Zwirble WT, Marshall JC, Bion J, et al. The Surviving Sepsis Campaign: results of an international guideline-based performance improvement program targeting severe sepsis. Crit Care Med. 2010;38: 367–74.
2. Khuri SF, Daley J, Henderson WG. The comparative assessment and improvement of quality of surgical care in the Department of Veterans Affairs. Arch Surg. 2002;137: 20–7.
3. Arriaga AF, Lancaster RT, Berry WR, Regenbogen SE, Lipsitz SR, Kaafarani HM, et al. The better colectomy project: association of evidence-based best-practice adherence rates to outcomes in colorectal surgery. Ann Surg. 2009;250:507–13.
4. Spanjersberg WR, Reurings J, Keus F, van Laarhoven CJ. Fast track surgery versus conventional recovery strategies for colorectal surgery. Cochrane Database Syst Rev. 2011:2:CD007635.
5. Ahmed J, Khan S, Gatt M, Kallam R, MacFie J. Compliance with enhanced recovery programmes in elective colorectal surgery. Br J Surg. 2010;97:754–8.
6. Gustafsson UO, Hausel J, Thorell A, Ljungqvist O, Soop M, Nygren J. Adherence to the enhanced recovery after surgery protocol and outcomes after colorectal cancer surgery. Arch Surg. 2011;146:571–7.

7. ERAS Compliance Group. The impact of enhanced recovery protocol compliance on elective colorectal cancer resection: Results from an international registry. Ann Surg. 2015;261(6):1153–59.

8. Cakir H, van Stijn MF, Lopes Cardozo AM, Langenhorst BL, Schreurs WH, van der Ploeg TJ, et al. Adherence to Enhanced Recovery after Surgery (ERAS) and length of stay after colonic resection. Colorectal Dis. 2013;15(8):1019–25.

21. Why Add an ERP to a Laparoscopic Case: The Colorectal Experience

Yanjie Qi and John R.T. Monson

The introduction of enhanced recovery after surgery was prompted by the increasing recognition that surgical stress caused by major surgery is a significant factor for postoperative morbidity and length of stay. As Kehlet points out in his 1997 paper, "the key pathogenic factor in postoperative morbidity, excluding failures of surgical and anesthetic techniques, is the surgical stress response with subsequent increased demands on organ function" [1]. This stress response manifests in a myriad of ways (pain, nausea, ileus, sleep disturbance, immobilization) that prevent timely recovery and discharge from hospital. The emphasis was made for a unifying, all encompassing team effort to prevent and treat these obstacles to recovery. This concept of multidisciplinary cooperation and well-defined patient care protocols has translated to the fast track protocols or enhanced recovery programs (ERP) that we have come to know. While this review focuses on colorectal surgery, the same principles are applicable across the spectrum of abdominal and thoracic procedures.

Core of ERP

Although there are institutional differences, the core of ERP remains the use of multimodal approach to reduce surgical stress, organ dysfunction, and postoperative morbidity. ERPs can be broken down into preoperative, intraoperative, and postoperative goals of care (Table 21.1). A key component of the preoperative phase is selection of

L.S. Feldman et al. (eds.), *The SAGES / ERAS®*
Society Manual of Enhanced Recovery Programs for
Gastrointestinal Surgery, DOI 10.1007/978-3-319-20364-5_21,
© Springer International Publishing Switzerland 2015

Table 21.1. Preoperative, intraoperative, and postoperative goals of care for ERP.

Preoperative	Intraoperative	Postoperative
1. Patient selection/ assessment	1. Neuraxial blockade (epidural vs. intrathecal)	1. Early removal of drains and lines
2. Patient education/ setting expectations	2. Goal based fluid administration (volume limited, use of esophageal Doppler)	2. Early mobilization
3. Planning of appropriate post-discharge support	3. Maintaining normothermia	3. Early oral intake
4. Selective mechanical bowel preparation	4. Sparing use of surgical drains	4. Routine prokinetics/ antiemetics
5. Carbohydrate loading	5. Removal of NGT in OR	5. "Balanced" analgesia, minimize narcotics
6. Preemptive analgesia		

patients. Those patients who are well nourished, relatively healthy, assigned ASA class 1 or 2 may benefit the most, although ERPs have been applied across the spectrum of patients and procedure complexity. More important than patient selection is the education of the individual regarding the treatment plan and postoperative expectations. Certainly, early mobilization and enteral nutrition goes against the traditional expectations of recovery from surgery. Providers and hospitals often also have a more conservative view of optimal postoperative care. In order for an ERP to be successful, it requires full "buy in" from the entire treatment team, including dieticians, nurses, surgeons, anesthesiologists, and other ancillary providers as well as hospital leadership. The other major elements of ERP are minimizing IV fluids, minimizing narcotics use, early removal of drains and tubes, early mobilization, and early enteral nutrition. Since its introduction in the mid-1990s by Kehlet, there have been multiple randomized control studies in colorectal patients reporting shorter lengths of stay, faster return of bowel function, and decrease in complication rates for ERPs compared to traditional perioperative care. A recent meta-analysis of 14 randomized controlled trials of colorectal operations showed that ERP shortened hospital stay (−2.28 days [95 % CI −3.09 to −1.47]), without increasing readmission rate. Additionally, ERPs were associated with a reduction in overall morbidity [relative ratio (RR)=0.60, (95 % CI 0.46–0.76)], particularly with respect to nonsurgical complications, i.e., respiratory and cardiovascular complications [RR=0.40, (95 % CI 0.27–0.61)] [2].

Laparoscopy and ERP

In a similar vein, since the early 1990s laparoscopy has been widely recognized to be associated with less pain, shorter postoperative ileus, improved pulmonary function, and shorter length of stay. Compared to other procedures, adoption was relatively slow for colorectal surgery due to oncologic concerns and issues associated with the learning curve such as bowel injury, conversion to open surgery, and longer operative times. Although the oncologic concerns have been put to rest, uptake of laparoscopic colectomy remains relatively low, with wide geographic variability. Similar to ERPs, systematic reviews and population datasets conclude that laparoscopy is associated with decreases length of stay, pain, ileus and overall complications compared to open surgery.

Since both laparoscopy and ERPs are associated with less surgical stress, better postoperative pain profiles, less postoperative ileus, and shorter length of stay, some practitioners advocated for the integration of laparoscopic colon resections within an enhanced recovery program. The benefits of this approach were not obvious to all. Some suggested that since laparoscopic colon resection already decreased postoperative pain and length of stay, the addition of an ERP would incur additional cost and complexity without significant return. Over the past decade, several randomized controlled trials have investigated the impact of the combination of an ERP with laparoscopy in colorectal surgeries.

In 2005, Basse et al. reported a small trial in Denmark comparing laparoscopic and open colectomies [3]. There were 30 patients in each arm undergoing either sigmoid colectomy or right colectomy for cancer or benign disease. A well-defined multimodal rehabilitation program was followed that included continuous epidural analgesia for 48 h, early oral feeding including protein drinks, active mobilization, and planned discharge on the second postoperative day. The type of surgery was blinded to the patient, the ward nurses, and the observer from the research team with use of a large opaque abdominal dressing. The dressing was not removed until a decision about discharge had been taken. The characteristics of the patients were comparable. However, the duration of surgery was significantly longer in the laparoscopic group: median 215 min versus 131 min. The measured outcomes included LOS, complications, postoperative fatigue and pain, reoperation, readmission, and some physiological measurements like pulmonary function tests and

CRP. The trial showed no differences in any of the measured outcomes. The study asserted that with appropriate blinding and strict adherence to ERP, there appears no additional benefit to laparoscopy. They concluded, "Functional recovery of a large variety of organ functions is fast but similar between laparoscopic and open procedures" [3].

Shortly after publication of the Basse article, King et al. contributed a similarly sized study of 60 colorectal cancer patients in the UK. The study had different inclusion criteria, including patients with rectal anastomoses (requiring a stoma), patients not living independently at home, and excluded those with benign disease. The clinical outcomes were length of stay (postoperative and including readmission), morbidity, and need for analgesia. The patient reported outcomes included sleep and fatigue. Patients who underwent laparoscopic surgery had a 32 % (7–51 %) shorter hospital stay than those having open surgery ($P = 0.018$) [4]. The median LOS of the laparoscopic group was 5.2 days, compared to 7.4 days in the open group. There were also fewer readmissions in the laparoscopic group (2 vs. 5 of open) and less OR blood loss. The operative time in the trial was similar between groups, 187 min for laparoscopic and 140 min for open approach. Additionally, the study looked at the economic differences between the two approaches. Operative costs were higher in patients randomized to laparoscopic surgery, due to increased OR time and the use of disposable laparoscopic equipment. These costs were more than offset by lower postoperative costs, such as reoperations and readmissions. The total cost of surgery was less for the laparoscopic approach by approximately £350. Though small in size, the UK trial suggests that use of laparoscopy within an ERP provides additional benefits compared to open surgery with respect to both by clinical outcomes and economic costs.

Several years later, results from the LAFA study, a Dutch multicenter randomized controlled trial, were published. The LAFA study assigned 427 subjects in nine centers to four treatment arms: Lap/Fast track, Lap/Standard, Open/Fast track, and Open/Standard. The primary outcome of the study was *total* postoperative hospital stay (THS), which included postoperative hospital stay (PHS) plus additional readmission days within 30 days of surgery. The secondary outcomes included PHS, overall morbidity, reoperation rate, readmission rate, and in house mortality. The THS and PHS for the Lap/Fast track group (5 days) were significantly shorter than the other treatment groups (6 or 7 days). The Open/Standard group had the longest length of stay, suggesting that benefits of ERP and laparoscopic surgery are additive, not overlapping [5]. The overall rates of morbidity, reoperation, readmission, and mortality were similar across all groups. The authors commented that not blinding the patients and providers to the type of surgery may be a source of bias, but asserted that strict discharge criteria had to be met and the primary outcome of the study was not influenced. They concluded that the optimal treatment for colectomy for cancer is a laparoscopic approach within an ERP system.

Most recently, the results of the British EnROL study were published [6]. This randomized controlled trial compared open versus laparoscopic surgery for colorectal cancer within an ERP. The study recruited 204 patients from 12 UK hospitals. The type of procedure was blinded to the patients and providers by a large abdominal dressing similar to the Basse study. Unlike previous trials, the primary outcome of the study was a patient-reported outcome measure of physical fatigue (MFI-20). The secondary outcomes included postoperative hospital stay, complications, reoperations, and readmissions. The study reports no difference in physical fatigue at 1 month based on the MFI-20 patient survey. There were significant difference between laparoscopy and open in length of primary hospital stay (5 vs. 6 days) and total length of hospital stay (5 vs. 7 days). There were no differences in complications, reoperation, or readmission rates. The authors conclude that laparoscopy for colorectal surgery within an established ERP is recommended over open procedures due to the decrease in LOS.

Vlug et al. published a follow up paper to the LAFA trial in which they examined the predictors of early recovery [7]. The LAFA trial database recorded adherence to 19 individual fast track care elements for each patient. With multivariate linear regression analysis, they reported that early advancement of oral intake, early mobilization, laparoscopic surgery, and female sex were independent determinants of early recovery. This data would be useful for institutions with limited resources that may not be able to apply all elements of an ERP. The goals with the highest impact factor would be to encourage early oral intake and early mobilization. Furthermore, it reinforced the concept that laparoscopic approach would be more likely to be result in early discharge and recovery.

Even with full implementation of an ERP, there is a cohort of patients whose hospital course runs longer than expected. Keller et al. compared patients who were hospitalized >4 days and those who were discharge prior to day 3 in a well-established ERP [8]. Not surprisingly, the group with longer hospitalizations had high rate of postoperative complications and 30-day reoperation rates. Patients in the early discharge group were younger, had lower BMI, lower ASA class and were less likely to have had previous abdominal surgery. In terms of intraoperative data, increased blood loss and increased operative time were associated with longer hospitalization. The study suggests that patients at risk for delayed discharge can be identified and that patients should be informed that they might not follow the usual course of recovery.

When designing and implementing an ERP, strategies for individual pathway elements may differ for open or laparoscopic surgery. One of the tenets of ERP is to use multimodal opiate-sparing analgesia, including neural blockade, acetaminophen and NSAIDs, in an effort to shorten postoperative ileus (see Chap. 13). While thoracic epidural is recommended for analgesia after open colorectal surgery in many guidelines, similar outcomes can be achieved with other modalities for laparoscopic colectomy, including spinal, patient-controlled analgesia, intravenous lidocaine or long-acting local anesthetics wound infusion. The use of transversus abdominis plane (TAP) blocks for postoperative pain control is also advocated as a relatively simple, surgeon-administered strategy. The benefits of adding IV acetaminophen and TAP blocks in patients undergoing elective laparoscopic colon resection by an experience laparoscopic surgeon in an established ERP were investigated in a case-matched series. The study reported a decrease in median LOS from 3.7 days to 2 days. It also demonstrated that the use of TAP blocks and IV acetaminophen were associated with a lower complication rate and no increase in readmissions [9].

Conclusion

Enhanced recovery programs are designed to address the obstacles of postoperative recovery. Laparoscopy has similar advantages as ERPs by decreasing the time to baseline functionality and length of stay. It seems to be the logical development for these two treatment modalities to be combined for even greater benefit. Despite the concern in the past that adding ERP to a laparoscopic procedure would not reap additional benefits, the latest studies have confirmed that length of stay is further decreased by the combination. In the era of constant pressure to maximize health care resource and minimize cost, the union of ERP with laparoscopy is both obvious and necessary.

Take Home Messages

- The main goal of enhanced recovery programs (ERP) is the reduction of surgical stress, organ dysfunction, and postoperative morbidity using a multimodal approach.
- ERP consists of many individual care elements implemented over the preoperative, intraoperative, and postoperative periods.
- The laparoscopic surgical approach has been incorporated as a component of ERP in multiple colorectal surgical programs.
- Recent studies have demonstrated the additional improvements in surgical outcomes and length of stay when laparoscopy has been integrated into successful ERPs.

References

1. Kehlet H. Multimodal approach to control postoperative pathophysiology and rehabilitation. Br J Anaesth. 1997;78(5):606–17.
2. Greco M, Capretti G, Beretta L, Gemma M, Pecorelli N, Braga M. Enhanced recovery program in colorectal surgery: a meta-analysis of randomized controlled trials. World J Surg. 2014;38(6):1531–41.
3. Basse L, Jakobsen DH, Bardram L, et al. Functional recovery after open versus laparoscopic colonic resection: a randomized, blinded study. Ann Surg. 2005;241(3):416–23.
4. King PM, Blazeby JM, Ewings P, et al. Randomized clinical trial comparing laparoscopic and open surgery for colorectal cancer within an enhanced recovery programme. Br J Surg. 2006;93(3):300–8.
5. Vlug MS, Wind J, Hollmann MW, et al. Laparoscopy in combination with fast track multimodal management is the best perioperative strategy in patients undergoing colonic surgery: a randomized clinical trial (LAFA-study). Ann Surg. 2011;254(6): 868–75.
6. Kennedy RH, Francis EA, Wharton R, et al. Multicenter randomized controlled trial of conventional versus laparoscopic surgery for colorectal cancer within an enhanced recovery programme: EnROL. J Clin Oncol. 2014;32(17):1804–11.
7. Vlug MS, Bartels SA, Wind J, et al. Which fast track elements predict early recovery after colon cancer surgery? Colorectal Dis. 2012;14(8):1001–8.
8. Keller DS, Bankwitz B, Woconish D, et al. Predicting who will fail early discharge after laparoscopic colorectal surgery with an established enhanced recovery pathway. Surg Endosc. 2014;28(1):74–9.
9. Keller DS, Stulberg JJ, Lawrence JK, Delaney CP. Process control to measure process improvement in colorectal surgery: modifications to an established enhanced recovery pathway. Dis Colon Rectum. 2014;57(2):194–200.

Part III
Examples of Enhanced Recovery Programs

22. Enhanced Recovery Programs for Colorectal Surgery: University Hospitals Case Medical Center

Benjamin P. Crawshaw, Karen M. Brady, and Conor P. Delaney

University Hospitals Case Medical Center, in Cleveland, Ohio, has been at the forefront of the development of enhanced recovery pathways (ERP) for over a decade. The Division of Colorectal Surgery has helped to carefully develop and investigate many elements that are now standard in ERPs at many institutions around the world. Utilizing a multidisciplinary approach to perioperative care, many patients can now be discharged home safely following colectomy in 24–48 h. The team, consisting of the attending surgeons, nurse practitioners, colorectal fellow, general surgical residents, enterostomal therapy nurses, and registered nurses, coordinate care within the guidelines of a well-established ERP to ensure the safest and most comfortable experience for patients. Through our work on enhanced recovery in the colorectal patient population, we have developed protocols that incorporate these principles to all abdominal surgery specialties including surgical oncology, gynecology oncology, general surgery, hepatobiliary, and urology. In this chapter, we provide an overview of our institute's ERP for colorectal surgery, beginning in the preoperative period and continuing through discharge and follow-up.

Preoperative Education

A critical aspect of any ERP is thorough patient education. Ensuring that patients are well prepared for the surgery and are aware of the milestones for discharge and recovery allows them to take an active role in the

L.S. Feldman et al. (eds.), *The SAGES / ERAS®*
Society Manual of Enhanced Recovery Programs for
Gastrointestinal Surgery, DOI 10.1007/978-3-319-20364-5_22,
© Springer International Publishing Switzerland 2015

process and increases adherence to the pathway. After a complete preoperative workup, we provide all patients with a comprehensive guide entitled "Your Guide to Abdominal Surgery." This guide, developed by our nurse practitioners and surgeons, explains all aspects of expected postoperative care and aims to be a reference for patients, their families, and caregivers to utilize before, during, and after their surgery and hospitalization. This guide covers all aspects of our ERP and relates, in layman's terms, what will occur after surgery so that the patient may anticipate what is to come.

Our guide is broken into several different sections and the table of contents is shown in Fig. 22.1. Preoperative information, such as bowel prep instructions, what to bring to the hospital, and a description of what to expect day to day during their hospital stay is provided. Various aspects of our ERP are described to patients, along with detailed information on topics such as postoperative pain control and how to use the patient controlled anesthesia (PCA), the importance of ambulation and instructions for the incentive spirometer, and details of how the patient may expect their diet to advance and their hospitalization to progress. Finally, information for care at home is included for education and reference. Topics include: prevention and diagnosis of dehydration; ostomy and drain care; ostomy output log; anticipatory information regarding common problems (nausea, pain, poor appetite); and indications to contact the doctor immediately (Fig. 22.2).

Preoperatively, all patients are seen within approximately 2 weeks by anesthesia for preoperative evaluation, medical optimization if necessary, and baseline labs including type and screen. All patients have an assessment of home support in anticipation of any home care needs that may be required at the time of discharge. To identify patients at risk, we use a Modified Frailty Score (Fig. 22.3) that has been correlated with hospital length of stay and need for additional home support. Patients undergoing operations with anticipated stoma creation are seen by our stoma team for education and planning. The stoma team will again see these patients the morning of surgery in the preoperative holding area for marking of the stoma site.

Perioperative Protocols

For all elective surgeries, patients are contacted by the surgeon's office several days before the scheduled procedure date. Time and date of the operation are confirmed and information on arrival time, parking, and preoperative instructions are provided.

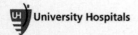 University Hospitals

This booklet explains what to expect when having abdominal surgery. It is a guide you can turn to before surgery, while in the hospital and after you go home. Inside are info sheets written by our experts at University Hospitals.

Bring this booklet with you on your surgery day so you can use it while you are in the hospital. If you have any questions after reading this, please speak with your surgeon or nurse.

Table of Contents

This info is a general resource. It is not meant to replace your doctor's advice. Ask your doctor or health care team any questions. Always follow their instructions.

This booklet was created by University Hospitals Department of General Surgery and University Hospitals Seidman Cancer Center Office of Patient and Public Education.

Fig. 22.1. Information packet table of contents. (©2015 University Hospitals Case Medical Center. Used with permission.)

Call your surgeon's office right away if you:

- Feel sick to your stomach or you are throwing up
- Have new or more pain not helped by your pain medicine
- Have a fever higher than 100° F
- Have new bleeding or bruising
- Have redness, swelling, warmth or firmness around your wound (incision) or drain site
- Have drainage from your wound or drain that changes color, looks thick or cloudy or smells bad
- Have pain, swelling, redness or warmth in your leg or arm
- Have chest pain or shortness of breath
- Have any other concerns or questions

If you have an ileostomy, you also need to call your surgeon if you:

- Have more than 1000 ml (milliliters) of stool output in 24 hours
- Feel weak, dizzy or more tired than normal

You may need to be seen in the clinic or go to the ER (emergency room) for these problems. You may need IV fluids to make up for the fluid loss.

- **If you do not have your surgeon's phone number, call 216-844-1000 to speak with the hospital operator. Ask for your surgeon's phone number or to connect you with his or her office.**

- **Call 9-1-1 if you have any problems that you think are an emergency.**

Fig. 22.2. Indications to call surgeon.

There are several standard protocols that we follow for patients in the days leading up to surgery. We utilize full mechanical bowel prep in the majority of cases, with the exception of right colectomies. The preferred bowel prep for most cases is a polyethylene glycol solution, along with oral neomycin and metronidazole, avoiding solid food the day before surgery. Additional preoperative oral medications include gabapentin 150–300 mg TID for 3 days prior to surgery, which has been shown to decrease postoperative pain. Finally, patients are instructed to drink a nutritional supplement the night before surgery (we use Boost Glucose Control®), though we have not noted any effect of this on bowel prep success.

On the day of surgery, patients are instructed to arrive at least 2 h prior to the schedule start of surgery. They are admitted to the hospital and brought to the preoperative holding area. In addition to standard preparation for the operating room, our patients follow several additional

Pre-operative Grade of Fitness (To be obtained during patient history)
Conor P. Delaney, MD, MCh, Ph.D

Unique ID: _____

Date of visit: _____

Care Setting: Inpatient   Outpatient

Scored by: _____

The CSHA Clinical Frailty Score (Circle the category that best describes the patient)			
	1. Very Fit	People who are robust, energetic, well-motivated, these people exercise regularly and are the most fit group for their age
	2. Well	People who have no active disease, but are less fit than category 1. Often they exercise or are seasonally active
	3. Well, with treated comorbid disease	Disease symptoms are well controlled compared to those in category 4, but are not regularly active beyond routine walking
	4. Vulnerable	Although not frankly dependent, often symptoms limit expectations. These people commonly complain of being "slowed up" or tired throughout the day.
	5. Mildly frail	These patients have more evident slowing, with limited dependence on others for instrumental activities of daily living. Often, mild frailty progressively impairs walking, shopping, meal preparation, and housework.
	6. Moderately frail	They require help for both instrumental and non-instrumental activities of daily living. These patients need help with all outside activities and dressing, bathing, and housekeeping inside the house
	7. Severely frail	Completely dependent on others for activities of daily and personal care or terminally ill and approaching end of life

Fig. 22.3. Modified Frailty Index. (Adapted from Frailty Index from Farhat et al. J Trauma Acute Care Surg, Volume 72, Number 6, with permission.)

Retrospective Grade of Fitness (To be calculated from medical records)
Conor P. Delaney, MD, Ph.D

Unique ID: _____

Date of visit: _____

Care Setting: Inpatient   Outpatient

Scored by: _____

11-Item Modified Frailty Index (1 point for each item present)	
1. History of Diabetes Mellitus	
2. History of either COPD or pneumonia	
3. History of Congestive Heart Failure	
4. History of Myocardial Infarction	
5. History of either prior PCIG, PCS, or angina	
6. History of Hypertension Requiring Medication	
7. History of either Peripheral Vascular Disease or Rest Pain	
8. History of Impaired Sensorium	
9. History of Transient Ischemic Attack	
10. Cerebrovascular Accident	
11. History of Cerebrovascular Accident with Neurological Deficit	
A. Total Patient Score	
B. Total Variables with Data Present	
Modified FI Score (A/B)	

Fig. 22.3. (continued).

protocols. A final dose of gabapentin is given orally 1–2 h before the scheduled start time. If additional bowel prep is required, a sodium phosphate enema (Fleet®) is administered. All patients without other contraindication receive subcutaneous injection of 5000 units heparin for thromboprophylaxis. Finally, Alvimopan 12 mg is given orally for all planned open colorectal cases and laparoscopic colorectal cases with a perceived high risk for conversion. If laparoscopic cases are not converted, Alvimopan is not given post-operatively.

Intraoperatively, patients receive standard perioperative antibiotics at induction and before incision, and then at appropriate recommended intervals. Steroid dependent patients receive a steroid pulse. We give all patients without renal impairment a single dose of 1000 mg IV acetaminophen intraoperatively, along with ketorolac 15–30 mg IV. If possible, we avoid abdominal drains, nasogastric tubes, and the use of epidurals (except in narcotic dependent laparotomies), as these have not been shown to improve outcomes after laparoscopic surgery and may negatively impact patient recovery. Fluid administration is left to the discretion of the anesthesia team, but we are currently exploring the utility and benefit of goal-directed fluid therapy with the use of noninvasive stroke volume measurement. Finally, abdominal wall nerve block is performed at the conclusion of all cases. We perform this through a transversus abdominus plane (TAP) block using a solution of 0.5 mg/kg 5 % Marcaine injected bilaterally into the TAP midway between the iliac crest and the costal margin at the anterior axillary line, as we have described in several recent publications.

At the conclusion of the case, patients are extubated at the discretion of anesthesia and brought to the recovery room for close monitoring before transfer to the regular nursing floor. Selective admission to the surgical intensive care unit for ongoing respiratory support or close postoperative monitoring is made on a case-by-case basis through discussion between the attending surgeon and attending anesthesiologist.

Postoperative Enhanced Recovery Pathways

Major Open Abdominal Cases

The ERP utilized for open abdominal cases is summarized in Table 22.1. Immediately postoperatively, all patients are placed on a morphine or hydromorphone PCA without basal dose. IV ketorolac is continued from the last intraoperative dose every 6 h around the clock for a total of ten doses. Due to cost impacting availability of IV acetaminophen within our hospital's formulary, we are using oral acetaminophen, 650–1000 mg every 6 h postoperatively, continued until discharge. Oral gabapentin is continued TID for all patients until the time of discharge. On postoperative day 2 (or as soon as the patient is tolerating clear diet), the PCA is stopped. Oral oxycodone 5 mg every 4 h prn is

Table 22.1. Open abdominal surgery ERP.

Postoperative/PACU	Post-op day 1	Post-op day 2	Post-op day 3	Post-op day 4	Post-op day 5
• Ketorolac 15–30 mg Q6 h ATC (*HOLD FOR POOR RENAL FUNCTION OR BLEEDING*) • Oral acetaminophen 650 mg every 6 h ATC once able to tolerating oral meds • Morphine or hydromorphone PCA (no basal dose) • Prophylactic antibiotics ARE NOT CONTINUED, unless specific therapeutic indication	• Heparin 5000 units SQ Q8, SCDs • Sips/chip, advance to clears as tolerated • CBC, BMP QOD, unless indicated • Maintenance IVF@ 50 cc/h • PCA Pump • Oral acetaminophen 650 mg Q6 h ATC • Ketorolac 15–30 mg Q6 h ×10 doses ATC (*hold for poor renal function, bleeding*) • Alvimopan 12 mg po BID ×14 doses, *if given preop* • Gabapentin 150–300 mg po TID, while in house (*hold for dizziness*) • OOB, ambulate 5× • DC Foley—unless otherwise indicated	• Heparin 5000 units SQ Q8 • SCDS • Clear liquids • Boost BID • Advance diet to soft if tolerating clears • DC Foley if not POD #1, (*document appropriately*) • DC PCA • Acetaminophen 650 mg po Q6 h ATC • Ibuprofen 800 mg po TID (*DC ketorolac*) • Oxycodone 5 mg po Q4 h prn • Hold IV • Narcotics, used for break through only	• Heparin 5000 units SQ Q8 • SCDS when in bed • Low Residue diet/ soft diet • If ostomy-remove rod if loose • Continue oral pain medications, prn • DC IV narcotic analgesia • CBC, BMC • OOB • Ambulate 5× day • Heplock IV (keep IVF if ostomy) • Initiate loperamide (if watery ileostomy output over 1000 ml. DC alvimopan if initiated) • PO medications/ resume appropriate home medications	• Heparin 5000 units SQ Q8 • SCDS when in bed • Advance diet to soft if not already, encourage oral intake • Continue oral pain medication, prn • DC IV narcotic analgesia • All meds to po • OOB • Ambulate 5× day • Ostomy—rod out, if not done on POD # 3 • If IV steroids—convert to oral prednisone	• Heparin 5000 units SQ Q8 • SCDS • OOB • Ambulate 5× day • CBC, BMP (*avoid routine labs if discharge planned for today*) • Discharge planning • DC alvimopan, gabapentin prior to discharge • Make follow-up appointment prior to discharge

- Steroid Taper-hydrocortisone if steroids within the last 6 months

- Chewing gum 1 stick TID prn
- PT assessment prn
- ET consult for new ostomy
- Ondansetron 4 mg IV Q6 h prn nausea
- Famotidine 40 mg IV Q6 GERD
- Zolpidem 5 mg QHS prn sleep

- CRP
- IVF @ KVO
- Start appropriate home medications
- OOB
- Ambulate 5× day
- Begin discharge planning to assess for barriers

- Discharge planning to assess barriers: initiate placement forms, begin precertification if needed for placement
- Assess suitability for discharge

- Discharge Planning assess for barriers
- *Discharge planning*: complete placement forms for home/HC/SNF based on needs

---

ATC around the clock, *DC* discontinue, *HC* home care, *IVF* intravenous fluids, *KVO* keep vein open (low flow rate), *OOB* out of bed, *PCA* patient controlled analgesia, *SCDs* sequential compression devices, *SNF* skilled nursing facility, *SQ* subcutaneously started, along with ibuprofen 800 mg TID after the final dose of ketorolac. IV narcotics are used on a case-by-case basis for severe breakthrough pain only, and are not routinely ordered as a standing PRN order. Patients are discharged home with prescriptions for oral acetaminophen, ibuprofen and oxycodone prn.

Patients are allowed sips of water and ice chips the night of surgery, and diet is advanced to clear fluids as tolerated on postoperative day 1, and to a soft/low residue diet on postoperative day 2. Nutritional supplement drinks are ordered twice daily beginning postoperative day 1 and continued until discharge. IV fluids are turned off as soon as the patient is tolerating fluids. Patients are encouraged to chew one stick of sugar-free gum three times a day. Alvimopan 12 mg twice daily is continued for patients that received a dose preoperatively and is discontinued with the return of flatus or stoma output. If needed, IV Ondansetron is used for postoperative nausea. For patients with a new stoma, the enterostomal therapy team is consulted on postoperative day 1 for additional education and instructions for the patient and family for management at home. Ileostomy output is titrated through the addition of Loperimide and Diphenoxylate/atropine (Lomotil) as needed. Home stoma supplies, including devices to measure daily output, are arranged prior to discharge. In addition, patients and families are educated on the signs and symptoms of dehydration and instructed how to adjust dosing of Loperamide and Lomotil to slow down output if needed.

We do not continue prophylactic antibiotics after surgery unless there is a specific indication. It is our practice to follow routine blood work (complete blood count, basic metabolic panel) every other day, beginning on postoperative day 1. Lab work is not ordered if discharge is anticipated later that day. A one-time blood draw for C-reactive protein is done on postoperative day 2, as increased CRP may be associated with complications or readmission and patients may be further assessed before discharge. Subcutaneous heparin and compression stockings are used during hospitalization. Urinary catheters are removed on postoperative day 1 (or 2 if unable on day prior, such as in frail elderly female patients having open surgery, in whom it is too uncomfortable to get onto a commode) unless otherwise indicated—for instance in those with concomitant partial cystectomy for locally invasive cancer, or concomitant bladder repair for fistula. Patients are encouraged to get out of bed for 2–3 h twice per day as tolerated after surgery, and nursing staff are trained to assist in ambulation around the unit five times daily. For patients on chronic steroids, an IV hydrocortisone taper is begun postoperatively and converted to oral prednisone for discharge.

Major Laparoscopic Abdominal Cases

The ERP for laparoscopic cases is shown in Table 22.2. Postoperative pain control for laparoscopic cases is similar to open cases, with the exception that a PCA is not used. Instead, oral oxycodone is initiated immediately, along with around the clock oral acetaminophen and IV ketorolac (which is only given for 24 h). IV Hydromorphone is used only as needed for breakthrough pain. Oral ibuprofen is begun similarly to open cases when IV ketorolac is stopped. Patients are again discharged home with prescriptions for oral ibuprofen, acetaminophen and oxycodone.

A clear liquid diet is ordered immediately following a laparoscopic case, and advanced to a soft diet as tolerated postoperative day 1. Nutritional supplements are again given twice a day, and patients are instructed to chew sugar-free gum three times a day. Alvimopan is not used postoperatively for any laparoscopic case. New stomas in laparoscopic cases are handled the same as those in open, with the assistance of the endostomal therapy team.

As with open patients, blood work is followed every other day and is not ordered on the day of planned discharge. Foley catheters are removed postoperative day 1 if present. No prophylactic antibiotics are continued unless otherwise indicated. Heparin is continued through discharge for thromboprophylaxis. Steroid taper is the same as in open cases.

Additional ERP Information

Postoperative fever is generally not evaluated in the first 48–72 h unless otherwise clinically indicated. In the event of suspected wound infection, routine cultures are not collected. One to two staples are removed from a dependent portion of the wound, and a 14-french mushroom catheter is placed for drainage if necessary. Blood transfusion is considered for hemoglobin <7 and is always at the discretion of the attending surgeon.

Discharge criteria for both open and laparoscopic cases are identical. Patients may be discharged when they are tolerating a diet, adequate pain control is achieved with an oral regimen, vital signs are stable, and any home going needs have been addressed. Ostomy output should have stabilized, and adequate home support is mandatory. Physical therapy evaluation is ordered for patients that may require rehabilitation center placement.

Table 22.2. Laparoscopic abdominal surgery ERP.

Postoperative/PACU	Post-op day 1	Post-op DAY 2	Post-op DAY 3
• Ketorolac 15–30 mg Q6 h ATC	• Heparin 5000 units sq Q8 h	• Heparin 5000 units sq Q8 h	• Heparin 5000 units sq Q8 h
• Acetaminophen 650 mg po Q6 h ATC	• SCDs daily	• SCDs daily	• SCDs daily
• Prophylactic antibiotics *ARE NOT CONTINUED*, unless specific therapeutic indication	• Clear liquids in am, advance to soft diet as tolerated	• Soft diet	• Soft diet
• Steroid Taper-hydrocortisone if steroid within the last 6 months	• Boost 1 can BID	• Continue oral acetaminophen 650 mg po Q6 h ATC	• CBC, BMP (avoid routine labs, if planning for discharge today)
• Clear liquid diet	• Maintenance IVF 10–50 cc/h	• OOB at least 4–6 h	• If ostomy: remove rod
	• Continue oral acetaminophen 650 mg po Q6 h ATC	• Ambulate 5× day	• Discharge planning
	• Gabapentin 150–300 mg TID (while in hospital—*HOLD FOR DIZZINESS*)	• CRP	• Make follow-up appointment prior to DC
	• Oxycodone 5 mg Q4 h break through pain, *HOLD IV*	• All medications to po, resume all home medications not already started as appropriate	*DISCHARGE MEDS*
	• Ibuprofen 800 mg po TID (*DC IV KETOROLAC*)	• Discharge planning, assess for barriers	– Acetaminophen 650 mg po Q6 h ATC
	• CBC, BMP, then QOD unless otherwise indicated	• Assess for suitability for discharge	– Ibuprofen 800 mg po TID
	• Start appropriate oral home meds		– Oxycodone 5 mg Q4–6 h prn (DC meds in reverse order)
	• OOB, ambulate 5× day		
	• DC Foley		
	• Chewing gum 1 stick TID		
	• Avoid alvimopan		
	• Discharge planning to assess barriers		
	• Assess Suitability for discharge		

ATC around the clock, *DC* discontinue, *HC* home care, *IVF* intravenous fluids, *KVO* keep vein open (low flow rate), *OOB* out of bed, *PCA* patient controlled analgesia, *SCDs* sequential compression devices, *SNF* skilled nursing facility, *SQ* subcutaneously.

Order Sets

In order to streamline the ordering of our ERP, we have created specific order sets within our electronic medical record system for each specific pathway. Examples of our open and laparoscopic order sets are shown in Figs. 22.4 and 22.5. Diet and blood tests are automatically

Fig. 22.4. Open order set PDF. (©2015 University Hospitals Case Medical Center. Used with permission.)

Abdominal Surgery - Major Open ERP

Contingency

Contingency

- ☑ Call Physician For: heart rate Less Than 60 bpm Greater Than 100 bpm
- ☑ Call Physician For: Respiratory rate Less Than 10 breaths per minute Greater Than 30 breaths per minute
- ☑ Call Physician For: BP, systolic Less Than 80mmHg Greater Than 170mmHg
- ☑ Call Physician For: BP, diastolic Greater Than 100mmHg
- ☑ Call Physician For: urine output Less Than 250 mL Over 8 hours
- ☑ Call Physician For: pulse-ox Less Than 92%
- ☑ Call Physician For: Saturated dressings or purulent drainage
- ☑ Call Physician For: Increase in baseline pain not brought on by activity in duration of 4 hours or greater

Respiratory

Respiratory

- ☑ Oxygen
  To Maintain SpO2 of: 92%
  Wean to room air
- ☐ Pulse Oximetry Every Shift
- ☐ Incentive Spirometry
  Q1H, While Awake

Diet

Diet

- ☑ NPO Routine
  Except Sips of Water
- ☑ Clear Liquid Diet Routine
  Special Instructions: Plus ordered supplement. Avoid carbonated beverages : Discontinue POD #2
- ☑ Diet Soft
- ☐ Oral Nutritional Supplements Routine
  Boost Plus, 2 Times a Day
  Special Instructions: Post Op Supplement
  CMC Only

Pharmacy

Anticoagulation

- ☐ Heparin SubCutaneous
  DOSE = 5,000 unit(s) SubCutaneous Every 8 Hours
- ☐ Enoxaparin SubCutaneous (LOVENOX)
  DOSE = 30 mg SubCutaneous Every 12 Hours
  Clinician Notes: For obese patients or those at high risk for DVT

Antiemetics

- ☐ Ondansetron Injectable (ZOFRAN)
  DOSE = 4 mg IntraVenous Push Every 6 Hours, PRN Nausea

Fig. 22.4. (continued).

Abdominal Surgery - Major Open ERP

Pharmacy

Analgesics

☐ Acetaminophen Tablet (TYLENOL)
DOSE = 650 mg Oral Every 6 Hours

☐ Ibuprofen Tablet (ADVIL, MOTRIN)
DOSE = 800 mg Oral Every 8 Hours, PRN Pain - Mod (4-6)
Clinician Notes: Start POD #2 : To be used in combination with narcotic analgesia

☐ Ketorolac Inj   (TORADOL)
DOSE = 15 mg IntraVenous Push Every 6 Hours, PRN Pain - Mod (4-6)
Clinician Notes: Discontinue on POD #2

☐ Oxycodone Immediate Release Tablet (OXYIR, ROXICODONE)
DOSE = 5 mg Oral Every 4 Hours, PRN Pain - Mod (4-6)
Clinician Notes: Start on POD #2

☐ Oxycodone Immediate Release Tablet (OXYIR, ROXICODONE)
DOSE = 10 mg Oral Every 4 Hours, PRN Pain - Severe (7-10)
Clinician Notes: Start on POD #2

Corticosteroids + Taper doses

☐ Hydrocortisone Na Succinate Injectable (SOLU-CORTEF)
DOSE = 100 mg IntraVenous Push Every 8 Hours
Stop After 3 Doses

H2 Receptor Antagonists

☐ Famotidine Tablet (PEPCID)
DOSE = 40 mg Oral At Bedtime
Clinician Notes: For patients with pre-op history of GERD

☐ Famotidine Injectable (PEPCID)
DOSE = 20 mg IntraVenous Push Every 12 Hours
Clinician Notes: For patients with pre-op history of GERD

Hypnotics

☐ Zolpidem Tablet (AMBIEN)
DOSE = 5 mg Oral At Bedtime, PRN Sleep

Misc Medications

☐ Gabapentin Capsule (NEURONTIN)
DOSE = 300 mg Oral 3 Times a Day

☐ Alvimopan Capsule (ENTEREG)
DOSE = 12 mg Oral 2 Times a Day
Stop After 14 Doses
Clinician Notes: May NOT use unless given preoperatively

PCA Order Set

☐ Patient Controlled Analgesia (PCA) Order Set

Pharmacy IV Fluids

IV Fluids

☑ Convert IV to Heparin Lock When Taking Oral Fluids Well Once

PLAIN Fluids

☐ Sodium Chloride 0.45% Infusion IV Bag Volume = 1,000 mL IntraVenous <Continuous>

☐ Sodium Chloride 0.9% Infusion IV Bag Volume = 1,000 mL IntraVenous <Continuous>

☐ Dextrose 5% in Water Infusion IV Bag Volume = 1,000 mL IntraVenous <Continuous>

Fig. 22.4. (continued).

Abdominal Surgery - Major Open ERP

Pharmacy IV Fluids

PLAIN Fluids

☐ Dextrose 5% - NaCL 0.2% Infusion IV Bag Volume = 1,000 mL IntraVenous <Continuous>

☐ Dextrose 5% - NaCL 0.45% Infusion IV Bag Volume = 1,000 mL IntraVenous <Continuous>

☐ Dextrose 5% - NaCL 0.9% Infusion IV Bag Volume = 1,000 mL IntraVenous <Continuous>

☐ Dextrose 5% - Lactated Ringers Infusion IV Bag Volume = 1,000 mL IntraVenous <Continuous>

☐ Lactated Ringers Infusion IV Bag Volume = 1,000 mL IntraVenous <Continuous>

Fluids with POTASSIUM 20 mEq/L

☐ Sodium Chloride 0.45% with Potassium CL 20 mEq Premix Fluid IV Bag Volume = 1,000 mL IntraVenous <Continuous>

☐ Sodium Chloride 0.9% with Potassium CL 20 mEq Premix Fluid IV Bag Volume = 1,000 mL IntraVenous <Continuous>

☐ Dextrose 5% with Potassium CL 20 mEq Premix Fluid IV Bag Volume = 1,000 mL IntraVenous <Continuous>

☐ Dextrose 5% - Lactated Ringers with Potassium CL 20 mEq Premix Fluid IV Bag Volume = 1,000 mL IntraVenous <Continuous>

☐ Dextrose 5% - NaCL 0.2% with Potassium CL 20 mEq Premix Fluid IV Bag Volume = 1,000 mL IntraVenous <Continuous>

☐ Dextrose 5% - NaCL 0.45% with Potassium CL 20 mEq Premix Fluid IV Bag Volume = 1,000 mL IntraVenous <Continuous>

☐ Dextrose 5% - NaCL 0.9% with Potassium CL 20 mEq Premix Fluid IV Bag Volume = 1,000 mL IntraVenous <Continuous>

Fluids with POTASSIUM 30 mEq/L

☐ Dextrose 5% with Potassium CL 30 mEq Premix Fluid IV Bag Volume = 1,000 mL IntraVenous <Continuous>

☐ Dextrose 5% - Lactated Ringers with Potassium CL 30 mEq Premix Fluid IV Bag Volume = 1,000 mL IntraVenous <Continuous>

☐ Dextrose 5% - NaCL 0.2% with Potassium CL 30 mEq Premix Fluid IV Bag Volume = 1,000 mL IntraVenous <Continuous>

☐ Dextrose 5% - NaCL 0.45% with Potassium CL 30 mEq Premix Fluid IV Bag Volume = 1,000 mL IntraVenous <Continuous>

Fluids with POTASSIUM 40 mEq/L

☐ Sodium Chloride 0.9% with Potassium CL 40 mEq Premix Fluid IV Bag Volume = 1,000 mL IntraVenous <Continuous>

☐ Dextrose 5% with Potassium CL 40 mEq Premix Fluid IV Bag Volume = 1,000 mL IntraVenous <Continuous>

☐ Dextrose 5% - Lactated Ringers with Potassium CL 40 mEq Premix Fluid IV Bag Volume = 1,000 mL IntraVenous <Continuous>

☐ Dextrose 5% - NaCL 0.2% with Potassium CL 40 mEq Premix Fluid IV Bag Volume = 1,000 mL IntraVenous <Continuous>

☐ Dextrose 5% - NaCL 0.45% with Potassium CL 40 mEq Premix Fluid IV Bag Volume = 1,000 mL IntraVenous <Continuous>

☐ Dextrose 5% - NaCL 0.9% with Potassium CL 40 mEq Premix Fluid IV Bag Volume = 1,000 mL IntraVenous <Continuous>

Fig. 22.4. (continued).

Abdominal Surgery - Major Open ERP

Laboratory and Blood Bank

POD #1

☑ Basic Metabolic Panel
Plasma/Serum Separator
1st AM Draw

☑ Complete Blood Count
Lavender EDTA
1st AM Draw

POD #2

☐ C Reactive Protein, Serum
Serum Separator
-Do Not Use Green Top Tube.
Clinician Instructions: POD #2
1st AM Draw

POD #3

☑ Basic Metabolic Panel
Plasma/Serum Separator
Clinician Instructions: POD #3
1st AM Draw

☑ Complete Blood Count
Lavender EDTA
Clinician Instructions: POD #3
1st AM Draw

POD #5

☐ Basic Metabolic Panel
Plasma/Serum Separator
Clinician Instructions: POD #5
1st AM Draw

☐ Complete Blood Count
Lavender EDTA
Clinician Instructions: POD #5
1st AM Draw

Other Consults

Consults

☐ Social Work Consult Once

☐ Consult Dietitian

☐ Consult Wound Care Nurse

☐ PT Evaluate/Treat   Delay Start Until:T

Quality Monitor:

☑ Monitor for Core Measures-SCIP T

Fig. 22.4. (continued).

ordered, while the remaining aspects of the ERP are selected as indicated by the ordering physician. All residents that rotate through our service are formally educated in our ERP and taught how to use the relevant order sets by the team's nurse practitioners.

UH University Hospitals	**Order Set Configuration - Selected Order Set Name**
Report Parameters:	Order Set Name: Abdominal Surgery - Major Laparoscopic ERP
Report Definition:	Displays the content of the Order Set requested. Does not include nested order set details.

Abdominal Surgery - Major Laparoscopic ERP

Clinical Instructions

Clinical Instructions
- Post operative fever is generally not evaluated for the first 48-72 hours, unless clinically indicated.
- Stress dose steroids should be considered for patients receiving steroids within the past 6 months.
- Check with Attending Surgeon for any majordeviations from the postoperative order set.
- Transfusions are generally reserved for hemoglobin less than 7. Please discuss with all attendings before ordering
  blood transfusions.
- LAP : Alvimopan should generally not be used with laparoscopic bowel resection outside the setting of a
  research trial or for a patient at high risk of conversion, with discontinuation if completed laparoscopically.

Nursing
Vital Signs
☑ Vital Signs Every 4 Hours

Activity
☑ Ambulate T, Routine, 5 Times a Day, Assistance Level: First time with RN, Restrictions: None, In hallways

☑ Out of Bed Ad Lib T, Routine, <Continuous>, Night of Surgery, Assistance Level: None, Restrictions: None

☑ Up in Chair T, Routine, 2 Times a Day, For 3 hours, Assistance Level: None, Restrictions: None

Interventions
☑ Compression Device, Sequential <Continuous> Until ambulating and at night time

☑ Surgical Incision Care Abdomen, <Continuous>, Dressing

☑ Chewing Gum 3 Times a Day
  Have patient chew gum for 1 hour.
☑ Intake & Output <Continuous>

☑ Urinary Catheter to Gravity, care of <Continuous>

☐ Discontinue / Remove urinary catheter in morning on POD #1

☑ Education, Incentive Spirometry

☑ Weight Daily 0600

Fig. 22.5. Lap order set PDF. (©2015 University Hospitals Case Medical Center. Used with permission.)

Abdominal Surgery - Major Laparoscopic ERP

Contingency

Contingency

- ☑ Call Physician For: heart rate Less Than 60 bpm Greater Than 100 bpm

- ☑ Call Physician For: Respiratory rate Less Than 10 breaths per minute Greater Than 30 breaths per minute

- ☑ Call Physician For: BP, systolic Less Than 80mmHg Greater Than 170mmHg

- ☑ Call Physician For: BP, diastolic Greater Than 100mmHg

- ☑ Call Physician For: urine output Less Than 250 mL Over 8 hours

- ☑ Call Physician For: pulse-ox Less Than 92%

- ☑ Call Physician For: Saturated dressings or purulent drainage

- ☑ Call Physician For: Increase in baseline pain not brought on by activity in duration of 4 hours or greater

Respiratory

Respiratory

- ☑ Oxygen
  To Maintain SpO2 of: 92%
  Wean to room air
- ☐ Pulse Oximetry Every Shift

- ☑ Incentive Spirometry
  Q1H, While Awake

Diet

Diet

- ☑ Clear Liquid Diet Routine
  Special Instructions: Plus ordered supplement. Avoid carbonated beverages : Discontinue POD #1
- ☑ Diet Soft

- ☑ Oral Nutritional Supplements Routine
  Boost Plus, 2 Times a Day
  Special Instructions: Post Op Supplement
  CMC Only

Pharmacy

Anticoagulation

- ☐ Heparin SubCutaneous
  DOSE = 5,000 unit(s) SubCutaneous Every 8 Hours
- ☐ Enoxaparin SubCutaneous   (LOVENOX)
  DOSE = 30 mg SubCutaneous Every 12 Hours
  Clinician Notes: For obese patients or those at high risk for DVT

Antiemetics

- ☐ Ondansetron Injectable   (ZOFRAN)
  DOSE = 4 mg IntraVenous Push Every 6 Hours, PRN Nausea

Analgesics

- ☐ Acetaminophen Tablet (TYLENOL)
  DOSE = 650 mg Oral Every 6 Hours

Fig. 22.5. (continued).

Abdominal Surgery - Major Laparoscopic ERP

Pharmacy

Analgesics

☐ Ibuprofen Tablet (ADVIL, MOTRIN)
DOSE = 800 mg Oral Every 8 Hours, PRN Pain - Mod (4-6)
Clinician Notes: Start POD #1 : To be used in combination with narcotic analgesia

☐ Ketorolac Inj   (TORADOL)
DOSE = 15 mg IntraVenous Push Every 6 Hours, PRN Pain - Mod (4-6)

☐ Oxycodone Immediate Release Tablet (OXYIR, ROXICODONE)
DOSE = 5 mg Oral Every 4 Hours, PRN Pain - Mod (4-6)
Clinician Notes: Start on POD #1

☐ Oxycodone Immediate Release Tablet (OXYIR, ROXICODONE)
DOSE = 10 mg Oral Every 4 Hours, PRN Pain - Severe (7-10)
Clinician Notes: Start on POD #1

Corticosteroids + Taper doses

☐ Hydrocortisone Na Succinate Injectable (SOLU-CORTEF)
DOSE = 100 mg IntraVenous Push Every 8 Hours
Stop After 3 Doses

H2 Receptor Antagonists

☐ Famotidine Tablet (PEPCID)
DOSE = 40 mg Oral At Bedtime
Clinician Notes: For patients with pre-op history of GERD

☐ Famotidine Injectable   (PEPCID)
DOSE = 20 mg IntraVenous Push Every 12 Hours
Clinician Notes: For patients with pre-op history of GERD

Hypnotics

☐ Zolpidem Tablet (AMBIEN)
DOSE = 5 mg Oral At Bedtime, PRN Sleep

Misc Medications

☐ Gabapentin Capsule (NEURONTIN)
DOSE = 300 mg Oral 3 Times a Day

PCA Order Set

☐ Patient Controlled Analgesia (PCA) Order Set

Pharmacy IV Fluids

IV Fluids

☑ Convert IV to Heparin Lock When Taking Oral Fluids Well Once

PLAIN Fluids

☐ Sodium Chloride 0.45% Infusion IV Bag Volume = 1,000 mL IntraVenous <Continuous>

☐ Sodium Chloride 0.9% Infusion IV Bag Volume = 1,000 mL IntraVenous <Continuous>

☐ Dextrose 5% in Water Infusion IV Bag Volume = 1,000 mL IntraVenous <Continuous>

☐ Dextrose 5% - NaCL 0.2% Infusion IV Bag Volume = 1,000 mL IntraVenous <Continuous>

☐ Dextrose 5% - NaCL 0.45% Infusion IV Bag Volume = 1,000 mL IntraVenous <Continuous>

☐ Dextrose 5% - NaCL 0.9% Infusion IV Bag Volume = 1,000 mL IntraVenous <Continuous>

☐ Dextrose 5% - Lactated Ringers Infusion IV Bag Volume = 1,000 mL IntraVenous <Continuous>

Fig. 22.5. (continued).

Abdominal Surgery - Major Laparoscopic ERP

Pharmacy IV Fluids

PLAIN Fluids

- ☐ Lactated Ringers Infusion IV Bag Volume = 1,000 mL IntraVenous <Continuous>

Fluids with POTASSIUM 20 mEq/L

- ☐ Sodium Chloride 0.45% with Potassium CL 20 mEq Premix Fluid IV Bag Volume = 1,000 mL IntraVenous <Continuous>
- ☐ Sodium Chloride 0.9% with Potassium CL 20 mEq Premix Fluid IV Bag Volume = 1,000 mL IntraVenous <Continuous>
- ☐ Dextrose 5% with Potassium CL 20 mEq Premix Fluid IV Bag Volume = 1,000 mL IntraVenous <Continuous>
- ☐ Dextrose 5% - Lactated Ringers with Potassium CL 20 mEq Premix Fluid IV Bag Volume = 1,000 mL IntraVenous <Continuous>
- ☐ Dextrose 5% - NaCL 0.2% with Potassium CL 20 mEq Premix Fluid IV Bag Volume = 1,000 mL IntraVenous <Continuous>
- ☐ Dextrose 5% - NaCL 0.45% with Potassium CL 20 mEq Premix Fluid IV Bag Volume = 1,000 mL IntraVenous <Continuous>
- ☐ Dextrose 5% - NaCL 0.9% with Potassium CL 20 mEq Premix Fluid IV Bag Volume = 1,000 mL IntraVenous <Continuous>

Fluids with POTASSIUM 30 mEq/L

- ☐ Dextrose 5% with Potassium CL 30 mEq Premix Fluid IV Bag Volume = 1,000 mL IntraVenous <Continuous>
- ☐ Dextrose 5% - Lactated Ringers with Potassium CL 30 mEq Premix Fluid IV Bag Volume = 1,000 mL IntraVenous <Continuous>
- ☐ Dextrose 5% - NaCL 0.2% with Potassium CL 30 mEq Premix Fluid IV Bag Volume = 1,000 mL IntraVenous <Continuous>
- ☐ Dextrose 5% - NaCL 0.45% with Potassium CL 30 mEq Premix Fluid IV Bag Volume = 1,000 mL IntraVenous <Continuous>

Fluids with POTASSIUM 40 mEq/L

- ☐ Sodium Chloride 0.9% with Potassium CL 40 mEq Premix Fluid IV Bag Volume = 1,000 mL IntraVenous <Continuous>
- ☐ Dextrose 5% with Potassium CL 40 mEq Premix Fluid IV Bag Volume = 1,000 mL IntraVenous <Continuous>
- ☐ Dextrose 5% - Lactated Ringers with Potassium CL 40 mEq Premix Fluid IV Bag Volume = 1,000 mL IntraVenous <Continuous>
- ☐ Dextrose 5% - NaCL 0.2% with Potassium CL 40 mEq Premix Fluid IV Bag Volume = 1,000 mL IntraVenous <Continuous>
- ☐ Dextrose 5% - NaCL 0.45% with Potassium CL 40 mEq Premix Fluid IV Bag Volume = 1,000 mL IntraVenous <Continuous>
- ☐ Dextrose 5% - NaCL 0.9% with Potassium CL 40 mEq Premix Fluid IV Bag Volume = 1,000 mL IntraVenous <Continuous>

Laboratory and Blood Bank

POD #1

- ☑ Basic Metabolic Panel
  Plasma/Serum Separator
  1st AM Draw
- ☑ Complete Blood Count
  Lavender EDTA
  1st AM Draw

Fig. 22.5. (continued).

Abdominal Surgery - Major Laparoscopic ERP

Laboratory and Blood Bank

POD #2

☐ C Reactive Protein, Serum
Serum Separator
-Do Not Use Green Top Tube.
Clinician Instructions: POD #2
1st AM Draw

POD #3

☐ Basic Metabolic Panel
Plasma/Serum Separator
Clinician Instructions: POD #3
1st AM Draw

☐ Complete Blood Count
Lavender EDTA
Clinician Instructions: POD #3
1st AM Draw

Other Consults

Consults

☐ Social Work Consult Once

☐ Consult Dietitian

☐ Consult Wound Care Nurse

☐ PT Evaluate/Treat Delay Start Until:T

Quality Monitor:

☑ Monitor for Core Measures-SCIP T

Fig. 22.5. (continued).

Summary

The implementation and continuous refinement of our ERP has allowed for expedited recovery and discharge following surgery in the vast majority of our patients. By creating and following the standardized pathways outlined above, both patients and providers may know what to expect in the perioperative period, and lays the groundwork for a safe and comfortable recovery.

Suggested Readings

1. Adamina M, Kehlet H, Tomlinson GA, Senagore AJ, Delaney CP. Enhanced recovery pathways optimize health outcomes and resource utilization: a meta-analysis of randomized controlled trials in colorectal surgery. Surgery. 2011;149:830–40.
2. Delaney CP, Brady K, Woconish D, Parmar SP, Champagne BJ. Towards optimizing perioperative colorectal care: outcomes for 1,000 consecutive laparoscopic colon procedures using enhanced recovery pathways. Am J Surg. 2012;203:353–5. discussion 355.

3. Favuzza J, Brady K, Delaney CP. Transversus abdominis plane blocks and enhanced recovery pathways: making the 23-h hospital stay a realistic goal after laparoscopic colorectal surgery. Surg Endosc. 2013;27:2481–6.

4. Krpata DM, Keller DS, Samia H, et al. Evaluation of inflammatory markers as predictors of hospital stay and unplanned readmission after colorectal surgery. Pol Przegl Chir. 2013;85:198–203.

5. Lawrence JK, Keller DS, Samia H, et al. Discharge within 24 to 72 hours of colorectal surgery is associated with low readmission rates when using Enhanced Recovery Pathways. J Am Coll Surg. 2013;216:390–4.

6. Tiippana EM, Hamunen K, Kontinen VK, Kalso E. Do surgical patients benefit from perioperative gabapentin/pregabalin? A systematic review of efficacy and safety. Anesth Analg. 2007;104:1545–56. table of contents.

7. Zhuang CL, Ye XZ, Zhang XD, Chen BC, Yu Z. Enhanced recovery after surgery programs versus traditional care for colorectal surgery: a meta-analysis of randomized controlled trials. Dis Colon Rectum. 2013;56:667–78.

23. Enhanced Recovery Programmes for Colorectal Surgery: The Guildford (UK) Experience

Timothy Rockall and Michael Scott

Enhanced recovery after surgery has been established for colorectal surgery in Guildford for over 10 years and has gone hand in hand with the introduction of minimally invasive surgery, which is critical for obtaining the very best results. The philosophy and the guidelines have become so well established that they amount to normal practice. The principal factor in the establishment of this system is the involvement of key personnel with the same aim. That aim is to ensure the optimal recovery of the patient with the avoidance of post-operative complications and rapid return to normal function and well-being. The key people who drive the process are the consultant surgeon, the consultant anaesthetist and the colorectal nurse specialist. The junior doctors, ward nurses, pain control team, physiotherapists also have their role and need to be integrated into the team approach. This is important because only with the best surgery and the best perioperative care will the best results be achieved. A good operation can be entirely undone by a poor anaesthetic and vice-versa.

There are of course many elements to the whole enhanced recovery programme (ERP) but it has to be recognised that independently some of these have a much more profound effect than others and some have a much stronger evidence base than others. The introduction of these processes in Guildford has been paralleled by research within the unit specifically aimed at determining the best fluid management protocols and the best analgesic modalities [1–6], which have in turn been incorporated into everyday practice [7]. These, together with minimally invasive

L.S. Feldman et al. (eds.), *The SAGES / ERAS®*
Society Manual of Enhanced Recovery Programs for
Gastrointestinal Surgery, DOI 10.1007/978-3-319-20364-5_23,
© Springer International Publishing Switzerland 2015

surgery, are considered the three pillars of success in our unit. In this chapter we describe the process of care in Guildford that enables us to achieve our published results [8–11].

Preoperative Care

Counselling

Counselling is a highly important aspect of introducing enhanced recovery principles to the patient, managing expectation and defining expected milestones in recovery. The general principles of the discussion are well established but are adapted to the operation being proposed, the social circumstances of the patient and their age and co-morbidity. It is important that these messages are delivered by senior members of both medical and nursing staff and given in a consistent manner—ideally as a joint consultation with the consultant surgeon and the nurse specialist. Consultation should also take place with the family members or carers present. It should be reinforced with written information provided in an easily understandable format. For patients undergoing elective colorectal resection and who are without major co-morbidity, the conversation revolves around the anticipated recovery plan and it is stressed that the programme is aimed at improving the quality of recovery and reducing the complication rate rather than being aimed at early discharge per se. Discussion would include all of the following.

- Admission time on the day of surgery
- Arrangements for bowel preparation at home where appropriate
- Stoma therapy consultation and training preoperatively if appropriate
- Proposed method of pain control and mechanisms for controlling breakthrough
- Arrangements for oral fluid and carbohydrate administration (Preload)
- Likely lines of access to be used and planned time of removal
- Plans for removal of urinary catheter
- Expected mobilisation milestones
- Expected discharge day
- Criteria for safe discharge for home

Information will be gained from the patient regarding the safety of the home environment and the levels of care and support available. Contact information for problems or concerns arising following discharge is also given to the patient.

For most patients they are informed that they will be able to drink free fluids on return to the ward following surgery. They will be offered a light evening meal on the day of surgery and a normal breakfast the following morning.

Patients are informed that it is anticipated that all lines and monitoring will be disconnected or removed on the morning following surgery—including intravenous access and urinary catheters. The exception to this is male patients undergoing low anterior resection who retain the urinary catheter for 48 h.

Patients are informed that discharge can occur as early as the first post-operative day as long as they fulfil the following criteria and that the average post operative hospital stay in our unit is 3 days.

Criteria for safe discharge to home

- Uncomplicated surgery
- Unremarkable abdominal findings
- Normal observations (vital signs)
- Tolerating free fluids
- Tolerating light diet
- No nausea or vomiting
- Pain controlled with regular oral analgesia
- Mobility confirmed by a supervised walk
- Patient happy to be discharged to home

Our philosophy is that the earlier the patients can return home, the more mobile they will be, the better they will eat and the better they will sleep—all factors that contribute to high-quality recovery and rapid return to the anabolic state [12, 13]. It also removes the patient from a potentially dangerous environment with the risk of hospital-acquired infection. There is strong emphasis on being able to contact clinicians or return to the hospital in the event of failure to make progress or developing complications. Readmission to hospital is not considered a failure of treatment but is in any case a rare event. There are certain "red flag" symptoms that patients are told they must return to hospital emergency department immediately which include sudden onset of severe abdominal pain, symptoms of obstruction, fever or rigors.

Nutrition

Fortunately it is relatively unusual for patients with colorectal disease to be severely malnourished compared to patients with upper gastrointestinal diseases. The focus of nutrition is on the immediate preoperative phase to avoid preoperative starvation and provide carbohydrate (CHO) load preoperatively and attenuate the catabolic response to surgery. The mechanism of delivering CHO in the form of a drink also delivers a fluid load that ensures the patients come to surgery well hydrated. We provide 800 ml of CHO the evening before surgery and a further 400 ml 2 h before surgery using PRELOAD (Vitaflo, UK).

Bowel Preparation

Mechanical bowel preparation is not routinely administered for patients undergoing colorectal resection. The bowel preparation protocol is determined by the planned surgery. Essentially, if a stapled anastomosis is to be fashioned trans-anally then a Phosphate enema is administered an hour prior to surgery to ensure the rectum and left colon are empty. It may also be self administered at home by the patient prior to admission. Full mechanical bowel preparation with stimulant and osmotic laxatives is reserved for patients having a rectal anastomosis with planned defunctioning loop ileostomy. For practical purposes this represents TME surgery for rectal cancer. This ensures that there is no bowel content between the stoma and the anastomosis. The Bowel preparation protocol is presented in Table 23.1.

Table 23.1. Bowel preparation protocol.

Right hemicolectomy	None
Extended Right hemicolectomy	None
Subtotal and ileo-rectal anastomosis	Phosphate Enema
Left hemicolectomy	Phosphate Enema
Sigmoid colectomy	Phosphate Enema
High anterior resection	Phosphate Enema
Low anterior resection with defunctioning ileostomy	Picolax® or Moviprep®
AP resection	None

Preoperative Assessment

All preoperative assessments including blood tests will have been carried out in a visit to the nurse led pre-assessment clinic. This will have included scrutiny of the patients' drugs, blood tests and ECG. Protocolised referral for cardiopulmonary exercise testing (CPET) in an anaesthetist led clinic is arranged if the exercise capacity threshold is below 4 METS. This is determined by questioning or a Shuttle Walk test.

Preoperative anaemia will be treated according to the cardiopulmonary status of the patient and staging of their cancer. Anticoagulants such as Warfarin or Clopidogrel are stopped and appropriate anticoagulation commenced depending on the indication. ACE inhibitors are not given the day of surgery.

Admission

Admission is arranged for approximately 2 h prior to surgery unless there is a specific indication to admit earlier such as in-patient bowel preparation or planned blood transfusion.

Perioperative Care

DVT Prophylaxis

All patients undergoing colorectal resection receive DVT prophylaxis. All patients are fitted with full-length graduated compression stockings unless contraindicated by vascular disease. Intra-operatively sequential calf compression is deployed. Post operatively the patients receive low molecular weight heparin such as 40 mg of Clexane (or equivalent) daily for 2 weeks and are taught to self-administer this once discharged. Patients at high risk of DVT may receive more prolonged administration. Patients who are normally anti-coagulated are reinitiated according to specific requirements after 48 h.

Anaesthetic

The aim of the anaesthetist is to provide anaesthesia with rapid awakening, good control of analgesia and minimal post-operative nausea and vomiting (PONV). The anaesthetist is also responsible for fluid therapy so that the patient's cardiac output is optimised, organs and tissues perfused and at the end of surgery is normovolaemic.

Standard induction of anaesthesia with Propofol 2–3 mg/kg and an opioid such as fentanyl 2–4 μg/kg or Alfentanyl 5–10 μg/kg followed by an appropriate dose of muscle relaxant should be administered followed by intubation with an oral endotracheal tube. We maintain neuromuscular blockade with a peripheral nerve stimulator (TOF or train of four watch) to a Post Tetanic Count of 2–4 to allow a lower pressure pneumoperitoneum. This appears to reduce pain post operatively but we are waiting the results of a randomised trial to confirm this in a more scientific manner.

Nasogastric tubes should not be routinely inserted unless there is gastric dilatation impairing surgery. If this is necessary, they can be removed at the end of the procedure.

Maintenance of anaesthesia should be with oxygen enriched air with a short acting volatile such as Sevoflurane or Desflurane titrated to effect. In the elderly a BIS monitor should be considered to deliver the minimal required dose and reduce the risk of post operative cognitive dysfunction.

Prophylaxis for PONV should be with a 5HT3 blocker such as Ondansetron 4 mg or Granisetron 1 mg. The addition of a small dose of Dexamethasone 4 mg may be beneficial but we are awaiting the DREAMS (Dexamethasone reduces emesis after major gastrointestinal) study to determine its safety in cancer surgery. If the patients are at high risk of PONV a target controlled Propofol Infusion should be considered.

Prophylactic antibiotics are given according to local policy and repeated as necessary up to 24 h.

The patient is warmed using a warm air blanket. Intravenous fluids are also warmed and the CO_2 gas used for pneumoperitoneum is warmed and humidified.

Intraoperative Analgesia

There are many options for analgesia for laparoscopic colorectal surgery. In our study on optimal analgesia in laparoscopic surgery thoracic epidural anaesthesia (TEA) did not confer the benefits seen in open surgery and instead tended to slow patients down after surgery as they were connected to pumps and had more problems with mobilising due to hypotension. Although it is possible to provide analgesia with the sole use of intravenous morphine we believe reducing the amount of morphine given is beneficial as larger doses increase the risk of ileus and affect sleep and well-being. The use of TAP (trans abdominus planus) blocks and local anaesthetic wound catheters are becoming increasingly used around the world however we have struggled with both efficacy and duration of analgesia. Our preferred method of providing analgesia is to use a spinal anaesthetic using a low volume (2–2.2 ml) of heavy bupivacaine 0.5 % with a dose of diamorphine dosed at 5 µg/kg (0.3–0.5 mg). Spinal anaesthesia is very safe and in our hands has very high efficacy. The diamorphine reduces opiate consumption in the postoperative period. We are often asked why we do not increase the dose of Diamorphine to try and avoid the use of morphine at all. We have found increasing the dose runs the risk of protracted nausea and vomiting so that patients cannot take oral multimodal analgesia or diet which then results in them getting further parenteral morphine and possibly further intravenous fluids, both of which increase the risk of post operative ileus. Our aim is to have the patient discharged to the ward comfortable, able to mobilise with minimal PONV. We do not see the need for a single dose of supplemental morphine in the PACU as a failure of the spinal. The patient groups more likely to need supplemental morphine are those that have had splenic flexure mobilisation or have a high extraction site.

Fluid Therapy and Haemodynamic Monitoring

It is essential to get fluid therapy correct as too little leads to complications and too much leads to increased complications and ileus. There is currently a lot of controversy over the use of additional monitoring using Minimally Invasive Cardiac Output (MICO) devices to guide fluid therapy (Oesophageal Doppler, LIDCO Rapid, Flotrac etc.). There has been little published data to support their use in laparoscopic surgery within an Enhanced Recovery Programme over a "zero balance" approach where the aim is to keep the patient normovolaemic with minimal increase in weight due to fluid excess. We believe that fluid therapy is about giving the right amount of fluid at the right time and to minimise the total volume given. This approach maintains vital organ and splanchnic perfusion but avoids the salt and water overload seen in many units. An individualised approach is important and to achieve this we use both clinical and haemodynamic parameters.

We deliver an individualised approach by using the Oesophageal Doppler during the operative period. This uses a soft oesophageal probe inserted after intubation. A doppler signal is emitted from the tip and a sensor measures the Doppler shift to determine red blood cell velocity in the descending aorta. When accurately focused many useful parameters are obtained such as peak velocity, stroke volume (through a nomogram for aortic diameter for age and height × stroke distance) and FTc (flow time corrected for systole). The oxygen delivery can be calculated and the performance of the heart in response to fluids and the physiological changes of Pneumoperitoneum and position of the patient during surgery. Although purists would argue against the absolute accuracy of these machines we find the numbers, waveforms and trends help identify the following physiological states: fluid responsiveness after commencement of intermittent positive pressure ventilation (IPPV), poor left ventricular performance in response to aortic loading during the Pneumoperitoneum, and hypovolaemia at the end of surgery once the patient is flat and Pneumoperitoneum released. We therefore fluid optimise prior to commencing surgery, monitor the left ventricular ejection and peak velocity during laparoscopy (and if it remains low consider further fluid boluses and whether the patient needs a higher level of care postoperatively) and fluid optimise at the end of surgery. We use a balanced crystalloid solution and total volumes given range widely but rarely exceed 30 ml/kg in total plus blood loss. The patients may need one or two more fluid boluses of 250mls in recovery depending on surgery but otherwise will receive a maximum of 1 litre of post operative intravenous fluids at a rate of 1ml/kg/hour until they tolerate oral diet.

Surgery

Set Up

The setup varies slightly according to the operation being undertaken. The positioning of the patient on the operation table is undertaken with consideration of both patient safety and optimising surgical access. Tilting of the patient both head down, head up and laterally means that the patient is at risk of movement on the operating table and causing injury.

To secure the patient on the operating table the following actions are undertaken.

1.   The patient's bare skin is placed in direct contact with either a non-slip mattress or a gel mat. This facilitates friction forces that prevent the patient sliding.

2. For left-sided resections where extreme head down tilt may be necessary—bilateral shoulder supports with thick gel blocks are placed in gentle contact with the shoulder. This is not necessary for right-sided resections.
3. A lateral support is placed over the deltoid muscle on the right for left-sided resections and on the left for right-sided resections. Gel padding is used.
4. Both arms are carefully wrapped at the sides once all venous and arterial access lines have been secured and protected.
5. For right-sided resections a strap is placed around the legs.
6. For left-sided resections or when perineal access is required the legs are placed in "yellow-fin" leg supports with the thigh at 180° to the abdominal wall and the knee bent at approximately 45°.
7. The legs are fitted with sequential compression stockings.
8. A urinary catheter is placed and secured.
9. A "Bair-hugger" warming blanket is positioned and secured prior to prepping the patient.

Surgical Principles

Whenever possible colorectal resection is undertaken using minimally invasive techniques. It is deemed necessary to perform an open laparotomy in a small minority of elective cases usually determined by considerations of the pathology. A higher proportion of emergency cases require open surgery because of the limitations of laparoscopy in these circumstances.

Surgery is conducted with these principles in mind

- Laparoscopic whenever feasible
- Experienced surgeon/supervisor to limit risk of conversion
- Minimising blood loss
- Minimising collateral damage
- Small extraction incisions placed transversely in the lower abdomen
- Short operating times
- Operating at low intra-peritoneal pressure where possible
- Meticulous and precise surgical technique

Whilst it is difficult to prove we believe that these principles of high-quality surgery are inevitably associated with the best outcomes when married with enhanced recovery and lead to less pain, less ileus and more rapid recovery of function.

Post-operative Care

Fluid/Diet

Oral fluids are commenced as soon as the patient is fully alert following surgery. It is feasible to commence fluids when the patient is still in the recovery unit and certainly within a few hours. The anaesthetist will have ensured that the patient is normovolaemic and well hydrated at the termination of surgery and IV fluids can be stopped immediately if the patient drinks satisfactorily.

A light diet is also commenced on the evening of surgery. The patient is encouraged to eat and would certainly expect to have a normal breakfast the morning after surgery.

Monitoring

Unless there is a specific indication for continuing monitoring any aspect of the patients physiology all lines are removed on the morning following surgery including IV access, central lines and arterial lines (if used), urinary catheter.

Intra-abdominal drains are not routinely used but when placed are usually there simply to drain excess irrigation fluid for example and is removed also at this time). Reasons to maintain monitoring of urine output would include patients with pre-existing renal failure. Urine output is not scrutinised in patients who have normal renal function and who have had an uncomplicated operation. Concern over renal function is better addressed by a simple blood test. There is a risk that reacting to a low urine output which is a normal physiological response to surgery in these circumstances leads to over-infusion of fluids with risk of ileus.

Mobilisation

The patient is actively encouraged to mobilise early after surgery. This is facilitated by minimally invasive surgery, good pain control and the removal of lines and catheters. The early removal of the catheter forces the patients to mobilise to the bathroom. Elderly and frail patients will require active nursing support to achieve this target. The concept of eating in a dining area away from the bed is also good in this regard where it is achievable.

Analgesia

The principle is to minimise the use of opiate analgesia. Whilst it is an excellent analgesic, it causes ileus and nausea, especially with increasing doses.

Most patients will have had a spinal injection of 2–2.2 ml of 0.5 % heavy Bupivacaine with a small dose of Diamorphine (0.3–0.5 mg) and so wake from surgery without pain. Additional morphine in recovery is required in upto 40 % of patients; however, with the addition of intrathecal opiates they rarely require opiates on the ward. Patients stay on average 2–4 h in recovery depending if they need supplemental morphine and after review by the anaesthetist. Our multimodal analgesic regime is based around regular Paracetamol (acetaminophen) 1 g four times a day with a regular NSAID such as Ibuprofen 400 mg three times a day, except where contraindicated and in this case replaced with regular Tramadol. Tramadol and Morphine are prescribed prn for breakthrough pain. Patients who have an epidural (usually open surgery or AP resection patients) have this in place for 48 h before returning to a similar regime. A PCA of morphine is sometimes used to good effect but always accompanied by regular oral Paracetamol (Acetaminophen) and NSAIDS and removed as soon as practicable.

Anti-emetics

Anti-emetics are administered as part of the general anaesthetic protocol. A combination of two antiemetics is most efficacious. Post operatively they are prescribed only on a PRN basis. Nausea should not be a contraindication to commencing diet but active vomiting clearly needs to be addressed.

Discharge Criteria

The whole team is motivated toward the two goals of reducing postoperative complications and minimising hospital stay. For the most part lack of bowel activity is not considered a contraindication to discharge and the criteria for assessing fitness for discharge is as follows.

- Pain controlled with oral analgesia (patient does not need to be pain free)
- Free of nausea and vomiting

- Tolerating free fluids
- Tolerating light diet
- Mobile
- Adequate home support
- Patient acceptability
- Passing urine normally

References

1. Day A, Smith R, Fawcett B, Scott M, Rockall T. The optimal fluid to use with an oesophageal Doppler monitor in laparoscopic colorectal surgery. Br J Surg. 2013;100:39.
2. Day A, Smith R, Fawcett B, Scott M, Rockall T. Does the choice of analgesia attenuate the stress response following laparoscopic colorectal surgery? Br J Surg. 2013;100:2.
3. Day A, Smith R, Jourdan I, Fawcett W, Scott M, Rockall T. Retrospective analysis of the effect of postoperative analgesia on survival in patients after laparoscopic resection of colorectal cancer. Br J Anaesth. 2012;109(2):185–90.
4. Levy BF, Fawcett WJ, Scott MJ, Rockall TA. Intra-operative oxygen delivery in infusion volume-optimized patients undergoing laparoscopic colorectal surgery within an enhanced recovery programme: the effect of different analgesic modalities. Colorectal Dis. 2012;14(7):887–92.
5. Levy BF, Scott MJ, Fawcett W, Fry C, Rockall TA. Randomized clinical trial of epidural, spinal or patient-controlled analgesia for patients undergoing laparoscopic colorectal surgery. Br J Surg. 2011;98(8):1068–78.
6. Levy BF, Tilney HS, Dowson HM, Rockall TA. A systematic review of postoperative analgesia following laparoscopic colorectal surgery. Colorectal Dis. 2010;12(1):5–15.
7. Levy BF, Scott MJ, Fawcett WJ, Day A, Rockall TA. Optimizing patient outcomes in laparoscopic surgery. Colorectal Dis. 2011;13 Suppl 7:8–11.
8. Levy BF, Scott MJ, Fawcett WJ, Rockall TA. 23-Hour-stay laparoscopic colectomy. Dis Colon Rectum. 2009;52(7):1239–43.
9. Day A, Smith R, Jourdan I, Rockall T. Laparoscopic TME for rectal cancer: a case series. Surg Laparosc Endosc Percutan Tech. 2012;22(2):e98–101.
10. Day AR, Smith RV, Jourdan IC, Rockall TA. Survival following laparoscopic and open colorectal surgery. Surg Endosc. 2013;27(7):2415–21.
11. Day AR, Middleton G, Smith RV, Jourdan IC, Rockall TA. Time to adjuvant chemotherapy following colorectal cancer resection is associated with an improved survival. Colorectal Dis. 2014;16(5):368–72.
12. Dowson HM, Ballard K, Gage H, Jackson D, Williams P, Rockall TA. Quality of life in the first 6 weeks following laparoscopic and open colorectal surgery. Value Health. 2013;16(2):367–72.
13. Dowson H, Cowie A, Ballard K, Gage H, Rockall T. Systematic review of quality of life following laparoscopic and open colorectal surgery. Colorectal Dis. 2008;10(8):757–68.

24. Setting Up an Enhanced Recovery Program Pathway for Bariatric Surgery: Current Evidence into Practice

Rajesh Aggarwal

Over the past two decades in particular, bariatric (or metabolic) surgery has increased in terms of its volume. Indeed, almost 180,000 cases were performed in the United States alone in 2013, comprised mostly of gastric banding (14 %), Roux-en-Y gastric bypass (34 %), and sleeve gastrectomy (42 %) [1]. This is not only a testament to the great demand of this type of surgery, in terms of patients who suffer from co-morbidities such as type II diabetes, sleep apnea, hypertension, and polycystic ovarian disease, but also to the fact that the surgery is considered a safe and viable option. Over the past 10 years, technical modifications such as changes to the anastomotic technique, and timing of thrombotic prophylaxis have led to the development of a safer laparoscopic technique [2]. Numerous prospective reports confirm extremely low rates of morbidity and mortality [3, 4].

With this in mind, it is timely to consider the next steps in the evolution of bariatric surgery, such as further reductions in complication rates and decreased length of hospital stay. The impact of clinical care pathways with respect to enhanced recovery programs has been strongly affiliated to colorectal surgery, and more recently have propagated almost all types of surgical practice [5]. It is with this background that it is important and relevant to consider the current scope, and future role of Enhanced Recovery After Surgery programs (ERPs) with respect to bariatric surgery.

L.S. Feldman et al. (eds.), *The SAGES / ERAS®*
Society Manual of Enhanced Recovery Programs for
Gastrointestinal Surgery, DOI 10.1007/978-3-319-20364-5_24,
© Springer International Publishing Switzerland 2015

Clinical Pathways in Bariatric Surgery

Whilst not under the name of ERP, the first publication to consider a clinical pathway for bariatric surgery was published in 2001, with respect to 28 patients, 12 of whom were recruited to a multidisciplinary clinical pathway [6]. The pathway involved patient education materials, standardized preoperative and postoperative orders, including early ambulation and oral diet, together with standardized discharge instructions. In comparison to the 16 patients who underwent standard care, there was a reduction in hospital stay of 3 days, similar complication and readmission rates, and a greater than 15 % decrease in resource utilization costs. In 2005, McCarty et al. published results of 2000 consecutive patients having undergone outpatient laparoscopic gastric bypass [7]. Of the 1699 (84 %) discharged within 23 h, 34 (1.7 %) were readmitted within 30 days, with low overall early (38, 1.9 %) and late (86, 4.3 %) complication rates, and only 2 (0.1 %) deaths. In this publication, the authors very much focus upon the perioperative period, in terms of analgesia, antiemetics, and surgical technique.

Whilst both of these studies reflect the impact of standardization of clinical processes, neither describes their approach with regard to adoption by other centers. More recently, in 2013, Lemanu et al. published a randomized controlled trial of enhanced recovery versus standard care after laparoscopic sleeve gastrectomy [8]. Of their 116 patients, 40 patients underwent the ERP protocol, and were compared to two other groups, i.e., a control group of 38 patients, and a historical cohort of a further 38 patients. What is of interest here is that the authors specifically defined the preoperative, intraoperative, and postoperative aspects of their ERP protocol (Table 24.1), including a summary of their discharge criteria. Their work was preceded by an extensive review of the current literature of bariatric and major abdominal surgery [9]. With regard to the clinical outcomes, the ERP group had a reduced length of stay (from 2 days to 1 day), with similar complication and readmission rates.

Discharge Criteria

An area of particular interest with the study from Lemanu et al. is with respect to the discharge criteria, which focus upon adequate pain relief, no wound disturbances, normal vital signs, uneventful technical procedure, patient ambulatory and tolerating free oral fluid by mouth [8].

Table 24.1. Components of bariatric enhanced recovery protocol.

Before surgery	Formal standardized preop. education
	Formal goal-setting session
	Tour of the ward
Morning of surgery	Clear oral fluids up to 2 h before surgery
	Carbohydrate drinks×2
During surgery	8 mg i.v. dexamethasone at induction of surgery
	Standardized anesthesia [1]
	Intraperitoneal local anesthesia [2]
	Avoidance of prophylactic nasogastric tubes and drains
After surgery	Early instigation of oral intake
	Mobilization 2 h after return to ward
	Standardized multimodal analgesia [3] and antiemesis [4]
	Standardized multimodal thromboprophylaxis [5]
After discharge	Telephone calls 1 day and 1 week after discharge
	2-week follow-up in clinic

Notes:
1. Induction agent (e.g., propofol), inhaled agent (e.g., sevoflurane), paralytic agent (e.g., rocuronium)
2. Bupivacaine 0.5 %
3. Acetaminophen PO or IV; Oxycodone PO or PR; Hydromorphone SC
4. Ondansetron IV
5. Mobilize 4 h after surgery; Sequential compression stockings; Heparin SC 7500 IU q12

Adapted from Lemanu DP, Singh PP, Berridge K, Burr M, Birch C, Babor R, MacCormick AD, Arroll B, Hill AG. Randomized clinical trial of enhanced recovery versus standard care after laparoscopic sleeve gastrectomy. Br J Surg. 2013 Mar;100(4):482–9; with permission

The discharge criteria are clearly defined, and unambiguous; further, they are supported by close patient follow-up after discharge, i.e., a phone call at 1 day and 1 week after leaving the hospital. It is imperative when building an ERP, to not only focus upon the processes of care within the hospital, but also upon standardization of the discharge criteria.

Compliance to ERP Components

A further aspect, which merits mention, is that the authors recorded compliance with components of the ERP protocol for the intervention and control groups [8]. This type of data is rarely seen, and shows interesting differences between the two groups. For example, all 100 % of the patients in the ERP group underwent preoperative education and a ward tour, compared to none of those in the control group. However, there were minimal differences between the two groups with regard to other factors, such as enoxaparin use, catheter removal, and avoidance of nasogastric tubes. This is important information for two purposes; firstly, to state that a number of the ERP components were already part of standard practice prior to the initiation of the trial, and secondly that there are areas which can achieve 100 % uptake with moderate effort, and minimal expense—such as a ward tour.

Which ERP Components Should I Start with?

So, the question that needs to be answered is with regard to which ERP components are of most importance, and thus require initial focus. A list of preoperative, intraoperative, and postoperative ERP components with regard to bariatric surgery are available in Table 24.2. Ideally, it is important to appraise the evidence for each criterion, which would lead to the development of an evidence-based ERP protocol for bariatric surgery. Whilst this has not been explicitly done, there is analogous work with respect to esophagectomy. Findlay et al. systematically reviewed the literature for all publications related to ERP and esophagectomy; they found six citations, which demonstrated favorable morbidity, mortality, and length of stay when compared with traditionally managed groups of patients [10]. However, they then continued to identify and define all the components of ERP for esophagectomy, and through systematic review of the evidence in esophagectomy or associated procedures, assigned evidence-based recommendations to each

Table 24.2. Processes of care to consider in ERP for bariatric surgery.

Preoperative	Intraoperative	Postoperative
Patient education	Orogastric tube	PACU duration
Preoperative assessment	Extubation	Oral intake
Date of admission	Leak test	Mobilization
Weight reduction		Antithrombotic therapy
Antithrombotic therapy		Incentive spirometry
Antibiotic therapy		Discharge criteria
Oral food intake		
Oral fluids		

component. For example, with regard to chest drains, their "use should be minimized; a single drain is as effective as two drains but less painful," and "delaying [oral] intake by routine anastomotic imaging is not recommended." Utilizing this type of methodology, with graded appraisal of the evidence, enables esophageal surgeons to make value judgments with regard to each component of the ERP pathway. Whilst it may not be too complex to develop and provide patients with an information brochure, post-discharge telephone calls may require a reorganization of staff responsibilities, and be more of a challenge.

Similarly, these types of processes to appraise the literature with regard to bariatric surgery can be performed. If the literature is absent, then at very least, data can be inferred from reports of analogous procedures.

Patient Information

The keys to development and implementation of an ERP-type patient care within bariatric surgery can be distilled into the following "take-home points." Firstly, patient education is critical, with respect to preoperative, intraoperative, and postoperative care. This can be done with the use of a booklet, DVD, or online material. The material needs to be easy to understand, and supported by simple diagrams and flow pathways. If the patient understands their expected care pathway, they are much more likely not only to engage in the pathway, but also to adhere to it. Postoperative tasks such as early mobilization, early oral fluid intake, and expected length of hospital stay should be provided to patients up front, so that they are truly active participants in their own care. Patients should also be aware of discharge criteria, as a target to aim toward. Whilst not described in the literature, an awareness of criteria that may raise concern with regard to a complication should also be made clear to patients, at the outset. Patients also like to share this information with their families, and should be encouraged to do so.

Standardization of Care Processes

From the clinical perspective, the greatest gain comes from standardization of preoperative, intraoperative, and postoperative processes. From anesthesia, to thrombotic prophylaxis and antibiotic therapy, to operative steps and equipment required. All of this serves to develop a uniform process of care, which means that anesthetic, nursing, and ward staff can develop a single standard of care [11]. This can also lead to reduced costs in terms of procurement, but also in terms of efficiency and subsequent productivity. The standardization of care also includes clear processes for management of complications, such as postoperative sepsis or bleeding [12]. Once again, this can reduce the risks of unnecessary investigations, and provide timely treatment for such patients.

Implementation and Outcomes Analysis

Implementation of a new pathway of care is challenging. The ideal manner is to engage the multidisciplinary stakeholders within the group early, so that when the pathway is launched, they have already all been involved. However, some degree of training is necessary, which at its simplest can be in the form of seminars, and at its most complex, can be through use of simulation-based training programs. When undertaking such a process to standardize and enhance care, it is critical to audit its implementation. A robust prospective registry should be maintained, and regularly monitored to ensure that new models of care continue to ensure patient safety.

References

1. http://asmbs.org/resources/estimate-of-bariatric-surgery-numbers. Accessed 21 Jan 2015.
2. McGrath V, Needleman BJ, Melvin WS. Evolution of the laparoscopic gastric bypass. J Laparoendosc Adv Surg Tech A. 2003;13:221–7.
3. DeMaria EJ, Pate V, Warthen M, Winegar DA. Baseline data from American Society for Metabolic and Bariatric Surgery-designated Bariatric Surgery Centers of Excellence using the Bariatric Outcomes Longitudinal Database. Surg Obes Relat Dis. 2010;6(4):347–55.
4. Longitudinal Assessment of Bariatric Surgery (LABS) Consortium, Flum DR, Belle SH, King WC, Wahed AS, Berk P, Chapman W, Pories W, Courcoulas A, McCloskey C, Mitchell J, Patterson E, Pomp A, Staten MA, Yanovski SZ, Thirlby R, Wolfe B. Perioperative safety in the longitudinal assessment of bariatric surgery. N Engl J Med. 2009;361(5):445–54.
5. Kehlet H. Multimodal approach to postoperative recovery. Curr Opin Crit Care. 2009;15(4):355–8.
6. Cooney RN, Bryant P, Haluck R, Rodgers M, Lowery M. The impact of a clinical pathway for gastric bypass surgery on resource utilization. J Surg Res. 2001;98(2):97–101.

7. McCarty TM, Arnold DT, Lamont JP, Fisher TL, Kuhn JA. Optimizing outcomes in bariatric surgery: outpatient laparoscopic gastric bypass. Ann Surg. 2005;242(4): 494–8. discussion 498–501.

8. Lemanu DP, Singh PP, Berridge K, Burr M, Birch C, Babor R, MacCormick AD, Arroll B, Hill AG. Randomized clinical trial of enhanced recovery versus standard care after laparoscopic sleeve gastrectomy. Br J Surg. 2013;100(4):482–9.

9. Lemanu DP, Srinivasa S, Singh PP, Johannsen S, Maccormick AD, Hill AG. Optimizing perioperative care in bariatric surgery patients. Obes Surg. 2012;22:979–90.

10. Findlay JM, Gillies RS, Millo J, Sgromo B, Marshall RE, Maynard ND. Enhanced recovery for esophagectomy: a systematic review and evidence-based guidelines. Ann Surg. 2014;259(3):413–31.

11. Aggarwal R. Better care in the operating room. World J Surg. 2014;38(12):3053–5.

12. Pucher PH, Aggarwal R, Qurashi M, Singh P, Darzi A. Randomized clinical trial of the impact of surgical ward-care checklists on postoperative care in a simulated environment. Br J Surg. 2014;101(13):1666–73.

25. Enhanced Recovery Pathways in Hepato-pancreato-biliary Surgery

Didier Roulin and Nicolas Demartines

In the last two decades enhanced recovery pathways (ERP) have been successfully implemented in various fields of surgery, notably in colorectal surgery where numerous meta-analyses have shown lower complication rates associated with reduced postoperative stay and diminished hospital costs [1, 2]. Following these encouraging results, ERP have been progressively implemented to hepato-pancreato-biliary (HPB) surgery, which is traditionally considered as high-risk surgery.

Review of the Current Literature

Although pancreatic surgery has become safer in high-volume specialized centers with a significant reduction of perioperative mortality to 5 %, reported morbidity rates still remain considerably high, ranging from 40 to 60 % with a postoperative length of stay ranging from 14 to 20 days after pancreaticoduodenectomy [3]. Delayed recovery is mainly due to pancreatic fistula and delayed gastric emptying. A recently published systematic review in pancreatic surgery found that ERPs were associated with both a significant decrease in length of stay of 2–6 days and a reduction in complications without increased mortality or readmission rate [3]. However, the occurrence of pancreatic fistula or delayed gastric emptying did not differ [3]. On the other hand, the pathways were heterogeneous and important data like time to functional recovery and compliance to the ERP elements were scarcely described. Therefore, future prospective studies based on the published guidelines for perioperative care for pancreaticoduodenectomy by the ERAS® Society are required in order to assess the proper impact of ERP on functional postoperative recovery [4].

L.S. Feldman et al. (eds.), *The SAGES / ERAS®*
Society Manual of Enhanced Recovery Programs for
Gastrointestinal Surgery, DOI 10.1007/978-3-319-20364-5_25,
© Springer International Publishing Switzerland 2015

ERP have also been recently implemented in liver surgery, which is associated with about 40 % morbidity, with specific complications like hemorrhage, biliary leakage, intra-abdominal abscess and liver failure. In a meta-analysis [5], hospital length of stay was reduced and functional recovery was accelerated without compromising morbidity or mortality rates, and readmission rates were similar. In a recent randomized controlled trial on ERP for open liver resection [6], the median time to be medically fit for discharge was reduced with the ERP from 6 to 3 days, as was overall length of stay (7 vs. 4 days). The medical complications were significantly reduced, while surgical complications were similar. The readmission rates and mortality remained unchanged but health related quality of life in the first month after surgery was significantly better in the ERP group. However, there is until today no standardized protocol, and the guidelines on liver resection perioperative care from the ERAS Society are pending.

Specific Items in ERP for Pancreatic and Liver Surgery

In the patient population undergoing HPB surgery, preoperative nutrition is a significant concern. A nutrition screening assessing the Nutritional Risk Score (NRS) [7] is routinely performed, and malnourished patients with a NRS ≥3 are referred to specific dietician consultation. As the majority of advanced HPB surgery is still performed by laparotomy, preoperative immunonutrition (Oral Impact®, Nestlé) is given for 7 days before the surgery, as this intervention may reduce the infectious complications rate [8].

In order to implement ERP in liver resection, there are two major elements requiring some adaptation from those applied in colorectal surgery: fluid management and prophylactic drainage. In liver surgery, a relative hypovolemia with a low central venous pressure less than 5 cm H_2O is maintained before and during liver resection, in order to minimize the amount of intra-operative blood loss. The blood pressure is controlled by vasopressors and blood transfusion when required. The central venous pressure can be lowered by the use of intravenous nitroglycerin during the liver resection. Once the resection is completed, euvolemia, as assessed by the central venous pressure, is restored by balanced crystalloid and colloid infusion, and hypoalbuminemia less than 20 g/L is compensated by intravenous albumin (20 %). For open liver surgery, a high thoracic epidural (T5–8) is placed and continued in the post-resection phase. Although not used in our center, a prophylactic drain placed close to the hepatic resection surface is still widely used, with the idea to prevent intra-abdominal collection, detect postoperative bleeding and bile leakage, as well as to drain ascites. However, a Cochrane Review did not show any statistically significant difference in terms of occurrence of postoperative infection or biloma or detection of bile leak and hemorrhage between the drain and no drain groups after elective liver resection [9]. Moreover, in a separate meta-analysis, there was a trend toward an increased rate of infected collections for drained patients [10]. There is currently no evidence to support the routine use of prophylactic drainage after liver resection. However, the use of abdominal drainage in order to prevent the accumulation of ascites, which can lead to ascitic leakage and wound dehiscence, remains debated in the current literature [11, 12]. Further trials are needed to assess its use in the specific group of cirrhotic patients.

In order to apply enhanced recovery principles to pancreatic surgery, and especially to pancreaticoduodenectomy, there are two main issues, which differ widely from colorectal ERP pathways: prophylactic drainage and postoperative nutrition. Following pancreatic resection, the use of prophylactic drains, placed in relation to both the biliary and pancreatic anastomoses, is still considered mandatory by many experts. Up to now there is only one randomized trial comparing prophylactic drainage vs. no drainage after pancreatectomy for pancreatic cancer [13]. This study found no significant difference in the mortality or the overall rate of complications whether intraperitoneal drains were present or not. Furthermore, drained patients were significantly more likely to develop an intra-abdominal collection or fistula (pancreatic and enterocutaneous). However, these data arise from a highly selected population of patients with pancreatic tumors treated in a specialized and experienced cancer center. In a meta-analysis comparing early vs. late drain removal, the incidence of pancreatic fistula was significantly lower in the early-removal group for patients at low risk of pancreatic fistula (amylase value in drains ≤5000 U/L at postoperative day 3) [14]. A recently published randomized multicenter trial comparing pancreaticoduodenectomy with or without routine drainage was interrupted by the data safety monitoring board because of increased mortality in the patients without drainage [15]. However, in this study all patients were randomized, irrespective of the pancreas consistency or the pancreatic duct size, and further trials specifically assessing the use of drainage in patients with higher risk of pancreatic fistula are warranted. Another intervention frequently used to prevent pancreatic fistula is somatostatin analogue, which reduces splanchnic blood flow and pancreatic secretion. In the current literature, somatostatin and its analogues do not reduce the rate of clinically significant fistula or overall morbidity and mortality [16] and are not systematically recommended [4]. Recently, new somatostatin analogues with longer half-life and broader binding profile such as pasireotide have been developed, and their use was found to be associated with a reduction of the rate of clinically significant pancreatic fistula following pancreatic resection in a randomized trial of 300 patients [17]. Further trials, with subgroup analyses specifically assessing the pancreatic texture and duct size, are necessary to evaluate the role of systematic somatostatin analogues in the prevention of postoperative pancreatic fistula.

Postoperative nutrition after a pancreatic resection is a key issue. A naso-gastric tube is routinely placed during surgery in order to evacuate air. However, there is high-level evidence that prophylactic nasogastric decompression increases the risk of pulmonary atelectasis and pneumonia and alters return of bowel function [18]. Therefore, the prophylactic use of nasogastric tube postoperatively should be avoided. In the postoperative period, a recent multicenter randomized controlled trial in patients undergoing major upper gastrointestinal and HPB surgery, including 82 pancreaticoduodenectomy, concluded that allowing early diet was safe for these patients and that enteral tube feeding did not confer benefit [19]. Therefore, patients should be allowed to gradually increase oral food intake over 3–4 days according to their tolerance. The use of enteral or parenteral nutritional should be reserved for patients developing major complications, with parenteral nutrition indicated only in those patients who cannot tolerate enteral nutrition [4]. A frequent complication after pancreaticoduodenectomy is delayed gastric emptying which can occur in up to a quarter of the patients. If prolonged delayed gastric emptying occurs, it may be necessary to insert a naso-jejunal feeding tube. In this case, supplemental nutrition should be established within ten postoperative days in order to resume a regular diet sooner [20].

Practical Implementation of ERP in Hepato-pancreato-biliary Surgery

Following successful implementation of ERP in elective and emergency colorectal surgery in our Department starting 2011 [21, 22], ERP was introduced in October 2012 for elective pancreas surgery and in

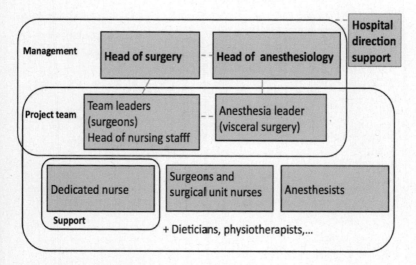

Fig. 25.1. Organization chart of enhanced recovery team.

June 2013 for elective liver surgery. Separate pathways were implemented for pancreaticoduodenectomy and spleno-pancreatectomy, as the latter, which does not include any digestive anastomosis, is less prone to delayed gastric emptying. For liver surgery, all different types of resection up to four segments were included in a single pathway. Based on the previously introduced ERP team for colorectal surgery, a similar group was organized (Fig. 25.1). Under the direction of the chair of the Department for Visceral Surgery, the three pillars of the ERP team were the surgeons, anesthesiologists, and nurses. For pancreas and liver, the surgeons in charge of the respective units were designed as leaders of the team and supported by two to three designated surgeons. The anesthesia leader was the same as for the colorectal ERP and also benefited from the support of other anesthetists. On the nurses' part, a dedicated ERP nurse was involved in each of these pathways. The administrative direction was involved from the beginning and played a substantial role in obtaining the required resources. In addition, nutritionists, physiotherapists, and stoma-therapists were also involved in regular ERP team meetings in order to monitor and improve our protocols, which are detailed on Table 25.1. Specific documentation including patient education booklets and logbooks where the patients record their own progress, anesthesia protocols, standardized care maps and medical orders, were established.

Table 25.1. Perioperative care elements for hepato-pancreato-biliary surgery.

	Liver resection	Duodenopancreatectomy
Preoperative counseling	Preadmission counseling (surgeon, dedicated nurse) + written information	
Preoperative biliary drainage	–	Endoscopic biliary drainage if serum bilirubin higher than 250 μmol/L
Preoperative smoking and alcohol consumption	Smoking and alcohol abstinence 1 month before surgery	
Preoperative nutrition	Nutritional status assessment by the dedicated nurse (NRS score) and referral to dietician if at risk (NRS ≥3)	
Oral bowel preparation	Avoidance of oral bowel preparation	
Fasting	Clear fluids until 2 h, solids 6 h before surgery	
Carbohydrate drinks	800 ml on evening and 400 ml 2 h before surgery	
Preanaesthetic medication	No long-acting sedative premedication	
Antithrombotic prophylaxis	LMWH 12 h before surgery and continued for 4 weeks after surgery	
	Intermittent pneumatic compression when in bed until POD 4	
Antimicrobial prophylaxis and skin preparation	Antibioprophylaxis: Cefuroxime 1.5 g + metronidazole 500 mg iv 30–60 min before incision	
	Skin preparation with a scrub of chlorhexidine-alcohol	
Analgesia	Thoracic epidural analgesia (T5–8) until POD 4	
	If no epidural: intravenous lidocaine or transversus abdominis plane block/wound infiltration	
PONV prophylaxis	Perioperative: Droperidol 1 mg iv and betamethasone 4 mg iv at the beginning of operation, ondansetron 4 mg iv at the end of operation	
	Postoperative: ondansetron 4 mg 3×/day and betamethasone 4 mg 1–2×/day if needed, until POD 3–5	
Hypothermia prevention	Active warming (cutaneous and perfusions warming) to maintain body temperature ≥36.1 °C	
Glycemic control	Perioperative intravenous/postoperative subcutaneous insulin if glycemia more than 10 mmol/L	

(continued)

Table 25.1. (continued).

	Liver resection	Duodenopancreatectomy
Intraoperative fluids	Before liver resection: – Minimal intravenous fluids (aim central venous pressure <5 cm H_2O), vasopressors During liver resection: – Venous vasodilatation with nitroglycerin to maintain low central venous pressure After liver resection: – Euvolemia restoration with balanced crystalloids and colloids if necessary	Balanced crystalloids 3–5 mL/kg/h. Goal directed crystalloids or colloid (according to pulse pressure variation/transesophageal doppler or minimally invasive cardiac output monitors)
Postoperative fluids	Balanced crystalloids 1000 ml during the first 24 h then 500 mL/day until POD 6	Balanced crystalloids 1000 ml during the first 24 h, then 500 mL/day until POD 4, and then 250 mL/day until POD 8
Nasogastric intubation	No routine postoperative gastric tube	
Abdominal drains	No routine abdominal drain	Perianastomotic drain removal on POD 3 if amylase content in drain less than 5000 U/L
Somatostatin analogues	–	Not used routinely
Bladder catheter	Removal on POD 3	
Nutrition	Free fluid and 2 nutritional supplements (300 kcal each) on day of surgery. Normal diet from POD 1 with 2 nutritional supplements per day	Free fluid and 2 nutritional supplements (300 kcal each) on day of surgery. Progressive realimentation from POD 1 with 2 nutritional supplements per day Pancreatic enzyme replacement therapy at each meal

(continued)

Table 25.1. (continued).

	Liver resection	Duodenopancreatectomy
Bowel movement stimulation	Oral Magnesium hydroxide 2×/day. Chewing gum at will	
Mobilization	First mobilization on the day of surgery, at least 6 h out of bed with 2 ward rounds per day thereafter	
	Incentive spirometry 4×/day	

NRS nutritional risk score, *POD* postoperative day, *LMWH* low molecular weight heparin, *PONV* postoperative nausea and vomiting

In the preoperative phase, immunonutrition is provided to all patients undergoing major open abdominal surgery. As this is done in outpatient clinic, a specific organization needs to be put in place. In our institution, the ERP dedicated nurse is in charge of this task. The immunonutrition supplement is given three times a day for 7 days before surgery. In our experience, this was well tolerated by the patients with a range of 15–20 doses ingested by each patient.

Our preliminary results in the implementation of ERP in pancreatectomy were assessed in a before/after design comparing the first 43 consecutive pancreaticoduodenectomy performed after ERP implementation with a historic control cohort of 43 patients operated immediately before implementation. Overall postoperative morbidity was 63 % with the ERP compared to 79 % in the control group ($p = 0.128$). Severe complications (Clavien grade of $\geq 3a$) occurred in 35 % and 44 %, respectively ($p = 0.51$), with fewer surgical and medical complications in ERP patients without reaching statistical significance. Postoperative median length of stay was significantly reduced from 20 days in the pre-ERP group to 14 days with ERP care ($p = 0.003$). In a preliminary subgroup analysis, the reduced length of stay seemed to be among patients with postoperative complications. The ERP implementation resulted in a significant change in the management of postoperative nutrition. As an illustration, prophylactic nasogastric tube use was reduced from 86 to 12 % with no modification in the reinsertion rate (37 % in the ERP group compared to 33 % in the traditional group) or occurrence of delayed gastric emptying (28 % vs. 40 %, $p = 0.36$). Another example of an important change in our practice was the use of somatostatin analogue. Its use was abandoned in the ERP group with no impact on the rate of pancreatic fistula (14 % vs. 28 %, $p = 0.18$). In October 2014, we compared 127 patients treated with the ERP with 61 non-ERP pancreaticoduodenectomy patients: length of stay was lower after ERP implementation (24 vs. 18 days, $p=0.055$) and morbidity in the ERP group was significantly lower (66 % in ERP, vs. 82 % in non-ERP, $p=0.02$).

For liver resection, in a preliminary comparison of 32 consecutive ERP patients with a control group of 71 patients operated on before ERP implementation, we found a significant reduction in length of stay, which decreased from 16 to 8 days ($p=0.004$). Postoperative complications were also decreased, from 35 % in the control patients to 16 % in the ERP patients ($p=0.032$). In October 2014, a comparison between 74 ERP vs. 78 non ERP liver resections confirmed both that the significant reduction in length of stay and complication rate were sustained.

Once the ERP for pancreatic and liver resection were implemented in our institution, all elective patients were systematically included without any exclusion criteria. According to our own experience, every patient can benefit from the ERP interventions, regardless of age or comorbidities. The standardized pathways (Table 25.1) are a starting point, and the individual items are adapted whenever required, according to the postoperative evolution. Postoperative complications that led to deviations from the proposed pathway generally concerned drains, nutrition, and supplementary investigations, and were adapted according to clinical evaluation. A recently published retrospective cohort study identified factors associated with "failure" of a HPB pathway [23], defined as length of stay in the intensive care unit (ICU) more than 24 h after surgery, unplanned admission to ICU within 30 days, readmission to the hospital within 30 days after surgery, reoperation for complications and/or 30-day mortality. Predictive factors of ERP failure were smoking, high preoperative alanine transaminase/glutamic-pyruvic transaminase concentration (defined as more than 67 IU/L in men and more than 55 IU/L in women), or postoperative complications. Therefore, smoking cessation before surgery seems to play an important role and the patients with high preoperative alanine transaminase may require specific attention.

Conclusion

The implementation of an ERP in HPB surgery is safe and feasible with a significant reduction of length of stay and postoperative complications, both for major pancreas and liver resection. Presently, many of the principles of HPB ERP are extrapolated from colorectal ERP. Therefore, implementation of ERP in HPB surgery based on previous experience in colorectal surgery is probably easier to achieve, as this was the case in our institution. However, there are distinct differences like the role of prophylactic drainage as well as the specific fluid management in liver resection, and the postoperative nutrition following pancreaticoduodenectomy. Further prospective cohort studies assessing the association of adherence to individual pathway items with functional recovery and outcome after HPB surgery are required. The development of laparoscopy for HPB surgery also needs specific assessment within ERP, as this might lead to some adaptations of the protocol. Moreover, the management of colorectal carcinoma patients with synchronous liver metastases might be influenced by the use of ERPs for liver and colon resections, as a quicker recovery might enable earlier adjuvant chemotherapy (Fig. 25.2). The occurrence of postoperative complications not only impedes the achievement of an enhanced recovery but also has an impact on long-term survival [24, 25]. As ERP reduces early postoperative complications in HPB surgery, it might also have a potential impact on long-term survival, but this still need to be specifically addressed.

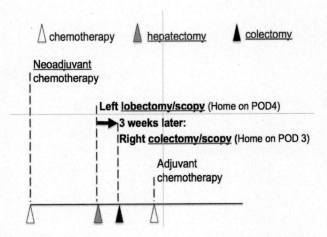

Fig. 25.2. Reverse treatment of colorectal carcinoma with synchronous liver metastasis within an enhanced recovery pathway (ERP). A 73-year-old female patient was diagnosed with a right colon carcinoma with synchronous left liver metastasis. After neoadjuvant chemotherapy, she successively underwent a left liver lobectomy followed by a right hemicolectomy, both within an ERP. After uneventful recovery, she then underwent adjuvant chemotherapy. *POD* postoperative day.

References

1. Greco M, Capretti G, Beretta L, Gemma M, Pecorelli N, Braga M. Enhanced recovery program in colorectal surgery: a meta-analysis of randomized controlled trials. World J Surg. 2014;38(6):1531–41.
2. Lee L, Li C, Landry T, Latimer E, Carli F, Fried GM, et al. A systematic review of economic evaluations of enhanced recovery pathways for colorectal surgery. Ann Surg. 2014;259(4):670–6.
3. Coolsen MM, van Dam RM, van der Wilt AA, Slim K, Lassen K, Dejong CH. Systematic review and meta-analysis of enhanced recovery after pancreatic surgery with particular emphasis on pancreaticoduodenectomies. World J Surg. 2013; 37(8):1909–18.
4. Lassen K, Coolsen MM, Slim K, Carli F, de Aguilar-Nascimento JE, Schafer M, et al. Guidelines for perioperative care for pancreaticoduodenectomy: Enhanced Recovery After Surgery (ERAS(R)) Society recommendations. World J Surg. 2013;37(2):240–58.
5. Coolsen MM, Wong-Lun-Hing EM, van Dam RM, van der Wilt AA, Slim K, Lassen K, et al. A systematic review of outcomes in patients undergoing liver surgery in an enhanced recovery after surgery pathways. HPB. 2013;15(4):245–51.
6. Jones C, Kelliher L, Dickinson M, Riga A, Worthington T, Scott MJ, et al. Randomized clinical trial on enhanced recovery versus standard care following open liver resection. Br J Surg. 2013;100(8):1015–24.
7. Kondrup J, Rasmussen HH, Hamberg O, Stanga Z, Ad Hoc ESPEN Working Group. Nutritional risk screening (NRS 2002): a new method based on an analysis of controlled clinical trials. Clin Nutr. 2003;22(3):321–36.
8. Cerantola Y, Hubner M, Grass F, Demartines N, Schafer M. Immunonutrition in gastrointestinal surgery. Br J Surg. 2011;98(1):37–48.
9. Gurusamy KS, Samraj K, Davidson BR. Routine abdominal drainage for uncomplicated liver resection. Cochrane Database Syst Rev. 2007;3, CD006232.
10. Petrowsky H, Demartines N, Rousson V, Clavien PA. Evidence-based value of prophylactic drainage in gastrointestinal surgery: a systematic review and meta-analyses. Ann Surg. 2004;240(6):1074–84. discussion 84–5.
11. Liu CL, Fan ST, Lo CM, Wong Y, Ng IO, Lam CM, et al. Abdominal drainage after hepatic resection is contraindicated in patients with chronic liver diseases. Ann Surg. 2004;239(2):194–201.
12. Fuster J, Llovet JM, Garcia-Valdecasas JC, Grande L, Fondevila C, Vilana R, et al. Abdominal drainage after liver resection for hepatocellular carcinoma in cirrhotic patients: a randomized controlled study. Hepatogastroenterology. 2004;51(56):536–40.
13. Conlon KC, Labow D, Leung D, Smith A, Jarnagin W, Coit DG, et al. Prospective randomized clinical trial of the value of intraperitoneal drainage after pancreatic resection. Ann Surg. 2001;234(4):487–93. discussion 93–4.
14. Diener MK, Tadjalli-Mehr K, Wente MN, Kieser M, Buchler MW, Seiler CM. Risk-benefit assessment of closed intra-abdominal drains after pancreatic surgery: a systematic review and meta-analysis assessing the current state of evidence. Langenbecks Arch Surg. 2011;396(1):41–52.

15. Van Buren II G, Bloomston M, Hughes SJ, Winter J, Behrman SW, Zyromski NJ, et al. A randomized prospective multicenter trial of pancreaticoduodenectomy with and without routine intraperitoneal drainage. Ann Surg. 2014;259(4):605–12.

16. Koti RS, Gurusamy KS, Fusai G, Davidson BR. Meta-analysis of randomized controlled trials on the effectiveness of somatostatin analogues for pancreatic surgery: a Cochrane review. HPB. 2010;12(3):155–65.

17. Allen PJ, Gonen M, Brennan MF, Bucknor AA, Robinson LM, Pappas MM, et al. Pasireotide for postoperative pancreatic fistula. N Engl J Med. 2014;370(21):2014–22.

18. Nelson R, Edwards S, Tse B. Prophylactic nasogastric decompression after abdominal surgery. Cochrane Database Syst Rev. 2007;3, CD004929.

19. Lassen K, Kjaeve J, Fetveit T, Trano G, Sigurdsson HK, Horn A, et al. Allowing normal food at will after major upper gastrointestinal surgery does not increase morbidity: a randomized multicenter trial. Ann Surg. 2008;247(5):721–9.

20. Beane JD, House MG, Miller A, Nakeeb A, Schmidt CM, Zyromski NJ, et al. Optimal management of delayed gastric emptying after pancreatectomy: an analysis of 1,089 patients. Surgery. 2014;156(4):939–46.

21. Roulin D, Blanc C, Muradbegovic M, Hahnloser D, Demartines N, Hubner M. Enhanced recovery pathway for urgent colectomy. World J Surg. 2014;38(8):2153–9.

22. Roulin D, Donadini A, Gander S, Griesser AC, Blanc C, Hubner M, et al. Cost-effectiveness of the implementation of an enhanced recovery protocol for colorectal surgery. Br J Surg. 2013;100(8):1108–14.

23. Lee A, Chiu CH, Cho MW, Gomersall CD, Lee KF, Cheung YS, et al. Factors associated with failure of enhanced recovery protocol in patients undergoing major hepatobiliary and pancreatic surgery: a retrospective cohort study. BMJ Open. 2014;4(7):e005330.

24. Petermann D, Demartines N, Schafer M. Severe postoperative complications adversely affect long-term survival after R1 resection for pancreatic head adenocarcinoma. World J Surg. 2013;37(8):1901–8.

25. Khuri SF, Henderson WG, DePalma RG, Mosca C, Healey NA, Kumbhani DJ, et al. Determinants of long-term survival after major surgery and the adverse effect of postoperative complications. Ann Surg. 2005;242(3):326–41. discussion 41–3.

Key References

Lassen K, Coolsen MM, Slim K, Carli F, de Aguilar-Nascimento JE, Schafer M, et al. Guidelines for perioperative care for pancreaticoduodenectomy: Enhanced Recovery After Surgery (ERAS(R)) Society recommendations. World J Surg. 2013;37(2): 240–58.

Coolsen MM, van Dam RM, van der Wilt AA, Slim K, Lassen K, Dejong CH. Systematic review and meta-analysis of enhanced recovery after pancreatic surgery with particular emphasis on pancreaticoduodenectomies. World J Surg. 2013;37(8):1909–18.

Coolsen MM, Wong-Lun-Hing EM, van Dam RM, van der Wilt AA, Slim K, Lassen K, et al. A systematic review of outcomes in patients undergoing liver surgery in an enhanced recovery after surgery pathways. HPB. 2013;15(4):245–51.

26. Enhanced Recovery Programs for Upper Gastrointestinal Surgery: How I Do It

Chao Li, Monisha Sudarshan, and Lorenzo E. Ferri

Esophagectomy is one of the most complex and high-acuity procedures performed. The mortality of esophagectomy has been estimated at 8 % across the USA (1–2 % in high-volume centers) and carries a morbidity rate of 30–60 %, an important fraction of which comprise cardiopulmonary complications [1, 2]. In high-volume centers, the morbidity and mortality after esophagectomy can be significantly reduced to acceptable levels (1–2 % mortality), and enhanced recovery programs may further improve these outcomes. Although enhanced recovery programs (ERPs) were initially developed in the context of lower acuity procedures such as colorectal resections, this experience is applicable across a variety of procedures, and there is demonstrable value in using a written, multimodal, evidence-based, step-by-step approach to standardizing perioperative care for complex procedures such as esophagectomy [3, 4].

In many centres, esophagectomy perioperative care has not changed significantly since the 1980s. Patients are routinely admitted to the intensive care unit directly from the operating theatre intubated and ventilated for 24–48 h. Nasogastric tubes are kept in for 1 week at which time a contrast esophagram is performed, only after which oral intake initiated. Urinary catheters are kept for the duration of the epidural (frequently 5–7 days) and chest tube drains are placed until oral feeding has started—all of which limit mobility. This results in a hospital stay in the 10–14-day range [5, 6].

In more recent years, rather than a move towards ERP, there has been in fact a paradigm shift in many centers in the entirely opposite direction—delaying any oral intake for up to 4 weeks [7].

L.S. Feldman et al. (eds.), *The SAGES / ERAS®*
Society Manual of Enhanced Recovery Programs for
Gastrointestinal Surgery, DOI 10.1007/978-3-319-20364-5_26,
© Springer International Publishing Switzerland 2015

Complex upper GI surgery presents us with unique challenges in the creation of such an ERP, not least of which is the willingness to change from such a traditional care model. As an example of such an application, we will introduce our ERP for perioperative esophagectomy care, which is a good representation at the most complex end of the spectrum of elective GI surgery.

Our Enhanced Recovery Program for Esophagectomy

History and Development

McGill's journey in implementing enhanced recovery programs commenced in 2001 with a postoperative ERP developed for foregut surgery focusing on laparoscopic paraesophageal hiatal hernia repair, Nissen fundoplication, and Heller myotomy [8]. Initial results indicated a decreased length of stay, decreased resource use, a decrease in complications, and excellent patient acceptance. This provided background experience with the implementation and assessment of standard pathways that could be transitioned into an ERP for esophagectomy, recognizing a need to improve postoperative care in complex surgeries. Although a standard order set for esophagectomy patients was introduced in 2005, it lacked the other vital components of enhanced recovery programs.

Implementation of clinical pathways requires the active participation and input of surgeons, anesthesia, nursing staff, and the preoperative clinic in the stages of its inception, revision, and execution.

A multidisciplinary surgical recovery team including a general surgeon, an anesthesiologist, nursing (inpatient and outpatient), physiotherapy, pharmacy, pain service, and nutrition expertise was tasked with the development of perioperative pathways. A full-time, care pathway coordinator was dedicated to the project to ensure efficiency. Esophagectomies, despite relative low annual volume compared to other procedures, accounted for the eighth highest use of hospital bed days in our tertiary care center, and was identified as a potential high-impact area for reduction of morbidity, mortality, and hospital resource use. The objectives of the developed ERP included enhanced recovery through early oral nutrition, epidural analgesia, minimizing the use and duration of drains, and ensuring early mobilization and compliance with spirometry and chest physiotherapy. All interventions were identified after thorough review of the medical literature to ensure evidence-based management. The team worked closely with front line providers of care in thoracic surgery (surgeons, nurses) to ensure clinical feasibility during creation and implementation of the pathway, as well as creation of a patient education booklet, pre-printed order sheets for physicians, and daily care maps for nurses (example order sheet and care map in Figs. 26.1 and 26.2).

Elements of the McGill University Esophagectomy Enhanced Recovery Program

Our initial enhanced recovery pathway for esophagectomy was implemented for all esophagectomy patients in June 2010 with an initial target of discharge on day 7. This pathway has evolved and undergone incremental changes over the years to each of its elements. The current pathway is described in Table 26.1 and has a target discharge of postoperative day 6.

Preoperative Nutritional Management

Poor preoperative nutritional status is a concern in this patient population, as esophageal cancer frequently presents with dysphagia and significant weight loss. All new diagnoses of esophageal cancer are seen by a dedicated upper GI cancer nutritionist on the first clinical visit to discuss strategies to maintain appropriate nutritional intake using protein-rich drinks. Patients with locally advanced adenocarcinoma (T3 or N1) and appropriate performance status are referred for neoadjuvant chemotherapy based on a multicenter phase II trial [9]. We have found that symptomatic patients generally respond rapidly to neoadjuvant treatment and dysphagia lessens frequently within 1 week of starting treatment, enabling better oral intake [10].

Patient Education

Core to the success of an enhanced recovery pathway is the education of the patient and the family starting in the preoperative setting. Informing the patient on the postoperative process and managing patient expectations increases compliance to the pathway. At a preoperative visit, the expected postoperative course is reviewed with the patient

Centre universitaire
de santé McGill

McGill University
Health Centre

| ☐ HME MCH | ☒ HGM MGH | ☐ HRV RVH |
| ☐ HNM MNH | ☐ ITM MCI | ☐ CL LC |

0726

**Chirurgie thoracique– Suivi systématique pour
Oesophagectomie
Ordonnances médicales postopératoires**

Page 3 de/of 7

Thoracic Surgery- Esophagectomy Care Pathway
Post-operative medical orders

Initiales du médecin Pour chaque ordonnance *Physician's Initials for each order*	ORDONNANCE DU MÉDECIN / *PHYSICIAN'S ORDERS*				Initiales de l'infirmier(ère) notées *Nurse's initials noted*
	Postoperative Day 2				
	Remove NGT after chest X-Ray reviewed by physician, (conduit not distended). Advance to sips of water after removal of NGT. Strict aspiration precaution: avoid eating if drowsy and maintain head of bed (HOB) elevated at 30 - 45° at all times, and avoid lying recumbent within 3 h of eating. MD to remove initial drsg then leave incision exposed to air.				
	Investigations and tests: (Physician to order in OACIS)				
	Chest X Ray "status post esophagectomy" CBC, Electrolytes and Creatinine (Chloride, Potassium, Creatinine, Sodium, HCO₃, Glucose) INR/PT/PTT, Ca, Mg				
	Additional orders not included in esophagectomy surgery care pathway:				
	Discontinue clinical pathway due to: ☐ Esophagectomy leak ☐ DVT ☐ Pneumonia ☐ Stay greater than 24 h in ICU ☐ Prolonged intubation ☐ Abdominal complication ☐ Cardiac complication ☐ Other				

	Nom en lettres moulées *Name in print*	Signature	N° Permis *License N°*	Heure *Time* 00:00	Date AAYY/MM/JD
Médecin *Physician*					

	Nom en lettres moulées et/ou Numéro de permis *Name in print and/or License Number*	Parapher / *Initial*	Heure *Time* 00:00	Date AAYY/MM/JD
Infirmier(ère) *Nurse*				
Pharmacien(ne) *Pharmacist*	N/A	N/A	N/A	N/A

Fig. 26.1. Example of pre-written postoperative medical orders for postoperative day 2 after esophagectomy.

using an easy to follow pictorial depiction of the pathway course covering activities, nutrition, drain management and pain control (Fig. 26.3 and http://www.muhcpatienteducation.ca/surgery-guides/surgery-patient-guides.html?sectionID=31). This educational process is

Centre universitaire
de santé McGill

McGill University
Health Centre

☐ HME / MCH   ☒ HGM / MGH   ☐ HRV / RVH
☐ HNM / MNH   ☐ ITM / MCI   ☐ CL / LC

Chirurgie Thoracique/
Suivi systématique pour eosophagectomie
Page 3 de/of 7
Thoracic Surgery /Esophagectomy Clinical Care Pathway

Standards of Care

	Postoperative day 2
Tests	• CBC, electrolytes and Creatinine, INR/PT/PTT, Ca, Mg. • Chest X Ray "status post esophagectomy".
Consults	• Nutritionist for nutritional education PRN.
Treatments/ Nursing care	• Assess and reinforce drsg q shift and PRN. Physician to change initial dressing. • Assess mental status, motor and sensory block q shift. • Assess quality of peripheral pulses, time of capillary refill. • Assess skin condition for redness, skin breakdown, irritation or signs of infection q shift - Braden scale. • Assist with Inspirometer 10 x q 1 h while awake. Start in the lower settings (400 – 800 cc/sec). Auscultate lungs q shift. Chest physiotherapy q 4 h. • Assist with mouth care q shift PRN. • NGT to LWS - Flush NGT q 6 h with 20 mL of water and may give medication via NGT. Record output in OACIS q shift. • Remove NGT after chest X-Ray reviewed by physician, (conduit not distended). • Irrigate feeding jejunostomy, if present, with 30 - 60 mL of water QID when not in use. • Initial dressing removed by physician • Keep AES until fully ambulating - remove for a.m. care. • If CT in situ- Maintain CT to –20cm suction. Call physician if output is greater than 100 mL/h x 2 h. Record output q shift in OACIS. • If large bore JP in situ - Maintain JP to bulb suction-record output in OACIS q shift. • Record BM on OACIS. • Record Weight on OACIS. • Take and record VS as per epidural policy; VS sheet including BP, HR, RR, T°, pain score at rest and movement, SpO₂. Physician to be notified if BP systolic is less than 100 mmHg or HR is greater than 110bpm or T° is greater than 38°C. •
Medications	• Assess pain according to pain scale 0-10; Give Pain medication via epidural infusion. Refer to epidural order sheet. • Restart patient's own medication as ordered by physician. • Titrate O₂ to maintain SpO₂ greater than 92%. D/C O₂ if SpO₂ level is greater than or equal to preop baseline.
Activity	• Assist patient in a chair 30 - 60 minutes- 3/day and ambulate half-length of hallway- 3/day (approx.35 m).
Nutrition/Diet /Hydration	• Consult nutritionist re: recommendation of rate increase for tube feeding. • Keep IV patent. Change IV peripheral site and/or central IV drsg - and all tubings as per IV. • Advance to sips of water after removal of NGT. • Record N/V on VS sheet, medicate as ordered PRN. • Strict aspiration precaution: avoid eating if drowsy, maintain HOB elevated at 30 - 45° at all times and avoid lying recumbent within 3 h of eating.

Patient and Family teaching/ Discharge teaching	• Reinforce PRN;
	  o DB and C exercises
	  o Pain control goals less than 4/10
	  o Use of inspirometer
	
	• Assess coping/anxiety and provide support PRN
	• Review "Path to Home Guide" as needed.

Imprimé par le service - DM-4413 (REV 2014/02/13) *CUSM Repro MUHC*

Fig. 26.2. Example of pre-written postoperative nursing care map for postoperative day 2 after esophagectomy.

Table 26.1. Summary of the elements of the enhanced recovery program for esophagectomy.

Pre- and intraoperative	
Nutritional management	• Routine nutritionist consultation at time of diagnosis and during neoadjuvant therapy • Fast-track neoadjuvant chemotherapy to enable greater oral intake [10]
Patient education	• Education booklet provided • Web-based interactive program provided • Pathway is reviewed with patient at preoperative visit
Analgesia	• Routine dual-thoracic epidural catheter insertion to cover abdominal land thoracic fields [12]
Fluid management	• Avoid fluid overload, balanced fluid administration— aim for (4–6 ml/kg/h)
Minimally invasive approach	• Selected for high-grade dysplasia or early clinical T1–T2 N0-stage cancer
Postoperative	
Intensive care unit	• Extubation in the operating room and observation in post-anesthesia care unit for 6 h • Avoidance of routine intensive care unit admission
Thoracic drainage	• Avoidance of rigid chest tubes and pleural drainage systems • Use of one large-capacity (400 ml), large-bore (19Fr) soft closed suction drain • Remove thoracic drain when full diet tolerated and drainage < 450 ml/24 h
Conduit decompression	• Nasogastric tube removed on postoperative day 2 if no conduit over-distension on X-ray
Urinary catheter	• Removed on postoperative day 1

Oral intake	• No routine surgical jejunostomy
	• Once nasogastric tube removed (postoperative day 2):
	  – Water on postoperative day 2
	  – Clear fluid diet on postoperative day 3
	  – Solid post-esophagectomy diet on postoperative day 5

Radiology	• Daily portable upright chest X-ray until removal of chest tube • No routine contrast esophagram prior to solid intake [18]
Mobilization	• Every postoperative day: incentive spirometry every hour when awake • Day 1: Sit in chair for 30 min 2 times, ambulate ½ length of hallway 2 times • Day 2: Sit in chair for 30 min 3 times, ambulate ½ length of hallway 3 times • Day 3: Sit in chair for 60 min 3 times, ambulate full length of hallway 4 times • Day 4–5: Sit in chair for 60 min for all meals (3 times), ambulate full length of hallway 4 times • Day 6: Discharge

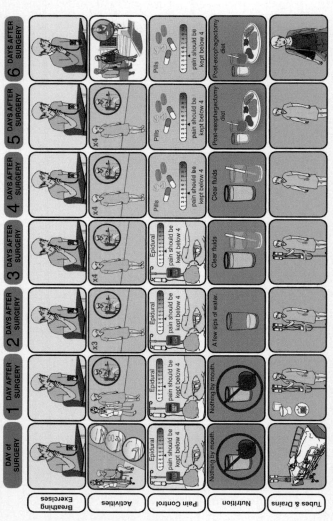

Fig. 26.3. Patient educational material with pictorial representation of expected esophagectomy pathway course. The full booklet is available at http://www.muhcpatienteducation.ca/surgery-guides/surgery-patient-guides.html?sectionID=31 (courtesy of McGill University Health Centre Patient Education Office, Montreal, QC, Canada.).

further enhanced by the presence of a comprehensive and interactive web-based care module that covers the entire patient trajectory for this complex disease (http://www.muhcpatienteducation.ca/cancer-guides/cedars-cancer-guides/esophageal-cancer.html?sectionID=25&guideID=24).

Minimally Invasive Approach

We use a selected approach to surgery that is dependent on both patient disease and patient performance status. For patients with a clinical T1 or T2 N0 disease or for patients with high grade dysplasia, we offer a minimally invasive approach which is advantageous in decreasing the surgical stress response and lessening postoperative pain. Although minimally invasive esophagectomy does not appear to reduce mortality or pulmonary complications, there is a trend towards decreased intraoperative blood loss and decreased length of stay [11]. For more advanced disease requiring a 2-fields approach, it is possible to respect oncologic principles by doing the intra-abdominal mobilization by laparoscopy but to create the conduit, resect the thoracic disease, and perform the anastomosis using an open approach.

Epidural Anesthesia

Effective pain control is the cornerstone of expedited recovery. It reduces the risk of pneumonia, promotes early mobilization and decreases dependence on narcotics. Since the Ivor Lewis and 3-hole esophagectomies involve multiple dermatomes, optimal pain control targets both thoracic and abdominal regions. We use a dual-epidural catheters technique (thoracic and abdominal) that is associated with improved analgesia, decreased rate of major postoperative complications and decreased length of stay, without increasing catheter-related adverse effects compared with single-catheter use [12].

Avoiding Intraoperative Fluid Overload

Intraoperative management that is rooted in judicious intraoperative fluid administration results in decreased morbidity and mortality. Transfusion of blood products has been associated with decreased long-term survival in esophagectomy patients, and this correlation is observed for other cancer surgeries as well [13]. Intraoperative fluid restriction facilitates extubation in the OR suite and also decreases pulmonary complications especially in the setting of thoracic surgery [14].

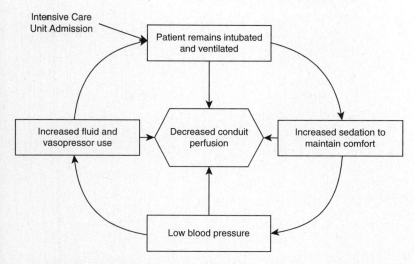

Fig. 26.4. The intensive care unit cycle after esophagectomy to be avoided.

Avoidance of Intensive Care Unit

In traditional care, patients are often transferred from the operating room to an intensive care unit where they remain intubated and ventilated for up to 2 days. Remaining intubated in the intensive care unit restricts recovery as patients are unable to communicate and mobilize on their own. Moreover, keeping patients ventilated often induces discomfort that leads to a vicious cycle of increasing sedation, decreased blood pressure, and eventual compensation with over-resuscitation or vasopressor use which may stress blood flow to the esophageal conduit (Fig. 26.4).

We avoid routine admission to the intensive care unit and aim for extubation at the end of the case. Immediately postop, patients are observed for up to 6 h in the post-anesthesia care unit before transfer to a dedicated thoracic surgery floor.

Thoracic Drainage

Multiple chest tubes are routinely used after thoracic surgery and the large size and rigidity of these drains not only limit mobility, but also induce significant pain. To ensure adequate chest drainage yet minimize discomfort we are now using soft, flexible, high-capacity closed suction

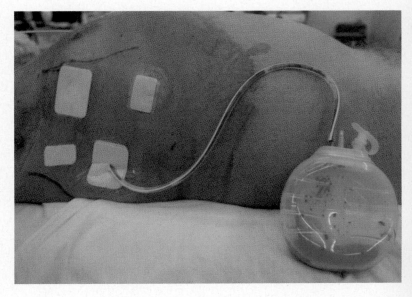

Fig. 26.5. Use of soft closed suction drainage after minimally invasive esophagectomy.

drains, as is increasingly seen post-thoracic surgery [15]. Increased patient comfort translates into higher rates of postoperative mobilization which is further enhanced by the lack of a cumbersome pleural drainage system (Fig. 26.5).

Conduit Decompression

Although the viewpoint of retaining the nasogastric tube in order to avoid gastric conduit distention and resultant anastomotic complications is universally shared, recent studies demonstrate that early removal of the NGT (within 48 h) is associated with fewer complications. The largest randomized controlled trial studying NGT duration and outcomes found no difference in pulmonary complications or anastomotic leakage if NGTs were removed on postoperative day 2 vs. 7 [16]. We routinely place a NGT during esophagectomy to aid in retracting the posterior wall of a hand-sewn anastomosis, thus facilitating completion of the anterior wall. This tube is removed on the second postoperative day, and is reinserted only should there be significant conduit distension on the daily routine chest X-ray (Fig. 26.6).

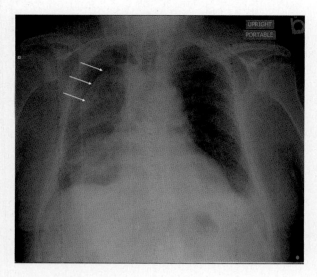

Fig. 26.6. Postoperative chest X-ray showing significant distension of esophageal conduit requiring reinsertion of nasogastric tube.

Urinary Catheter

Early removal of the urinary catheter functions as another integral component in our pathway and contributes to decrease rates of urinary tract infection. We have adopted this early removal even in the presence of using dual-epidural catheters and have found no statistical increase in rates of re-catheterizations when a protocol based on urinary volume monitoring using ultrasound is used. In a randomized trial performed in our institution, early catheter removal not only contributed to decreased urinary tract infections but this group also had an overall shorter length of stay in comparison with the standard group (when the urinary catheter remains until the epidural catheter is removed) [17].

Oral Feeding and Contrast Esophagram

Traditionally, oral feeding is delayed until the nasogastric tube is removed at 1 week, followed by contrast esophagram to assess the integrity of the anastomosis. Depending on the results of the esophagram, the decision to start oral feeds is made. Some centers may even elect to delay oral intake for 3–4 weeks, using a jejunostomy feeding tube in the interim. We have investigated the utility and prognostic ability of a contrast esophagram and found that its routine use has little clinical impact with a sensitivity of less than 50 % [18]. Therefore we proceed with early removal of the nasogastric tube and early feeding with clinical judgment guiding the use of further investigation for anastomotic leaks. Our postoperative nutritional plan therefore allows water after removal of the nasogastric tube on day 2, advances to a clear fluid diet for days 3 and 4, and follows with a solid post-esophagectomy diet on day 5.

Feeding jejunostomy is routinely used in many North American centers. However, complications related to jejunostomies are not minor and occur at a rate of approximately 10 % (higher than our institutional anastomotic leak rate), with re-laparotomy reported in up to 3 % of patients [19]. Therefore we avoid routine placement of feeding jejunostomies and use them only in selected patients. Instead we advanced to an oral diet (liquids) after removal of the nasogastric tube on day 2.

Institutional Results

We performed a retrospective before-and-after analysis including all patients undergoing esophagectomy for cancer or high-grade dysplasia from June 2009 to December 2011 [4]. A 7-day multidisciplinary enhanced recovery program was introduced in June 2010 (and has since been revised to a 6-day target—see Fig. 26.3). Patients undergoing pharyngo-laryngo-esophagectomy and emergency surgeries were excluded.

There were 47 patients operated on before implementation of the enhanced recovery program and 59 after for a total of 106 patients. These patients were well matched with respect to age, gender, preoperative body mass index, comorbidities, type of surgery, and stage of disease. On univariate analysis, overall length of hospital decreased by 2 days from a median of 10 [9–17] days to 8 [7–17] days after ERP implementation (Table 26.2). There was no difference in overall morbidity (62 % prior vs. 59 % after), especially with respect to anastomotic leakage (11 % vs. 14 %), pulmonary complications (32 % vs. 24 %), and readmissions (6 % vs. 5 %). The decrease in length of stay was mostly for patients with no complications or minor complications. Prior to the ERP, only 6 % of patients were discharge by postoperative day 7 (our target date). In the first 6 months of implementation, only 15 % of patients were discharged by postoperative day 7 whereas this increased

Table 26.2. Summary of clinical outcomes before and after implementation of an enhanced recovery program for esophagectomy.

	Traditional care ($n=47$)	Enhanced recovery ($n=59$)
Length of stay[a]	10 [9–17]	8 [7–17]
No complication[a]	8 [8–9]	7 [7–8]
Minor complication[a]	11 [9–15]	8 [7–10]
Major complication	19 [15–47]	21 [13–33]
Overall morbidity	29 (62 %)	35 (59 %)
Pulmonary complication	16 (32 %)	13 (24 %)
Readmissions	3 (6 %)	3 (5 %)
Weighted mean cost (CAN$)[a]	$22,835	$20,169

[a]Statistically significant difference ($p<0.05$)
Adapted from Lee L, Li C, Robert N, Latimer E, Carli F, Mulder DS, et al. Economic impact of an enhanced recovery pathway for oesophagectomy. Br J Surg. 2013;100(10):1326–34; Li C, Ferri LE, Mulder DS, Ncuti A, Neville A, Lee L, et al. An enhanced recovery pathway decreases duration of stay after esophagectomy. Surgery. 2012;152(4):606–16, with permission

to 42 % subsequently. On multivariate analysis, implementation of our enhanced recovery program was associated with an 18 % decrease in length of stay, adjusting for age, gender, surgical approach, and postoperative complications.

Using the same population, we estimated the cost for each patient during their hospital stay [3]. Using deviation-based cost modeling, patients were divided into "on course" (LOS < 50th percentile, minor or no complication), "minor deviation" (LOS 50th to 75th percentile, minor or no complication), "moderate deviation" (LOS > 75th percentile and minor or major complication), or "major deviation" (any patient with a major complication requiring intervention or intensive care use) cohorts. After implementation of the ERP, significant cost differences were found for patients in the "on course" (CAN$-742) and "minor deviation" (CAN$-4120) categories for an average cost saving of CAN$-2666 per patient.

Conclusion

There are specific organizational challenges in formulating an ERP for upper GI surgery. The postoperative course comprises a longer time period and has many more elements than the usual enhanced recovery program. Directives relative to radiological testing and timing of removal of nasogastric and chest drains are also present which would not be necessary in other types of abdominal surgeries. Nonetheless we have found the esophagectomy pathway to be safe and effective in decreasing length of stay and costs without increase in morbidity or readmissions.

References

1. Birkmeyer JD, Stukel TA, Siewers AE, Goodney PP, Wennberg DE, Lucas FL. Surgeon volume and operative mortality in the United States. N Engl J Med. 2003; 349(22):2117–27.
2. Park DP, Welch CA, Harrison DA, Palser TR, Cromwell DA, Gao F, et al. Outcomes following oesophagectomy in patients with oesophageal cancer: a secondary analysis of the ICNARC Case Mix Programme Database. Crit Care. 2009;13 Suppl 2:S1.
3. Lee L, Li C, Robert N, Latimer E, Carli F, Mulder DS, et al. Economic impact of an enhanced recovery pathway for oesophagectomy. Br J Surg. 2013;100(10):1326–34.
4. Li C, Ferri LE, Mulder DS, Ncuti A, Neville A, Lee L, et al. An enhanced recovery pathway decreases duration of stay after esophagectomy. Surgery. 2012;152(4):606–16.
5. Zehr KJ, Dawson PB, Yang SC, Heitmiller RF. Standardized clinical care pathways for major thoracic cases reduce hospital costs. Ann Thorac Surg. 1998;66(3):914–9.
6. Swisher SG, Hunt KK, Carmack Holmes E, Zinner MJ, McFadden DW. Changes in the surgical management of esophageal cancer from 1970 to 1993. Am J Surg. 1995;169(6):609–14.
7. Tomaszek SC, Cassivi SD, Allen MS, Shen KR, Nichols FC, Deschamps C, et al. An alternative postoperative pathway reduces length of hospitalisation following oesophagectomy. Eur J Cardiothorac Surg. 2010;37(4):807–13.
8. Ferri LE, Feldman LS, Stanbridge DD, Fried GM. Patient perception of a clinical pathway for laparoscopic foregut surgery. J Gastrointest Surg. 2006;10(6):878–82.
9. Ferri L, Ades S, Alcindor T, Chasen M, Marcus V, Hickeson M, et al. Perioperative docetaxel, cisplatin, and 5-fluorouracil (DCF) for locally advanced esophageal and gastric adenocarcinoma: a multicenter phase II trial. Ann Oncol. 2012;23(6):1512–7.
10. Cools-Lartigue J, Jones D, Spicer J, Zourikian T, Rousseau M, Eckert E, et al. The management of dysphagia in esophageal adenocarcinoma patients undergoing neoadjuvant chemotherapy: can invasive tube feeding be avoided? Ann Surg Oncol. 2015; 22(6):1858–65.
11. Sudarshan M, Ferri L. A critical review of minimally invasive esophagectomy. Surg Laparosc Endosc Percutan Tech. 2012;22(4):310–8.
12. Brown MJ, Kor DJ, Allen MS, Kinney MO, Shen KR, Deschamps C, et al. Dual-epidural catheter technique and perioperative outcomes after Ivor-Lewis esophagectomy. Reg Anesth Pain Med. 2013;38(1):3–8.
13. Komatsu Y, Orita H, Sakurada M, Maekawa H, Hoppo T, Sato K. Intraoperative blood transfusion contributes to decreased long-term survival of patients with esophageal cancer. World J Surg. 2012;36(4):844–50.

14. Neal JM, Wilcox RT, Allen HW, Low DE. Near-total esophagectomy: the influence of standardized multimodal management and intraoperative fluid restriction. Reg Anesth Pain Med. 2003;28(4):328–34.

15. Ishikura H, Kimura S. The use of flexible silastic drains after chest surgery: novel thoracic drainage. Ann Thorac Surg. 2006;81(1):331–3.

16. Mistry RC, Vijayabhaskar R, Karimundackal G, Jiwnani S, Pramesh C. Effect of short-term vs prolonged nasogastric decompression on major postesophagectomy complications: a parallel-group, randomized trial. Arch Surg. 2012;147(8):747–51.

17. Zaouter C, Kaneva P, Carli F. Less urinary tract infection by earlier removal of bladder catheter in surgical patients receiving thoracic epidural analgesia. Reg Anesth Pain Med. 2009;34(6):542–8.

18. Cools-Lartigue J, Andalib A, Abo-Alsaud A, Gowing S, Nguyen M, Mulder D, et al. Routine contrast esophagram has minimal impact on the postoperative management of patients undergoing esophagectomy for esophageal cancer. Ann Surg Oncol. 2014;21(8):2573–9.

19. Weijs TJ, Berkelmans GH, Nieuwenhuijzen GA, Ruurda JP, Soeters PB, Luyer MD. Routes for early enteral nutrition after esophagectomy. A systematic review. Clin Nutr. 2015;34(1):1–6.

27. Department-Wide Implementation of an Enhanced Recovery Pathway

Lawrence Lee

There is abundant data supporting the clinical effectiveness of enhanced recovery pathways (ERP) [1–4]. By combining multiple evidence-based interventions into a single multidisciplinary care package involving all perioperative phases, ERPs shorten hospitalization and reduce complications [1]. In essence, ERPs represent a knowledge translation strategy to help get evidence into practice. Yet these pathways are complex, as they may contain up to 20 different perioperative elements, many of which are contrary to traditional surgical practice. Recent surveys of perioperative management practices for bowel resection in the USA reported that management remained fairly "conventional" for a large proportion of procedures, as the majority of cases in those studies still underwent bowel preparation and less than half received preoperative patient education [5, 6]. Like any significant change in practice, creating a culture of "enhanced recovery" requires vision, commitment, energy, planning, and (ideally) institutional support. Consensus must be achieved between all of involved care providers, and personnel must also be trained. A dedicated multidisciplinary team is ideal [7] to synthesize the existing evidence into a practical and usable care pathway, as well as implement the pathway and perform continuous quality improvement. Substantial dedication is required from the multidisciplinary team members and a learning curve should be expected [7, 8]. A simple written pathway or standard order set is not enough to constitute "enhanced recovery," as compliance to many elements may be poor, even in the presence of a dedicated ERP team [9]. But ultimately the improved results that have been seen with the ERP across diverse institutions and procedures provide substantial motivation for use and evidence that these pathways work.

L.S. Feldman et al. (eds.), *The SAGES / ERAS®*
Society Manual of Enhanced Recovery Programs for
Gastrointestinal Surgery, DOI 10.1007/978-3-319-20364-5_27,
© Springer International Publishing Switzerland 2015

The decision to adopt an ERP can either originate from the clinicians at the grassroots level, or as a directive from upper management. We favor the former, but these two approaches are not mutually exclusive. Often, a local clinical champion, a surgeon, or anesthesiologist who recognizes the benefits of this approach initiates the ERP. This local clinical champion then recruits like-minded individuals to form an ERP steering committee, which oversees the development and initiation process. In this setting, support from administration is vital to ensure that the steering committee is given the adequate authority and ideally resources that are necessary to successful overcome barriers to implementation. Similarly, the involved stakeholders at the ground level must support a top-down approach to ERP adoption. There is no "right" way to implement an ERP; however, there are several strategies that should be adopted to provide the highest chance of successful implementation. This chapter provides an overview of the implementation process, focusing on these strategies. Our own institutional experience is described, and examples of our bowel surgery standard order sets, as well as other accompanying material, are provided.

Steering Group

The role of the steering group is crucial for successful implementation. Studies have shown that projects are more likely to succeed with a clearly defined change management team and approach [10]. This group is usually composed of clinical leaders from all relevant stakeholder groups. Surgeons and anesthesiologists usually lead the group, but it is important to include nursing from all perioperative phases, as well as other allied health professionals such as physiotherapists and nutritionists. The multidisciplinary nature and the inclusion of credible leaders (especially nursing) are paramount, as this will ensure that the proposed changes are compatible with local realities. It is crucial that the steering group understands the needs and perspectives from all groups that affect patient care. For instance, one of the pathway elements at our institution was to have the patient be transferred immediately to the chair upon arrival to the surgical ward; however upon audit, compliance to this element was low. The reason was eventually traced to the transfer practice between the post-anesthesia care unit and the ward, in particular the role of the patient transport department. Adherence improved once the difficulties faced by this group were resolved.

The role of the steering group is to develop or adopt a preexisting pathway, identify barriers to implementation, obtain consensus and support from all relevant stakeholder groups, schedule a timeline for implementation, in particular a firm launch date, and perform continuous audit and feedback. It is extremely helpful to include an ERP coordinator within the steering group, as this person will educate frontline staff, coordinate between the various stakeholder groups, and ensure that the changes proposed by the steering group are actually put into practice. Depending on the availability of local resources, the ERP coordinator can be re-assigned from a previous position, such as the preoperative clinic, or a new position can be created.

At our institution, our first experience was initiated in 2005 by an anesthesiologist working with colorectal surgeons and the ward nurse manager to develop an ERP for selected patients undergoing laparoscopic colon surgery [11]. To bring the benefits of the ERP approach to a wider variety of patients and scale up to ensure institutional benefits, a multidisciplinary group consisting of surgeons, anesthesiologists, nurses, physiotherapists, nutritionists, and clinical epidemiologists was formally established as the Surgical Recovery (SURE) Program with a full-time dedicated ERP nurse specialist in October 2008. We found that the inclusion of an epidemiologist or a medical librarian is useful to help identify and filter through large amounts of relevant literature. This team was tasked with the development, implementation, and monitoring of processes that may improve patient recovery after major surgery through collaboration with clinical leaders across different surgical subspecialties. Since its creation, this group has successfully developed and implemented pathways for multiple procedures beyond colorectal surgery, such as esophagectomy [12], prostatectomy [13], pulmonary resection, hip/knee arthroplasty, nephrectomy, hepatectomy [14], and others.

The principles of enhanced recovery may be applied to other procedures other than in colorectal surgery. There is an increasing amount of data to demonstrate the effectiveness of ERPs in other procedures, such as liver and gastric resections [14, 15]. Given the substantial investment that is required to set up an ERP, it would be resource efficient if the local expertise that is established in the implementation of an initial pathway be used to develop ERPs for other procedures in the same setting. In this manner, required resources may be amortized over a larger number of patients, and may be offset by the potentially larger scale improvements in outcomes.

Change Management

Traditionally perioperative care has been delivered within "silos" of service; that is, physicians and other healthcare providers tended to work solely within their own domain of expertise, with minimal to no collaboration with other specialties. ERPs require the dismantling of these artificial boundaries to provide full multidisciplinary care of the patient as he or she goes through each perioperative phase. Consensus must be reached by all of the involved stakeholders in all perioperative phases, including nursing, anesthesia, surgery, and other ancillary personnel. This is often the most difficult and time-consuming step, as it often necessitates that certain healthcare providers cede control over aspects of care traditionally under their control. Even if healthcare providers are aware of the best current evidence and are willing to change, departures from long-standing practices are difficult. This becomes especially difficult if the local environment is not conducive to change.

Implementing change can rarely be performed in a single step; rather, a well-planned iterative process incorporating multiple interventions aimed at specific obstacles is usually required [16]. These barriers to change can be classified into three main categories: social, professional, and organizational [17]. It is useful to identify and understand potential barriers to change so that they are targeted with the appropriate interventions. Social barriers represent the reluctance of the involved stakeholders to change their long-standing practices in favor of the new change, either because of obsolete knowledge or disagreements with the evidence. For instance, many surgeons are still hesitant to begin oral intake in the immediate postoperative period, despite level 1 evidence demonstrating the safety and benefits of this approach [6, 18]. Examples of professional barriers are when physicians may not have the necessary skillset that is required of the change proposal. New techniques may need to be learned (for instance, minimally invasive procedures for surgeons or fluid-directed therapy and neural blockade analgesia for anesthesiologists). Finally, organizational barriers relate to limitations in available resources, financial constraints, or lack of time. In particular, there is much concern about whether ERPs will increase nursing workload; however it appears that this is largely unfounded [19]. Clearly, different obstacles to change require different solutions. Social barriers may be overcome by the inclusion of credible leaders to convince the other stakeholders of the benefits of such an approach. Involvement of key stakeholders and obtaining consensus is key to solving professional barriers. Finally, support from administration may be especially helpful to overcome organizational barriers.

Implementation of Enhanced Recovery Pathways

The adoption of an ERP into clinical practice can be divided into three different steps: development, implementation, and evaluation (Fig. 27.1).

Development

The first step is to decide whether to develop an ERP from scratch, or adopt a preexisting one. There are many published examples of ERP for various types of procedures [14, 15, 20, 21], in addition to ERAS

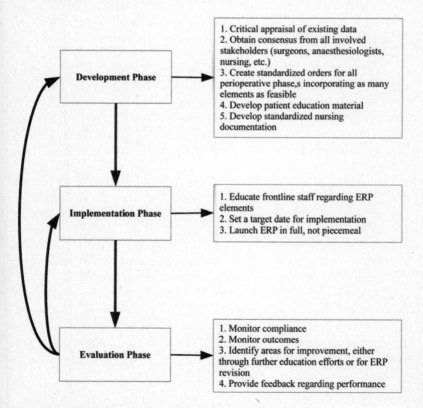

Fig. 27.1. Enhanced recovery pathway implementation process.

The content of the figure boxes:

Development Phase
1. Critical appraisal of existing data
2. Obtain consensus from all involved stakeholders (surgeons, anaesthesiologists, nursing, etc.)
3. Create standardized orders for all perioperative phase,s incorporating as many elements as feasible
4. Develop patient education material
5. Develop standardized nursing documentation

Implementation Phase
1. Educate frontline staff regarding ERP elements
2. Set a target date for implementation
3. Launch ERP in full, not piecemeal

Evaluation Phase
1. Monitor compliance
2. Monitor outcomes
3. Identify areas for improvement, either through further education efforts or for ERP revision
4. Provide feedback regarding performance

Society best practice guidelines for perioperative care [22–25]. However, the local practice environment, organizational culture, and availability of resources must be taken into consideration as they may influence specific pathway elements. Guidelines for perioperative care may include more than 20 different elements, and implementation of a pathway that is not feasible within a local setting is likely to fail. The necessity and feasibility of each pathway elements should be evaluated for local settings. Nevertheless, existing pathways may serve as a starting point. An example of the bowel surgery ERP at our institution is shown in Table 27.1. It is at this point that consensus must be obtained from all of the relevant stakeholders for what will be included in the pathway and how these elements will be operationalized. Potential barriers to implementation must also be identified, and the appropriate actions taken to remedy them.

Prior to undertaking an ERP, an audit strategy should be discussed and baseline data should be collected for benchmarking. This is continued throughout the development and implementation periods to provide information to the steering committee. There is nothing like reliable data to motivate quality improvement projects. An outcome of interest to all stakeholders should be selected. Length of stay and readmissions are convenient intra-institutional markers that correlate with organ recovery, complications, and cost and are easy to collect. Ideally, adherence to process measures, occurrence of common complications (ileus, SSI, nausea/vomiting, UTI), time to be medically fit for discharge, and patient-reported outcomes would also be collected [26].

Once the ERP elements are decided, specific ERP material must also be created. This includes procedure-specific patient education material (see Fig. 26.3), pathway order sets, and dedicated nursing documentation (Fig. 27.2a, b). In particular, efforts should be made to create clear patient education material. It is important that these educational materials be written in a manner that can be easily understood by patients. At our institution, booklets were created for each ERP, in consultation with the hospital Patient Education Office, and were written to target a low health literacy level [27]. These booklets are generously illustrated, and contained procedure descriptions, preoperative optimization to be undertaken by the patient, detailed day-by-day expectations and goals, and post-discharge instructions.

Table 27.1. Sample multimodal perioperative care pathway for bowel surgery.

Preoperative assessment and optimization

- Evaluation of medication compliance and control of risk factors: hypertension, diabetes, COPD, smoking, alcohol, asthma, CAD, malnutrition, anemia
- Psychological preparation for surgery and postoperative recovery: explanation of perioperative pathway, diet and ambulation plan, presence of drains, expectation about duration of hospital stay (3-4 days)
- Physical preparation with exercises at home
- Surgical considerations: operative approach (laparoscopic vs. open)
- Oral bowel preparation for rectal resections with planned ileostomy only
- Stoma teaching as needed

Day of surgery

- Drink clear fluids with carbohydrates up to 2 h prior to operation unless risk factors are present (history of GERD, previous difficult intubation, diabetes, achalasia, morbid obesity, neurological disease, pregnancy)

Preinduction

- Administer long-acting sedative medication, and antibiotic and DVT prophylaxis

Intraoperative management

Anesthetic management

- Induce with propofol, give short-acting opiates (fentanyl) for analgesia, consider adjuvants for analgesia (beta blockers or lidocaine), administer rocuronium or desflurane
- Prevent PONV with dexamethasone, ondansetron, or droperidol
- Restrict intraoperative fluids (6 ml/kg/h)
- Insert epidural catheter for postoperative analgesia
- Keep patient warm

Surgical care

- Provide incisional anesthesia with local anesthetic at beginning and end of procedure. If laparoscopic: keep abdominal insufflation as low as possible (12 mmHg); maximize the use of small (5 mm) trocars. Minimize incision length if open surgery
- Remove NG tube prior to extubation

(continued)

Table 27.1. (continued)

Postoperative strategy

Day of surgery (postoperative day 0)

- Discontinue IV fluids upon arrival to surgical ward
- Gum chewing for 30 min TID
- Full fluid diet and 1 can of nutritional supplementation beverage to ensure at least 1 L of oral intake
- Ensure at least 2 h out of bed (sitting in chair)
- Avoidance of opioid analgesia

Postoperative day 1

- Discontinue urinary drainage catheter
- Gum chewing for 30 min TID
- Advance diet as tolerated. Ensure 1 can of nutritional supplementation beverage with each meal (target total volume of 2 L during the day)
- Ensure patient is out of bed for at least 8 h during the day. Walk length of hallway with assistance TID
- Avoidance of opioid analgesia

Postoperative day 2

- Gum chewing for 30 min TID
- Diet as tolerated. Ensure 1 can of nutritional supplementation beverage with each meal (target total volume of 2 L during the day)
- Ensure patient is out of bed for at least 8 h during the day. Walk length of hallway with assistance TID
- Commence epidural stop test at 6 AM. If stop test positive, remove epidural catheter at 10 AM
- Avoidance of opioid analgesia

Postoperative day 3

- Gum chewing for 30 min TID
- Diet as tolerated. Ensure 1 can of nutritional supplementation beverage with each meal (target total volume of 2 L during the day)
- Ensure patient is out of bed for at least 8 h during the day. Walk length of hallway with assistance TID
- Avoidance of opioid analgesia
- Discharge before lunch if discharge criteria met (adequate analgesia with oral analgesics, absence of fever and N/V, voiding, able to handle activities of daily living, passing flatus, wound check)
- Schedule follow-up appointment in clinic 2 weeks after surgery

a

Chirurgie Générale
Suivi systématique pour chirurgie colorectale
NORMES DE FICHES DE COLLECTE DE DONNÉES ET AVQ

Page 4 de/of 10
POD 0

General Surgery
Colorectal Care Pathway
ASSESSMENT AND ADL FLOWSHEET STANDARDS

Clinical pathway is initiated by physician order and implemented through nursing protocol.
Pathway outlines standards of care. Any deviation, complication or activity NOT accomplished should be initialed, documented with rationale in progress Notes and problems on the Plan Thérapeutique Infirmier (PTI).

	Postoperative day 0	
Tests		
Consults	Ostomy patients: Enterostomal Therapy nurse consulted regarding ostomy system fitting for discharge	
Treatments/ Nursing care	Assess and reinforce dressing q shift and PRN Assess and record on ADL flowsheet for abdominal distension, bowel sounds, passing flatus and bowel movement. Assess mental status, motor strength q shift Assess quality of peripheral pulses, time of capillary refill Assess respiratory pattern and lung expansion Assess skin condition for redness, skin breakdown, irritation or signs of infection q shift Assist patient to use inspirometer 10 x q 1h while awake- start in the lower settings (200-400mL/sec) - auscultate lungs q shift - DB&C q 1h while awake Assist with mouth care q shift PRN Consult A.N.M or N.M. or social worker or patient flow coordinator for complex discharge planning and initiate PTI. Urinary catheter to straight drainage - call physician if urine output is less than 120 mL over 4 hours monitor and record output q shift on I&O sheet - Urinary catheter care as per nursing protocol Keep AES until fully ambulating - remove for AM care. Remind patient to chew gum for 30 minutes during evening PRN Take and record VS q 4h on OACIS including BP, HR, RR, T°, pain score at rest and movement, O₂ saturation (SpO₂)- notify physician if HR greater than 120 bmp, BP lower than 80/50 or T° greater than 38°C	
Medications	Assess pain according to pain scale 0-10; Record pain level on OACIS, or on "Documentation related to administration and surveillance of short-acting opioids. If patient taking opioids. Refer to the acute pain service orders for epidural or PCA usage and follow monitoring standards. Restart patient's own medication as ordered by physician-reconcile medication at admission.	
Activity	Assist to get up in chair in PM as tolerated	
Nutrition/Diet /hydration	IV TKVO on arrival to floor Record any nausea and vomiting (N&V) medicate as ordered PRN After patient's arrival to floor start patient on full fluid diet (approximately 1 L) and 1 nutritional supplement Keep IV patent-change IV peripheral site and all tubings as per IV nursing protocol	
Patient and Family teaching/Discharge teaching	Reinforce PRN; o DB&C exercises o Pain control goals less than 4/10 o Use of inspirometer	Assess coping/anxiety and provide support Review "Path to Home Guide" as needed

Fig. 27.2. Example of nursing documentation. (**a**) Nursing standards for postoperative day 0. (**b**) Nursing documentation tool for postoperative day 0 (courtesy of McGill University Health Centre, Montreal, Quebec, Canada).

b

Chirurgie Générale
Suivi systématique pour chirurgie colorectale
FICHES DE COLLECTE DE DONNÉES ET AVQ

Page 3 de/of 10
JOURNÉE POST-OPÉRATOIRE/POST-OP DAY (POD) 0

General Surgery
Colorectal Care Pathway
ASSESSMENT AND ADL FLOWSHEET

Clinical pathway is initiated by physician order and implemented through nursing protocol.
Pathway outlines standards of care. Any deviation, complication or activity NOT accomplished should be initialed, documented with rationale in progress Notes and problems on the Plan Thérapeutique Infirmier (PTI).

Mental status/neuro				Respiratory				Circulatory				VS/pain control			
D	E	N		D	E	N		D	E	N		D	E	N	
			Patient oriented to person, place and time				Patient does deep breathing and coughing (DB&C) and uses inspirometer q 1h while awake with assistance PRN				AES are on D: Y/N E: Y/N N: Y/N				q 4 h x 24 h- all within acceptable limits Refer to OACIS
			Level of sedation evaluated and recorded.				Regular respiratory pattern				Peripheral pulses of feet and hands are palpable, strong, and Regular. No tingling or numbness				Pain level maintained less than 4/10 and recorded
			Sensation is equal and normal bilaterally				Chest wall expansion equal on both sides. Is not using accessory muscles.				Capillary refill is less than or equal to 2 seconds				Epidural ☐ yes ☐ no -patent and infusing well and site intact
			Motor strength is equal and normal in all limbs				No cough or secretions				No chest pain, no palpitations				PCA ☐ yes ☐ no -patent and infusing well and site intact
							Air entry (A/E) is clear bilaterally with no adventitious sounds heard								

G/I				G/U				Diet /hydration				Skin integrity			
D	E	N		D	E	N		D	E	N		D	E	N	
			Abdomen is soft				Urinary catheter ☐ yes ☐ no				IV to keep vein open on arrival to floor. Next site change				IV site intact with no signs of infection (no redness, not warm, not painful)
			Abdomen without tenderness				if yes, Urinary catheter to straight drainage maintaining adequate urine output greater or equal to 120 mL over 4 hours				Patient started on full fluids and one nutritional supplement				Initial incisional dressing is dry and intact (D&I)
			No nausea												
			No vomiting												
Ostomy Patients								Patient chewed gum for 30 minutes this evening				Skin is warm, dry No cyanosis, no edema			
			ET nurse consulted regarding ostomy system fitting for discharge				If no, patient urinating within 6 hours postop- no complaints of postop urinary retention.				Mouth care done PRN				Skin is intact with no redness and no pressure sores noted.
							Urine is clear and yellow				PO well tolerated. D: Y/N E: Y/N N: Y/N (N/A)				
Bowel sounds present D: Y/N E: Y/N N: Y/N															
Passing flatus D: Y/N E: Y/N N: Y/N															
Bowel movement D: Y/N E: Y/N N: Y/N															

Tests/investigations				Activities				Family				
D	E	N		D	E	N		D	E	N		
							With assistance - Patient up in chair as tolerated - 2-4 hours after arrival to ward.				Patient and family refer to "A Guide to Bowel Surgery"	
											Patient and family appear to be coping well with surgery -Calm and cooperative -Listens attentively to information	

Nurse's signature;	Days	Evening	Night
Date(YYYY/MM/DD):			

Fig. 27.2. (continued)

Implementation

Once the development of a suitable pathway is complete, the implementation phase involves educating the involved stakeholders of the new ERP management strategies, including preoperative clinic, operating room, post-anaesthesia care unit, and ward nurses, as well as allied health professionals. These education efforts should include a brief introduction to the key principles of ERP, and outline the entire perioperative pathway, rather than just specific portions. Significant changes should be highlighted and evidence for the change provided. Each stakeholder group should be made aware of their contributions to the ERP, and how it affects the total care of the patient. All of the relevant documents must also be at hand, so that frontline staff may familiarize themselves with the new changes. There should be no surprises once the ERP is formally introduced. It is important to also include other personnel that do not provide direct patient care, but may affect patient care indirectly. For example, the admitting personnel had to be educated to no longer inform patients to begin nil per os as of midnight before their surgery, as this was contradictory to the ERP education material and had been causing confusion amongst patients. These education efforts should be spearheaded by the steering group, in particular the clinical leaders in each specialty and the ERP coordinator. Having institutional data available to highlight areas for improvement is invaluable, as people tend to have an inaccurate picture of how current care differs from best practice or outcomes.

A clear timeline for the implementation process should also be laid out, including a firm launch date for which the ERP is put into practice. We recommend this approach over piecemeal integration of several pathway elements at a time, as this may engender frustration amongst users over a perceived lack of improved outcomes [28]. Process measures and outcome data should be collected for a cohort of patients prior to formal ERP introduction.

Evaluation

After ERP implementation, the multidisciplinary steering group should continue to monitor compliance and outcomes, and provided feedback to the respective healthcare staff according to performance. It is important that process measures are constantly audited. The learning curve period after initial ERP implementation may last up to 1 year [28].

In particular, initial compliance may be poor, especially for elements that run contrary to longstanding practices [29]. Given these early experiences, there has been some concern that protocol compliance and outcomes may not be replicated outside of a randomized trial. However, even if protocol adherence is lower in real-life practice, important beneficial outcomes may still be achieved [30]. Nevertheless, improved adherence will likely result in better outcomes [9, 31]. It is useful to demonstrate both up-to-date adherence and outcome data to the frontline staff, as this will positively reinforce and combat any continued doubt towards the ERP. It is also critical to listen to feedback from staff in order to understand where barriers and challenges remain.

Several different audit tools have been developed specifically to monitor process measures for ERPs. In particular, the ERAS Society Interactive Audit Tool includes standardized data collection and allows for comparison across participating centres [32]. Another option includes the American College of Surgeons' National Surgical Quality Improvement Program, which now includes ERP process measures in the colorectal specific module. Institutions are increasingly relying on their own electronic medical records to retrieve data. In our early experience, we collected information about hospital stay and reasons for delayed discharge in a shared excel file through our hospital intranet, initiated by the preoperative clinic nurse and completed weekly by the ward nurse managers. This allowed for useful information to be relayed back to frontline providers to promote adherence with the pathway. Regardless of the audit tool, it is important that areas of weakness identified during audit be acted upon, through either targeted educational efforts or organizational changes or whole-scale revisions of the ERP. Once an ERP is implemented, it is not recommended to continuously add new elements piecemeal. Rather, each pathway should undergo revision at predetermined time intervals (e.g., every 2 years) to ensure that updated best practices are included, as well as changes dictated by the local practice environment. It is also likely that with experience, ERPs can become progressively more complex.

Summary

This chapter has summarized the necessary steps and highlighted the important strategies for successful ERP implementation. ERP may represent significant change from traditional perioperative practices, and many barriers to change may exist. Strong clinical leadership, consensus from all involved stakeholders, and cooperation across specialties are required given the complexity of an ERP. Local realities should always be taken into consideration. Important elements for the development, implementation, and evaluation of an ERP were also provided.

References

1. Zhuang CL, Ye XZ, Zhang XD, Chen BC, Yu Z. Enhanced recovery after surgery programs versus traditional care for colorectal surgery: a meta-analysis of randomized controlled trials. Dis Colon Rectum. 2013;56(5):667–78.
2. Findlay JM, Gillies RS, Millo J, Sgromo B, Marshall RE, Maynard ND. Enhanced recovery for esophagectomy: a systematic review and evidence-based guidelines. Ann Surg. 2014;259(3):413–31.
3. Kagedan DJ, Ahmed M, Devitt KS, Wei AC. Enhanced recovery after pancreatic surgery: a systematic review of the evidence. HPB (Oxford). 2015;17(1):11–6.
4. Malviya A, Martin K, Harper I, et al. Enhanced recovery program for hip and knee replacement reduces death rate. Acta Orthop. 2011;82(5):577–81.
5. Delaney CP, Senagore AJ, Gerkin TM, et al. Association of surgical care practices with length of stay and use of clinical protocols after elective bowel resection: results of a national survey. Am J Surg. 2010;199(3):299–304. discussion 304.
6. Kehlet H, Buchler MW, Beart Jr RW, Billingham RP, Williamson R. Care after colonic operation—is it evidence-based? Results from a multinational survey in Europe and the United States. J Am Coll Surg. 2006;202(1):45–54.
7. Kehlet H, Wilmore DW. Multimodal strategies to improve surgical outcome. Am J Surg. 2002;183(6):630–41.
8. King PM, Blazeby JM, Ewings P, et al. The influence of an enhanced recovery programme on clinical outcomes, costs and quality of life after surgery for colorectal cancer. Colorectal Dis. 2006;8(6):506–13.
9. Maessen J, Dejong CH, Hausel J, et al. A protocol is not enough to implement an enhanced recovery programme for colorectal resection. Br J Surg. 2007;94(2): 224–31.
10. Eisenbach R, Watson K, Pillai R. Transformational leadership in the context of organizational change. J Change Manag. 1999;12(2):80–9.
11. Carli F, Charlebois P, Baldini G, Cachero O, Stein B. An integrated multidisciplinary approach to implementation of a fast-track program for laparoscopic colorectal surgery. Can J Anaesth. 2009;56(11):837–42.
12. Li C, Ferri LE, Mulder DS, et al. An enhanced recovery pathway decreases duration of stay after esophagectomy. Surgery. 2012;152(4):606–14. discussion 614-606.
13. Abou-Haidar H, Abourbih S, Braganza D, et al. Enhanced recovery pathway for radical prostatectomy: implementation and evaluation in a universal healthcare system. Can Urol Assoc J. 2014;8(11-12):418–23.

14. Jones C, Kelliher L, Dickinson M, et al. Randomized clinical trial on enhanced recovery versus standard care following open liver resection. Br J Surg. 2013; 100(8):1015–24.

15. Lemanu DP, Singh PP, Berridge K, et al. Randomized clinical trial of enhanced recovery versus standard care after laparoscopic sleeve gastrectomy. Br J Surg. 2013; 100(4):482–9.

16. Grol R. Personal paper. Beliefs and evidence in changing clinical practice. BMJ. 1997;315(7105):418–21.

17. Grol R, Grimshaw J. From best evidence to best practice: effective implementation of change in patients' care. Lancet. 2003;362(9391):1225–30.

18. Reissman P, Teoh TA, Cohen SM, Weiss EG, Nogueras JJ, Wexner SD. Is early oral feeding safe after elective colorectal surgery? A prospective randomized trial. Ann Surg. 1995;222(1):73–7.

19. Sjetne IS, Krogstad U, Odegard S, Engh ME. Improving quality by introducing enhanced recovery after surgery in a gynaecological department: consequences for ward nursing practice. Qual Saf Health Care. 2009;18(3):236–40.

20. Delaney CP, Zutshi M, Senagore AJ, Remzi FH, Hammel J, Fazio VW. Prospective, randomized, controlled trial between a pathway of controlled rehabilitation with early ambulation and diet and traditional postoperative care after laparotomy and intestinal resection. Dis Colon Rectum. 2003;46(7):851–9.

21. Vlug MS, Wind J, Hollmann MW, et al. Laparoscopy in combination with fast track multimodal management is the best perioperative strategy in patients undergoing colonic surgery: a randomized clinical trial (LAFA-study). Ann Surg. 2011;254(6): 868–75.

22. Cerantola Y, Valerio M, Persson B, et al. Guidelines for perioperative care after radical cystectomy for bladder cancer: Enhanced Recovery After Surgery (ERAS(®)) society recommendations. Clin Nutr. 2013;32(6):879–87.

23. Nygren J, Thacker J, Carli F, et al. Guidelines for perioperative care in elective rectal/pelvic surgery: Enhanced Recovery After Surgery (ERAS(®)) Society recommendations. World J Surg. 2013;37(2):285–305.

24. Gustafsson UO, Scott MJ, Schwenk W, et al. Guidelines for perioperative care in elective colonic surgery: Enhanced Recovery After Surgery (ERAS(®)) Society recommendations. World J Surg. 2013;37(2):259–84.

25. Lassen K, Coolsen MM, Slim K, et al. Guidelines for perioperative care for pancreaticoduodenectomy: Enhanced Recovery After Surgery (ERAS®) Society recommendations. World J Surg. 2013;37(2):240–58.

26. Feldman LS, Lee L, Fiore Jr J. What outcomes are important in the assessment of Enhanced Recovery After Surgery (ERAS) pathways? Can J Anaesth. 2015; 62(2):120–30.

27. Health Literacy in Canada: a healthy understanding. 2008. http://www.ccl-cca.ca/pdfs/HealthLiteracy/HealthLiteracyReportFeb2008E.pdf. Accessed 23 Oct 2012.

28. Carter F, Kennedy RH. Setting up an enhanced recovery programme. In: Francis N, editor. Manual of fast-track recovery for colorectal surgery. London: Springer; 2012.

29. Polle SW, Wind J, Fuhring JW, Hofland J, Gouma DJ, Bemelman WA. Implementation of a fast-track perioperative care program: what are the difficulties? Dig Surg. 2007;24(6):441–9.

30. Ahmed J, Khan S, Gatt M, Kallam R, MacFie J. Compliance with enhanced recovery programmes in elective colorectal surgery. Br J Surg. 2010;97(5):754–8.

31. Feroci F, Lenzi E, Baraghini M, et al. Fast-track colorectal surgery: protocol adherence influences postoperative outcomes. Int J Colorectal Dis. 2013;28(1):103–9.

32. ERAS Interactive Audit System. http://www2.erassociety.org/index.php/login-gateway. Accessed 15 Aug 2012.

28. The ERAS® Society

Olle Ljungqvist and Kenneth C.H. Fearon

The Enhanced Recovery After Surgery and Perioperative Care Society (ERAS; www.erassociety.org) was formed in January of 2010 in Amsterdam and a few months later that year formally registered as a not-for-profit multiprofessional, multidisciplinary academic medical society. The Society aims to improve perioperative care by developing science and research in the field, developing and promoting education and implementation of evidence-based perioperative care programmes. The ERAS Society was started as a network of doctors and nurses involved in different disciplines in surgical practice, anaesthesia and intensive care.

The ERAS Study Group

The ERAS Society was born out of a collaborative network in Northern Europe. Ken Fearon from Edinburgh and Olle Ljungqvist from Stockholm met at a conference outside London in 2000 and decided to start collaboration with some other groups interested in perioperative care. Ken had good contacts with Maarten von Meyenfeldt and Cornelius Dejong in Maastricht, the Netherlands and Olle had similar good relations with Henrik Kehlet in Copenhagen, Denmark and Arthur Revhaug in Tromsö, Norway. These leaders were invited to a small conference in London early the next year to discuss the prospects of further developing what was then often referred to as fast track surgery, and probably first mentioned in cardiac surgery [1]. These ideas in cardiac surgery had been further developed by Henrik Kehlet who described a multimodal approach to improve the rate of recovery after colonic

L.S. Feldman et al. (eds.), *The SAGES / ERAS®*
Society Manual of Enhanced Recovery Programs for
Gastrointestinal Surgery, DOI 10.1007/978-3-319-20364-5_28,
© Springer International Publishing Switzerland 2015

surgery [2]. Kehlet's work had been developed from the use of epidurals for pain relief and stress reduction. All participants had a keen interest in the stress response to surgery, nutrition and metabolism and the role that manipulating aspects of the stress response may have on outcomes after surgery. The Maastricht group had shown the effectiveness of nutritional support on outcomes in surgery, Tromsö had implemented early post-operative food and studied anabolic factors, Edinburgh had done studies on cancer and nutrition, and Stockholm had presented the idea of fluid and carbohydrate loading instead of overnight fasting and the role of insulin resistance in recovery.

Together the ERAS Group set out to put metabolism and nutrition back on the agenda for surgery and anaesthesia. The group started to hold regular meetings and began to review the literature available for perioperative care that could make a difference for improving outcomes and recovery. A very important aspect for the group was how to name the process of improvement. It was felt that "Fast track" had a negative cling to it by focussing on "fast" rather than the patient. The group there-fore decided to change the name of the process to Enhanced Recovery After Surgery—ERAS, and that is how the word was invented. This placed the focus on the patient's recovery and by improving recovery secondary gains could be achieved such as shorter length of stay and financial savings. However, for the group and later the ERAS Society, the focus remains with patient outcomes first and foremost. A key aspect throughout this work has been the involvement of nursing and other disciplines making the work truly multidisciplinary and involving these disciplines in the academic work has broadened the reach to all parties involved in patient care. Dothe Hjort-Jacobsen from Copenhagen, and Jose Maessen from Maastricht have been forerunners in this work.

Using colorectal surgery as their model, the group documented their own patterns of care and outcomes using either traditional care or the "ERAS programme" [3]. It was evident to the group that none of them were doing the ideal perioperative care programme. While Kehlet's group was closest to the ideal protocol, the others were further from it, and all units were doing things differently. They also surveyed specific aspects of perioperative care as practised at that time in five different European countries [4] and showed marked diversity of practice. For example, some patients were fed immediately after surgery whereas oth-ers were fasted routinely for 3 days! To try and unify management, the group then developed an evidence-based consensus perioperative care protocol with about twenty different elements [5].

It was decided to have all units move to using the "ideal ERAS" protocol and to study the process of change. This way it was thought that the units could support each other to overcome some of the obstacles that were presented. To support the project a common database was developed to document the results and audit the change. Once the data was reviewed a second revelation was made: it became clear that what was actually performed in the respective clinics was not what the leads had thought, and the units had problems and issues to deal with that they had not known before. It was also obvious that having a protocol was not going to be enough to make the change to an ideal care pathway [6]. Continuous data was the only way to truly know what was ongoing in the perioperative care path.

Using data and working together, progress was made and the units improved their outcomes successively, this time addressing the true issue that needed to be dealt with and not what were the perceived problems. Data was the key to drive change. Dr. Jonatan Hausel at Ersta hospital in Stockholm was the main creator behind initial database. This was the forerunner to the later developed ERAS® Interactive Audit System.

At around that time the Dutch group had the opportunity to work with professional change management experts in the Kwaliteitsinstituut CBO in the Netherlands. Using the protocol and the experiences from the ERAS study group and combining it with modern change management principles they ran a series of three consecutive implementation programmes each lasting 1 year and including 33 hospitals in the Netherlands (i.e. one third of all hospitals nationwide). These were very successful and showed that the principles of the ERAS protocol had a major impact and helped the units to reduce length of hospital stay by 3 days [7]. This occurred as the compliance with the ERAS Study group protocol was raised from around 45 % to 75 %.

From the early start of the group, research was high on the agenda and several papers including randomised trials of individual elements of the protocol (e.g. [8]) and Ph.D. theses were produced from the work of the group. Some of the key papers that came form the group were the reports on better outcomes with improved compliance with the protocol [9], which is actually a test of the guidelines. While testing of guidelines may seem very basic for any Medical Society to do, such testing is actually not performed commonly. For the ERAS Study Group, however, this work gave support to the ideas that the group were developing. In a meta analysis published in 2010 [10] it was shown for the first time, that applying the principles of ERAS actually had major impact on post-operative complications. An almost 50 % reduction in complications after colorectal surgery was found in that analysis. This was the first time that such evidence had been presented. Previously the focus had been on shortening of length of stay. While the principles had been developed in colorectal surgery there was also a movement exploring these principles in other surgical domains (see below).

The group expanded over time and Robin Kennedy from St Marks joined with his focus on laparoscopic colorectal surgery as an addition to the knowledge base, while Dileep Lobo from Nottingham brought expertise in fluid management, and the Berlin group with Claudia Spies and Arne Feldheiser strengthened the academic input from anaesthesia for the group. During the first 10 years the Study group had generous support from initially Nutricia, the Netherlands, and later from Fresenius-Kabi, Germany with unrestricted grants.

The ERAS Society

As the ERAS Study Group developed and experience accrued, it became obvious that ERAS was right at the heart of the needs of perioperative care in general. ERAS was leading to better care resulting in faster recovery of the patient/return to autonomy as well as a major reduction in post-operative complications. The information gathered showed that there was a need for a movement to begin to secure that best practice was gathered into guidelines, that the guidelines were being employed in practice and that perioperative care was constantly being improved and updated.

A key element of the work ahead was the need for a multiprofessional, multidisciplinary approach to the improvement of care and its implementation. This basis for improvement was to be employed in every aspect of ERAS; research, education and implementation. ERAS contained concepts that could be transferred to all types of surgery of any magnitude. This was obvious not only to the ERAS Study group but to all developers of perioperative care and thus the interest in ERAS was rising in a multitude of surgical domains. ERAS showed that recovery time was shortened and this reduced hospital stay, partly due to reduced complications but also a reduction in readmissions. This allowed for substantial savings of resources and costs [11]. This is key in the current health care development as the cost for health care has grown more than the Gross Domestic Product per year in many countries in the Western world in recent years, a development that is unsustainable.

The ERAS Society Organisation

It was decided that when starting the ERAS Society it would be built in stages. Realising that it takes time and effort to build a structure with specific aims, it would be necessary to allow for the foundation elements to be set up over a period of time with stability in the leadership. It was also felt that a structure allowing for strategic planning on a continuous basis would be of benefit in a world where health care is constantly changing.

The core members of the ERAS Study Group formed the Society and the key members of this group formed the Board of the Society with the mission to formulate overall strategic goals. In the initial years the Board would also appoint the Executive Chairman who would be given the task to build the core of the Society by appointing his own committee of executives for approval. An Executive Committee was formed with appointments to manage the treasury, secretarial duties, education and science. In addition a web master, Javier Fabra of the University of Zaragoza Spain, alongside a Web Editor and a Nurses section lead RN Dorthe Hjort Jacobsen were appointed. Apart from this core in the Executive Committee, appointments were made for specific task groups mainly directed to the formation of groups working in different domains in surgical disciplines and anaesthesia. With these pillars the ERAS Society started its existence and in its first 5 year existence has developed to a leading society for the multidisciplinary, multiprofessional approach to perioperative care.

ERAS in the World

Despite the interest and growth around the ERAS concept, the majority of care worldwide during the development of the ERAS Study Group/Society was still dominated by traditional practice, long recovery times and high complication rates. Modern care was not in use. As stated previously, this became even more evident when major surveys were performed by the group in Northern European countries that were regarded as leading in perioperative care [4]. The ERAS Study Group felt it had some important experiences and insights that would be useful to bring to surgery in general. In the UK the NHS started a national campaign to implement ERAS principles and the group supported this concept with ideas, experiences and knowledge.

But apart from this initiative and the Dutch experience, both supported by the ERAS study group, very little was done on a large scale for the implementation of ERAS.

The ERAS Study Group's basic interest was research and development, but it was also felt that moving the evidence found in research to practice was to be a key component of the mission for the group going forward. At the same time it was obvious that the group needed to establish resources to be able to make a serious effort to move implementation forward. The data base was a good tool for audit and research but could be further developed and could also serve as a tool during implementation if developed further. However, unfortunately at this particular moment in time the group did not have sufficient financial resource to do this and had to seek other means to move the implementation project forward.

Building Partnerships

Around that time STING, (Stockholm Innovation and Growth) alongside Karolinska Development, two major incubator organisations in Stockholm proposed to the ERAS Study Group to form a start-up company that could manage the IT for the database and develop a system for Interactive Audit for an implementation programme. This company could also serve to administrate the implementation programme for the group. Olle Ljungqvist was asked to start the company that would service the group and develop the IT side of the project. He started the company, Encare AB, in 2009 and for the sake of efficiency also became a Board member of the company to represent the Society. To minimise conflict of interest Olle was asked to report directly to the Chairman of the ERAS Society Board, subsequently the interests of the Society have been represented by other members of the Executive Committee who report directly to the Chairman of the Board. At the same time, the ERAS Study Group decided that it was time to build a much larger academic network and involve many more colleagues. To do so it was decided to start the Enhanced Recovery After Surgery Society for perioperative Care (The ERAS Society). Again the Society received an unrestricted grant from Nutricia to allow the start-up of the Society. The Society start-up was decided in Amsterdam in January 2010 and the formal registration as a not-for-profit multiprofessional, multidisciplinary medical academic society was done in Sweden in May 2010. The ERAS Society has had a formal agreement with Encare AB to service the Society for its implementation programme since the start of the Society.

The Congress Start Up

Another important task for the Society was to create a dedicated congress. The congress was to be based on the concepts of the ERAS philosophy—everyone involved in the care of the patient should come together. MCI was chosen as the service provider to partner development of the Congress. Like the service-provider relationship with Encare, this relationship has proved to be very successful. The first multiprofessional, multidisciplinary world ERAS congress was held in October 2012 in Cannes, France and attracted just over 200 delegates from 28 countries. The majority of lectures were held in just one lecture hall with all attendees assembled together. Only the late afternoon session was divided for anaesthesia and surgery and split to two lecture halls. The latter was the only major criticism received afterwards and for this reason the entire programme was held in only one lecture hall during the 2nd world congress of ERAS in Valencia, Spain (2014). This time, the attendance was more than doubled and the number of countries represented almost 40 from six continents. An introductory course for ERAS teams was held just before the congress and proved to be very much appreciated. Industrial interest had also grown substantially for the second event. Alongside these international events, the ERAS Society has also supported a number of regional and national events in many countries.

Research Developments

The core of the ERAS Society lies with the development of perioperative care and research is the foundation for this work. Just about all groups involved at the heart of the Society are involved in research and a lot of the more recent research information on ERAS comes from units working inside the ERAS Society. Whilst the early work was developed in a smaller group, with the expansion of the Society, and the engagement of many more units with the database, the Society is now in the process of developing improved research tools within the database, the ERAS Interactive Audit System. This will allow a much broader participation and larger patient volumes. The ERAS Interactive Audit System is prepared for all kinds of studies. The research structure being developed will have full transparency and users of the system will be welcome to submit proposals for studies using data in the database. A committee will review any study proposals and novel questions will be given the opportunity to be addressed using the system and published on behalf of the contributors of the data. The idea is to have all study protocols displayed alongside the investigators on the ERAS Society website as well as in Trials.com.

Education

The ERAS Society has developed a basic course for the introduction of ERAS to hospitals interested in starting ERAS in their own institution. This course will be run in conjunction with the ERAS congress on an annual basis and it is directed to multidisciplinary and multiprofessional teams. In addition, this introductory course has been run at national events in different countries and will continue to do so. The Society is working on a series of videos for education on the website. These will initially be of an introductory type and aimed at different disciplines and professionals. The Nurses section will play a special role in this educational series.

Guidelines

The ERAS Society has issued guidelines in a variety of surgical domains (www.erassociety.org). In 2012 the first 3 guidelines were published jointly in World Journal of Surgery and Clinical Nutrition: colonic resection, rectal surgery and pancreatic resections. These were followed by Guidelines in Cystectomy in 2013 in Clinical Nutrition, and for Gastric resections in the British Journal of Surgery in 2014. There are a number of groups working on similar guidelines in other surgical procedures in urology, gynaecology, orthopaedics, thoracic surgery, ENT (ear nose and throat) and oesophageal resections. The guidelines are written by leaders in their respective domains, people who have been involved in developing ERAS in their field. Once the guidelines are set, the plan is to have the individual elements and outcomes transferred to the ERAS Interactive Audit System, where they can be tested and validated. This will form the basis for further development of ERAS principles in different areas of surgery.

ERAS Implementation Programmes

Based on the initial experiences using the ERAS protocol in the Dutch series, the ERAS Society has further developed its implementation programmes. This has been done in collaboration with Qulturum, Jönköping, Sweden, a world-renowned group in quality improvement and change management in health care. The Implementation programmes are taught by ERAS and change management experts and administrated by Encare AB, the implementation service partner for the ERAS Society. Hospitals from Norway, Sweden, England, Switzerland, France and Canada have so far been trained successfully in this system, and there are a number of other countries where these implementation programmes are being set up. Similarly, the number of surgical domains included in these programmes is also expanding from being based on colorectal procedures to now also include cystectomy, nephrectomy, major gynaecology and pancreatic resections.

Networking

The ERAS Society is networking with a number of national organisations interested in collaboration around Enhanced Recovery. There are already a few national ERAS-like Societies in the world and the ERAS Society has established or is in the process of establishing collaborations with them. At the same time, in countries with no such Society structure in place, the ERAS Society is initiating collaborations based in the Centres of Excellence that are set up. These units have good ERAS structures in place, are trained by the ERAS Society to serve as teachers of ERAS in the ERAS Implementation programmes and they serve as leaders in their own countries or regions in ERAS care. Theses centres will form ERAS Society Chapters, which will be an integral part of the ERAS Society and its network. A similar agreement will be in place with the National Societies as well. For an updated view of the development of the ERAS Society network, please check the web site: www.erassociety.org.

In addition to these arrangements, the Society is open to collaborations with other Medical Societies. The ERAS Society has received the official endorsement from the Swedish Surgical Society already as a sign of collaboration. This manual on ERAS produced in collaboration with SAGES is another clear example of collaboration between Societies.

Future Developments

It is likely that the demands for ERAS will increase rapidly in the years to come. The economic savings that it brings alongside improved outcomes will be an important factor driving this development. The challenge for the Society is to keep up with the development. In addition, the ambition of the Society is to be able to provide larger and better data to further develop the knowledge and the basis for guidelines. To do this, a large expansion of the users of the database will be important. At the same time, many users on the same system will allow for faster transformation of change, especially if the system is built to facilitate such change. Although the Society started from a small group of people, it has now grown into and is continuing to grow into a large network of experts working side by side in a similar fashion to improve knowledge and ultimately optimal care for and with surgical patients. Even so there will be a need for a broad collaboration among many stakeholders in medicine and surgery together with the patients to tackle the challenge facing us; bringing better care to more people at a lower cost. The ERAS Society will tackle this challenge by developing knowledge, helping colleagues to receive the knowledge, empowering the patient's knowledge and education with the use of shared decision environments and make use of it by continuously updating and changing practice at a faster pace.

Acknowledgments The authors are grateful for the comment and review made by the members of the first Board of the ERAS Society: professors Maarten von Meyenfeldt, Arthur Revhaug and Cornelius Dejong. The authors also recognise the instrumental work made by many young colleagues and ERAS coordinators/ERAS nurses contributing to the development of the ERAS Group and later the ERAS Society, not least by their academic work. None mentioned, none forgotten.

References

1. Engelman RM, et al. Fast-track recovery of the coronary bypass patient. Ann Thorac Surg. 1994;58:1742–6.
2. Kehlet H. Multimodal approach to control postoperative pathophysiology and rehabilitation. Br J Anaesth. 1997;78(5):606–17.
3. Nygren J, et al. A comparison in five European centres of case mix, clinical management and outcomes following either conventional or fast-track perioperative care in colorectal surgery. Clin Nutr. 2005;24(3):455–61.
4. Lassen K, et al. Patterns in current perioperative practice: survey of colorectal surgeons in five northern European countries. BMJ. 2005;330(7505):1420–1.

5. Fearon KC, et al. Enhanced recovery after surgery: a consensus review of clinical care for patients undergoing colonic resection. Clin Nutr. 2005;24(3):466–77.
6. Maessen J, et al. A protocol is not enough to implement an enhanced recovery programme for colorectal resection. Br J Surg. 2007;94(2):224–31.
7. Gillissen F, et al. Structured synchronous implementation of an enhanced recovery program in elective colonic surgery in 33 hospitals in The Netherlands. World J Surg. 2013;37(5):1082–93.
8. Hendry PO, et al. Determinants of outcome after colorectal resection within an enhanced recovery programme. Br J Surg. 2009;96(2):197–205.
9. Gustafsson UO, et al. Adherence to the enhanced recovery after surgery protocol and outcomes after colorectal cancer surgery. Arch Surg. 2011;146(5):571–7.
10. Varadhan KK, Lobo DN. A meta-analysis of randomised controlled trials of intravenous fluid therapy in major elective open abdominal surgery: getting the balance right. Proc Nutr Soc. 2010;69(4):488–98.
11. Roulin D, et al. Cost-effectiveness of the implementation of an enhanced recovery protocol for colorectal surgery. Br J Surg. 2013;100(8):1108–14.

29. SAGES SMART Enhanced Recovery Program

Liane S. Feldman

The goal of surgical innovation should be to improve recovery for our patients. What if, some day, major abdominal surgery could be done without pain, ileus, cognitive disturbance, complications, and fatigue? If this is attained, then resource use and costs will decrease too, achieving higher value care for patients. The last decades have seen incredible advances in surgical techniques with a move toward minimally invasive approaches. Yet despite these advances, complications for some procedures remain high, with 21–45 % of patients experiencing complications after cancer resections. There are significant variations between centers in perioperative processes, complications, and duration of hospital stay, even for uncomplicated patients. Full recovery, even for relatively "minor" procedure like ambulatory laparoscopic cholecystectomy, takes longer than we think.

Guidelines for Perioperative Care

Minimally invasive surgery is an important strategy to reduce the metabolic impact of surgery and improve recovery. However, there are multiple other developments outside the traditional of the surgeon that may have a large impact on the surgical stress response and ultimately on outcomes. These include afferent neural blockade, pharmacologic interventions, fluid management, psychological preparation, exercise and nutritional interventions. Guidelines from the ERAS® Society on optimal perioperative management include over 20 evidence-based interventions that have been shown to improve outcomes. Most are "strong" recommendations, meaning they are supported by high-level evidence. They

L.S. Feldman et al. (eds.), *The SAGES / ERAS®*
Society Manual of Enhanced Recovery Programs for
Gastrointestinal Surgery, DOI 10.1007/978-3-319-20364-5_29,
© Springer International Publishing Switzerland 2015

involve the entire trajectory of surgical care, preoperative, intraoperative, and postoperative, and all stakeholders—patients, nurses, anesthesiologists, surgeons, and other team members. Several recommendations challenge tightly held surgical traditions around drain management, bowel preparation, intravenous fluids, and fasting. Enhanced recovery pathways, as described in this manual, integrate these various interventions into a standardized perioperative care pathway. The goal is to reduce surgical stress, support early return of normal functioning, reduce complications, and ultimately improve full recovery after major surgery. The use of an ERP is associated with reduced hospital stay and 30 % reduction in the risk of overall complications, without increasing mortality, major complications or readmissions. The effects are similar across different surgical disciplines and for laparoscopic and open surgery. The use of laparoscopy facilitates many other elements of an ERP, and the optimal approach is to combine the two. The Enhanced recovery approach is cost-effective compared to conventional perioperative management, even when implementation and management costs are taken into account.

Implementation of ERPs

However, adoption of ERPs into routine surgical practice has been slow. The most common perceived barrier is resistance to change and lack of knowledge about best practices. First of all, a large number of care elements must be addressed, which is intimidating. Even when clinicians are aware of evidence-based interventions, it is estimated that it takes 17 years to translate evidence into practice; it probably takes even longer to get unhelpful or even harmful care, like routine prolonged fasting, *out* of practice. The multimodal aspect of the ERP approach is also a challenge. Traditional perioperative care divides us into expertise silos and surgeons do not usually know of advances in anesthesia or nursing care for example. One of the key paradigm shifts with ERPs is from a provider-centric system where surgeons, anesthesiologists, and nurses function within expertise silos characterized by significant variability between practitioners and institutions, to one that is patient-centered with integration of each step of perioperative care into a cohesive pathway around the surgical patient.

There is not a "one-size fits-all" approach, but rather will vary somewhat depending on resources, skills and other hard realities between institutions. For example, depending on the institution, the introduction of multimodal analgesia for colon surgery may include thoracic epidural, transversus abdominis plane (TAP) block, spinal, or patient-controlled analgesia. The key is the creation of a multidisciplinary team dedicated to the ERP paradigm, open examination of current practice, and coming to consensus on the application of procedure-specific evidence-based care. Individual surgeons, anesthesiologists, nurses, or administrators cannot do this alone. The introduction of an ERP requires a team approach. But where does the team get information skills and tools to begin to create, implement and audit an ERP? There is no advantage to each team starting from a blank page, when a great deal of information is already available from experienced centers.

SAGES and Enhanced Recovery

The Society of American Gastrointestinal and Endoscopic Surgeons (SAGES) has long played a key role in educating and supporting surgeons to adopt innovative surgical techniques to improve surgical outcomes. SAGES recognizes that the best outcomes will result from combining laparoscopic surgery with optimal perioperative care. SAGES is introducing the SMART ("Surgical Multimodal Accelerated Recovery Trajectory") program. The Mission is to promote the integration of Enhanced Recovery care principles as a cornerstone of minimally invasive surgery to improve safety, efficiency, and outcomes of GI surgery.

SAGES SMART enhanced recovery will include:

- A web-based warehouse for educational resources related to best practices in perioperative care for GI surgery, with a focus on minimally invasive surgery, and including implementation strategies and case studies which will be accessible through the SAGES web portal
- Unique educational content delivered through postgraduate courses and the annual SAGES meeting
- Research in ERP implementation and outcomes, particularly where knowledge gaps related to laparoscopic surgery are identified
- Strategies to support patient education and self-management, even after hospital discharge
- Development of unique patient reported outcome measures developed to estimate recovery, especially after hospital discharge.

Conclusion

If the goal of modern surgical techniques like minimally invasive surgery is ultimately to improve recovery for patients, surgeons should be involved in leading the integration of evidence-based interventions from all phases of perioperative care into a cohesive care plan to optimize outcomes. Through the SMART program, SAGES is committed to promoting the coordinated activity of surgeons, anesthesiologists, and nurses to enhance the value of minimally invasive GI surgery.

Take Home Messages

- Both laparoscopic surgery and enhanced recovery perioperative care plans improve surgical outcomes
- The best results are when laparoscopic surgery is integrated into an ERP
- Teams need help to create, introduce, audit, and revise ERPs
- SAGES is a GI surgery specialty society with a particular interest in laparoscopic surgery. SAGES SMART enhanced program aims to promote and support knowledge and adoption of enhanced recovery principles in GI surgery, with a particular focus on minimally invasive surgery.

Suggested Readings

1. Porter ME, Lee TH. The strategy that will fix health care. Harv Bus Rev. October 2013;1–19.
2. Nicholson A, Lowe MC, Parker J, Lewis SR, Alderson P, Smith AF. Systematic review and meta-analysis of enhanced recovery programmes in surgical patients. Br J Surg. 2014;101(3):172–88.
3. Vlug MS, Wind J, Hollmann MW, Ubbink DT, Cense HA, Engel AF, et al. Laparoscopy in combination with fast track multimodal management is the best perioperative strategy in patients undergoing colonic surgery: a randomized clinical trial (LAFA-study). Ann Surg. 2011;254:868–75.
4. Kehlet H. Fast-track surgery—an update on physiological care principles to enhance recovery. Langenbecks Arch Surg. 2011;396(5):585–90.

12 Postoperative Ileus: Prevention and Treatment

Martin Hubner, Michael Scott,
and Bradley Champagne

L.S. Feldman et al. (eds.), *The SAGES / ERAS®*
Society Manual of Enhanced Recovery Programs for
Gastrointestinal Surgery, DOI 10.1007/978-3-319-20364-5,
pp. 133–146, © Springer International Publishing Switzerland 2015

DOI 10.1007/978-3-319-20364-5_30

The publisher regrets that the figure caption for figure 12.1 is missing a credit line in the original publication of the print and online versions. The following credit line was added to the caption of figure 12.1 on page 136.

The credit line should read:

"With permission from Chowdhury AH, Lobo DN. Fluids and gastrointestinal function. Current Opinion in Clinical Nutrition and Metabolic Care 14:469–476 © 2011 Wolters Kluwer Health | Lippincott Williams & Wilkins 1363-1950".

The online version of the original chapter can be found at
http://dx.doi.org/10.1007/978-3-319-20364-5_12

Index

L.S. Feldman et al. (eds.), *The SAGES / ERAS®*
Society Manual of Enhanced Recovery Programs for
Gastrointestinal Surgery, DOI 10.1007/978-3-319-20364-5,
© Springer International Publishing Switzerland 2015